Contemporary Topics in Molecular Immunology

Volume 6

Contemporary Topics in Molecular Immunology

A Continuation Order Plan is available for this series. A continuation order will bring delivery of each new volume immediately upon publication. Volumes are billed only upon actual shipment. For further information please contact the publisher.

Contemporary Topics in Molecular Immunology

Volume 6

EDITED BY

R. R. Porter

University of Oxford
Oxford, England

and

G. L. Ada

Australian National University
Canberra City, Australia

Springer Science+Business Media, LLC

The Library of Congress cataloged the first volume of this title as follows:

Contemporary topics in molecular immunology. v. 2–
New York, Plenum Press, 1973–

v. illus. 24 cm.

Continues Contemporary topics in immunochemistry.

1. Immunochemistry—Collected works. 2. Immunology—Collected works.

QR180.C635 574.2'9'05 73–648513
ISSN 0090–8800 MARC–S

Volume 1 of this series was published under the title *Contemporary Topics in Immunochemistry*

Library of Congress Catalog Card Number 73-648513

ISBN 978-1-4684-2843-8 ISBN 978-1-4684-2841-4 (eBook)
DOI 10.1007/978-1-4684-2841-4

Originally published by Plenum Press, New York in 1977
Softcover reprint of the hardcover 1st edition 1977

Contributors

Robert William Baldwin *Cancer Research Campaign Laboratories*
University of Nottingham
Nottingham, England

Celso Bianco *The Rockefeller University*
New York, New York

Michael J. Crumpton *National Institute for Medical Research*
London, England

Raymond A. Dwek *Department of Biochemistry*
Oxford University
Oxford, England

Arthur K. Kimura *Department of Immunology*
University of Uppsala Biomedical Center
Uppsala, Sweden

C. Milstein *Medical Research Council Laboratory of Molecular Biology*
Cambridge, England

Victor Nussenzweig *Department of Pathology*
New York University School of Medicine
New York, New York

T. H. Rabbitts *Medical Research Council Laboratory of Molecular Biology*
Cambridge, England

Richard Adrian Robins *Cancer Research Campaign Laboratories*
University of Nottingham
Nottingham, England

David Snary *National Institute for Medical Research*
London, England

Hans Wigzell *Department of Immunology*
University of Uppsala Biomedical Center
Uppsala, Sweden

Alan F. Williams *MRC Immunochemistry Unit*
Department of Biochemistry, Oxford University
Oxford, England

Preface

The distinction between molecular immunology and immunobiology is necessarily arbitrary. The most rapid progress is usually made in the blurred area between the two, when the chemist is aware of the full significance of the biological problems, and the biologist is alert to the contribution that a knowledge of molecular structure can be made to their solution. The range of scientific disciplines able to contribute to research in immunology, which this approach brings, is reflected in the present volume.

Protein chemists worked out the arrangement of the polypeptide chains and the amino acid sequences of antibodies and X-ray crystallographers the three dimensional structure, but more precise definition of the amino acid side chain positions in the combining site is required for an understanding of the subtleties of antibody specificity. That this can be achieved with physical techniques such as nuclear magnetic resonance has been shown by R. A. Dwek, and in his chapter he summarizes these results with a minimum of technical detail. The immune response has been shown to be dependent on complex cellular interactions and further progress will be facilitated by investigation of the molecular basis of these interactions. This necessitates study of the structure and organization of the molecules in the surfaces of lymphocytes and other cells. The histocompatibility antigens are found in most, if not all, nucleated cells but appear to have a special role in immune reactions in that their structural genes are closely linked to genes governing the immune responses. Though great difficulties are met in isolating sufficient material for structural studies, much progress is being made and Crumpton and Snary summarize present knowledge of the human histocompatibility antigens. More likely to play a role in cell–cell interaction are those antigens confined to particular cell types—the so-called differentiation antigens—and a possible candidate in the lymphocytes is Thy 1 which, in the mouse, is found on thymus cells and circulating T cells and not B cells, but which is also found in brain tissue. A closely related antigen is found in the rat, but with a somewhat different tissue distribution and it is present in sufficient amounts for isolation in milligram quantities. A. F. Williams discusses the general aspects of lymphocyte differentiation antigens, and his own work on the characteristics of Thy 1 from rat tissues. Tumor antigens, discussed by Baldwin and Robins, are far more complex and hence far less well defined than the histocompatibility and Thy 1 antigen and this chapter gives a clear assessment for the biochemist of current knowledge in the field.

The origin of the multiple genes coding for the large number of variable regions found in the antibodies in any individual animal has long been a source of controversy. Initial attempts to estimate the numbers of these structural genes by nucleic acid hybridization techniques led to conflicting results, but refinements of the methods used, and particularly careful purification and characterization of the messenger RNA used, has led to agreement that the numbers of variable region structural genes is likely to be small. Milstein and Rabbitts describe and evaluate these recent data.

The two chapters by Nussenzweig and Bianco and Kimura and Wigzel have less biochemical content than the others as the accessibility of the topics discussed to biochemical methods is only just being reached. The first discusses the interaction of immune complexes and lymphocytes, together with the involvement of complement components, and is clearly relevant to lymphocyte interaction in the immune response. The second is concerned with the resultant cytotoxicity of T cells, which again is likely to be determined by the T cell membrane structure.

This is a wide range of topics, though their interrelation is apparent, and the authors have met admirably our request to describe their own recent work in relation to that of others rather than to attempt comprehensive reviews of each subject.

G. A.
R. R. P.

Contents

Induction of Tumor-Immune Responses and Their Interaction with the Developing Tumor

Robert William Baldwin and Richard Adrian Robins

Cytotoxic T Lymphocyte Membrane Components: An Analysis of Structures Related to Function

Arthur K. Kimura and Hans Wigzell

Structural Studies in Solution on the Combining Site of the Myeloma Protein MOPC 315

Raymond A. Dwek

Department of Biochemistry, Oxford University
South Parks Road, Oxford, OX1 3QU, England

I. INTRODUCTION

One of the great triumphs of structural immunologists is that many of the ideas of structure and function, now verified by X-ray studies, had been proposed on the basis of chemical data. These ideas included the basic two-chain immunoglobulin structure, the location of the antigen-binding site, and the concept of domain structure. These features are summarized in Fig. 1, for an IgG molecule.

In 1959, Porter showed that under controlled conditions, it is possible to split the IgG molecule into Fab and Fc fragments. The Fab fragment was shown to have a molecular weight of 50,000 and retain antigen-binding activity. Further studies (Inbar *et al.*, 1972) have now shown that the Fab fragment itself can be split, yielding an Fv fragment of molecular weight 25,000, again with full hapten affinity.

The structural basis for these observations has been established through amino acid sequence studies on both normal immunoglobulins and myeloma proteins. These have led to the basic picture of a polypeptide chain structure consisting of two pairs of heavy and light chains joined by disulfide bonds. Each chain has regions of homology, termed *domains*, 110–120 residues long. The light chain has two such regions, the heavy chain four, making up a total molecular mass of 150,000. The amino acid sequence of the *N*-terminal region of these chains is variable—varying from one antibody molecule to another—whereas the sequence of the rest of the chain is identical within a given subclass

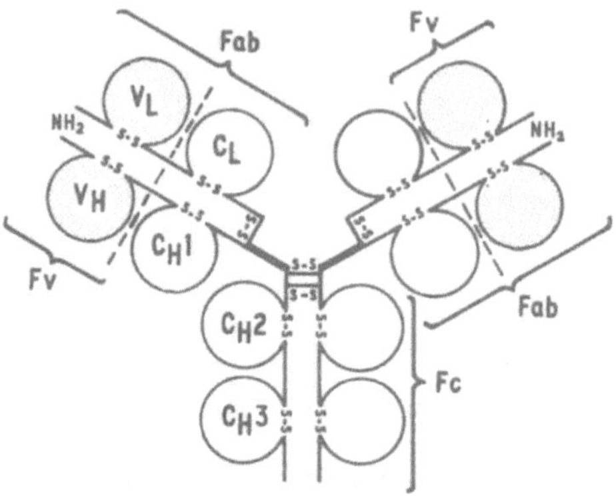

Figure 1. Schematic representation of immunoglobulin (IgG) molecule. The light (L) chains (mol. wt. 25,000) are divided into two homology regions, V_L and C_L. The heavy (H) chains (mol. wt. 50,000) are divided into four homology regions, V_H, C_H1, C_H2 and C_H3. The C_H1 and C_H2 are joined by a "hinge" region indicated by a heavier line. In an IgA molecule such as the MOPC 315 myeloma protein, the interchain S–S bonds in the Fab regions are absent.

or subtype. This variable region contains the antibody combining site. The important statistical analysis of the amino acids in this region in a number of different myeloma proteins by Wu and Kabat (1970) has firmly established the idea that within the variable region are certain hypervariable sequences of amino acids, and we now know that it is such sequences that provide the basis for antibody specificity. Thus, in the light chain, residues around 24-34, 50-55, and 89–96 were hypervariable, while in the heavy chain, hypervariability involved mainly residues 31-35, 50-65, and 95-102.

Within the domain, which is the basic building block of an immunoglobulin molecule, the X-ray crystallographic studies have shown that the basic structural unit of amino acids is the *immunoglobulin fold* (Poljak *et al.*, 1973; Amzel *et al.*, 1974; Schiffer *et al.*, 1973; Epp *et al.*, 1974; Poljak, 1975; Segal *et al.*, 1974; Davies *et al.*, 1975a,b). This fold consists of two layers of antiparallel β-pleated sheets. One of these layers has three hydrogen-bonded antiparallel strands; the other layer has four. The intradomain disulfide bond is located at the center of each domain, and connects the middle section of the three-chain layer with a parallel strand in the other layer (Fig. 2). A notable feature of this arrangement is that the invariant tryptophan lies very close to the disulfide bond. While Fig. 2 shows the schematic representation of one polypeptide chain, the arrangement of two chains in the Fab molecule is shown in Fig. 3. It can be seen that in the C region, the four stranded layers of each chain form the interface with the three stranded layers on the outside of the molecule. In the V region, however, the reverse arrangement of the layers obtains, with the four stranded layers on the outside.

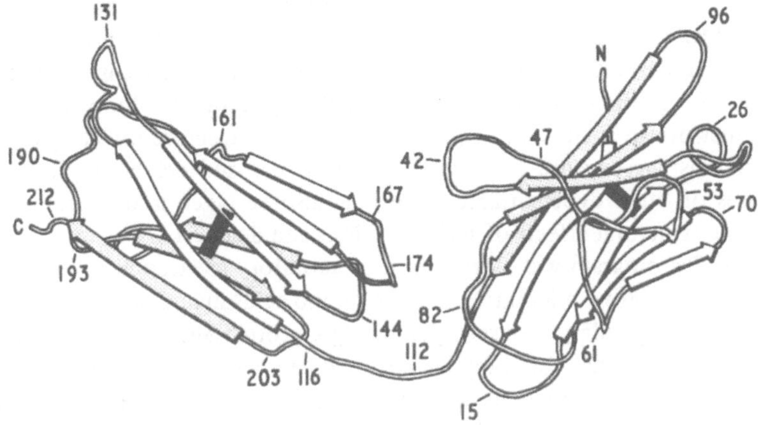

Figure 2. Schematic representation of the immunoglobulin fold of one chain as observed in the Bence-Jones protein Mcg. Arrows indicate the direction of the polypeptide chain. In both domains, white arrows represent stretches of extended chain lying in one plane, stippled arrows represent stretches lying in the other. Disulfide bonds are indicated as black bars connecting the two planes in each domain. Reprinted with permission from Schiffer *et al.* (1973). Copyright by the American Chemical Society.

The concept of the immunoglobulin fold as the basic structural unit has led to the suggestion that the variable region may be regarded as consisting of a rigid framework, with a particular hydrogen-bonding scheme, to which the hypervariable regions or loops are attached. Since these hypervariable loops involve at most 15 residues, and since the configurations of several of these loops are known from the X-ray crystal studies, it has been suggested (Poljak *et al.*, 1973; Poljak, 1975; Davies *et al.*, 1975a,b) that it is feasible to construct, by model-building, the hypervariable regions and thus the binding sites of different immunoglobulins from their known amino acid sequences.

The model-building method involves using the main chain coordinates of one or more of the corresponding fragments determined by X-ray analysis. The se-

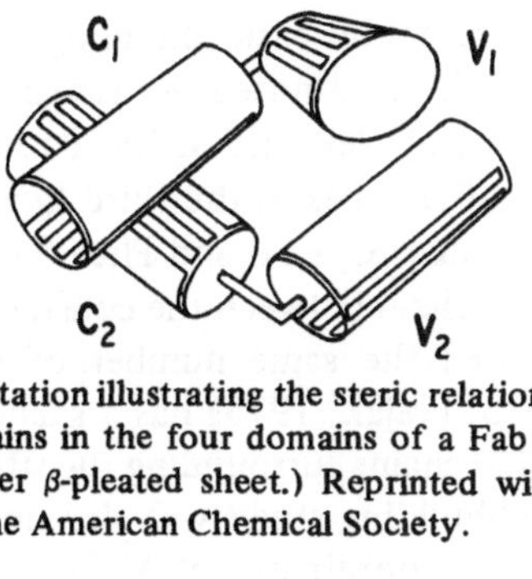

Figure 3. Schematic representation illustrating the steric relationship of the immunoglobulin folds of two polypeptide chains in the four domains of a Fab molecule. (The parallel bars represent the 4-stranded layer β-pleated sheet.) Reprinted with permission from Schiffer *et al.* (1973). Copyright by the American Chemical Society.

quences of these fragments are compared with those of the fragment for which the structure is required, so that they can be aligned for maximum sequence homology and structural analogy. The model is constructed using the immunoglobulin fold as the basic framework, with the hypervariable loops attached to this framework in such a way as to leave the basic structure unchanged except when it must be because of amino acid insertions and deletions. The known structures of other hypervariable loops may also be taken into account in estimating the structural effects of such insertions and deletions.

In 1973 a program was started in this laboratory to attempt to identify and to obtain the relative orientations of the amino acids in and near the combining site of the Dnp-binding mouse myeloma IgA protein MOPC 315. Attempts to obtain suitable crystals for X-ray analysis had been unsuccessful and a technique capable of giving comparable information in *solution* is therefore required. Nuclear magnetic resonance (NMR) is such a technique; however, structural determinations of proteins by NMR are still at a very early stage and the problems of resolution and assignment of peaks to individual amino acids are still very major ones, especially in the absence of a crystal structure (see, for example, Dwek 1973). In fact the largest protein where significant structural details had been determined using NMR was lysozyme (MW ~ 14,000 daltons) and this had been considerably aided by a knowledge of the crystal structure. Thus the extension of the NMR technique even to the Fv fragment (MW ~ 25,000 daltons) from MOPC 315 represented a major hurdle. New methodology had to be devised and our approach was to be based essentially on using the results from a variety of physical techniques in conjunction with NMR studies. The initial step, though, was to use the concept of the immunoglobulin fold to enable a structure prediction of the combining site to be made, and then to refine this using all the physical data. By concentrating mainly on the combining site contact residues, many of the problems normally encountered in a complete structural determination of the whole fragment would be eliminated.

The suggestion by Poljak *et al.* (1973) that Fab′ New could be used as a basic structural framework to predict the structure of the combining site of MOPC 315 was thus most timely and provided an important step forward for the NMR studies. Quite apart from use of the basic immunoglobulin fold in any structure prediction, Poljak *et al.* (1973) also noted the striking degree of homology between the (light) L(λ) chains of New and MOPC 315. In particular, each chain contains an equal number of residues in the third hypervariable region between the constant amino acid residues Cys 90 and Phe 98 (Table I). The third hypervariable region of the heavy chain between the constant residues Cys 96 and Trp 108 (Table II) also included the same number of residues. The model that emerges (Poljak *et al.*, 1973; Poljak, 1975) has a shallow combining site with a high density of aromatic side chains surrounding the site.

A more detailed model-building study was also undertaken by Padlan *et al.* (1976), using essentially the coordinates of McPC 603, but also most of the

Table I. Alignment of V_L Sequences

McPC 603[a]	1	Asp - Ile - Val - Met - Thr - Gln - Ser - Pro - Ser - Ser
MOPC 315[b]	1	Pca - Ala - Val - Val - Thr - Glu - Glu - - Ser - Ala
New[c]	1	Pca - Ser - Val - Leu - Thr - Gln - Pro - Pro - - Ser
	11	Leu - Ser - Val - Ser - Ala - Gly - Glu - Arg - Val - Thr
	10	Leu - Thr - Thr - Ser - Pro - Gly - Gly - Thr - (Val Ile)
	10	Val - Ser - Gly - Ala - Pro - Gly - Gln - Arg - Val - Thr
	21	Met - Ser - Cys - Lys - Ser - Ser - Glx - Ser - Leu - Leu
	20	Leu - Thr - Cys - Arg - Ser - Ser - Thr - Gly - Ala - Val
	20	Ile - Ser - Cys - Thr - Gly - Ser - Ser - Ser - Asn - Ile
	27d	Asx - Ser - Gly - Asx - Glx - Lys - Asx - Phe - Leu - Ala
	30	- - - Thr - Thr - Ser - Asn - Tyr - Ala - Asn
	27c	- - - Gly - Ala - Gly - Asn - His - Val - Lys
	35	Trp - Tyr - Glx -(Glx)- Lys - Pro - Gly - Glx - Pro - Pro
	37	Trp - Ile - Glx - Glx - Lys - Pro - Asx - His - Leu - Phe
	34	Trp - Tyr - Gln - Gln - Leu - Pro - Gly - Thr - Ala - Pro
	45	Lys - Leu - Leu - Ile - Tyr - X - X - X - X - X
	47	Thr - Gly - Leu - Ile - Gly - Gly - Thr - Ser - Asp - Arg
	44	Lys - Leu - Leu - Ile - Phe - His - Asn - Asn - Ala - Arg
	55	X - X - Gly - Val - Pro - Ala - Arg - Phe - Ser - Gly
	57	Ala - Pro - Gly - Val - Pro - Val - Arg - Phe - Ser - Gly
	61	- - - - - - - Phe - Ser - Val
	65	Ser - Gly - Ser - Arg - Thr - Asp - Phe - Thr - Leu - Thr
	67	Ser - Leu - Ile - Gly - Asp - Lys - Ala - Ala - Leu - Thr
	64	Ser - Lys - Ser - Gly - Ser - Ser - Ala - Thr - Leu - Ala
	75	Ile - Asx - Pro - Val - Glx - Ala - Asx - Asp - Val - Ala
	77	Ile - Thr - Gly - Ala - Glx - Thr - Glx - Asp - Asp - Ala
	74	Ile - Thr - Gly - Leu - Gln - Ala - Glu - Asp - Glu - Ala
	85	Thr - Tyr - Phe - Cys - X - X - X - X - X - X
	87	Met - Tyr - Phe - Cys - Ala - Leu - Trp - Phe - Arg - Asx
	84	Asp - Tyr - Tyr - Cys - Gln - Ser - Tyr - Asp - Arg - Ser
	95	- X - X - X - Phe - Gly - Gly - Gly - Thr - Lys
	97	- His - Phe - Val - Phe - Gly - Gly - Gly - Thr - Lys
	94	- Leu - Arg - Val - Phe - Gly - Gly - Gly - Thr - Lys
	104	Ley - Glu - Ile - Lys - Arg
	106	Val - Thr - Val - Leu - Gly
	105	Leu - Thr - Val - Leu - Arg

[a] McPC 603 sequence from Segal *et al.* (1974); since only the first 49 residues are known, the residues given for the rest of the sequence are those that occur most frequently in mouse κ chains (Davies *et al.*, 1975b).

[b] MOPC 315 sequence from Dugan *et al.* (1973).

[c] New sequence from Poljak *et al.* (1973); numbering according to Wu and Kabat (1970) to maximize structural homology.

Table II. Alignment of V_H Sequences

McPC 603[a]	1	Glu	Val	Lys	Leu	Val	Glu	Ser	Gly	Gly	Gly
MOPC 315[b]	1	Asp	Val	Gln	Leu	Gln	Glu	Ser	Gly	Pro	Gly
New[c]	1	Pca	Val	Gln	Leu	Gly	Glu	Ser	Gly	Pro	Glu
	11	Leu	Val	Gln	Pro	Gly	Gly	Ser	Leu	Arg	Leu
	11	Leu	Val	Lys	Pro	Ser	Gln	Ser	Leu	Ser	Leu
	11	Leu	Val	Arg	Pro	Ser	Gln	Thr	Leu	Ser	Leu
	21	Ser	Cys	Ala	Thr	Ser	Gly	Phe	Thr	Phe	Ser
	21	Thr	Cys	Ser	Val	Thr	Gly	Tyr	Ser	Ile	Thr
	21	Thr	Cys	Thr	Val	Ser	Gly	Ser	Thr	Phe	Ser
	31	Asp	Phe	Tyr	Met		Glu	Trp	Val	Arg	Gln
	31	Ser	Gly	Tyr	Phe	Trp	Asn	Trp	Ile	Arg	Gln
	31	Asn	Asp	Tyr	Tyr		Thr	Trp	Val	Arg	Gln
	40	Pro	Pro	Gly	Lys	Arg	Leu	Glu	Trp	Ile	Ala
	40	Phe	Pro	Gly	Asn	Lys	Leu	Glu	Trp	Leu	Gly
	40	Pro	Pro	Gly	Arg	Gly	Leu	Glu	Trp	Ile	Ala
	50	Ala	Ser	Arg	Asn	Lys	Gly	Asn	Lys	Tyr	Thr
	50	Phe	Ile	Lys	Tyr	Asp	Gly	-	-	-	Ser
	50	Tyr	Val	Phe	Tyr	His	Gly	-	-	-	Thr
	58b	Thr	Glu	Tyr	Ser	Ala	Ser	Val	Lys	Gly	Arg
	57	Asx	(Tyr	Gly)	Asx	Pro	Ser	Leu	Lys	Asn	Arg
	57	Ser	Asp	Thr	Asp	Thr	Pro	Leu	Arg	Ser	Arg
	68	Phe	Ile	Val	Ser	Arg	Asp	Thr	Ser	Gln	Ser
	68	Val	Ser	Ile	Thr	Arg	Asp	Thr	Ser	Glu	Asn
	68	Val	Thr	Met	Leu	Val	Asn	Thr	Ser	Lys	Asn
	78	Ile	Leu	Tyr	Leu	Gln	Met	Asn	Ala	Leu	Arg
	78	Gln	Phe	Phe	Leu	Lys	Leu	Asp	Ser	Val	Thr
	78	Gln	Phe	Ser	Leu	Arg	Leu	Ser	Ser	Val	Thr
	88	Ala	Glu	Asp	Thr	Ala	Ile	Tyr	Tyr	Cys	Ala
	88	Thr	Glx	Asx	Thr	Ala	Thr	Tyr	Tyr	Cys	Ala
	88	Ala	Ala	Asp	Thr	Ala	Val	Tyr	Tyr	Cys	Ala
	98	Arg	Asn	Tyr	Tyr	Gly	Ser	Thr	Trp	Tyr	Phe
	98	Gly	Asp	Asn	Asp	His	-	-	Leu	Tyr	Phe
	98	Arg	Asx	Leu	Ile	Ala	-	-	Gly	Cys	Ile
	106	Asp	Val	Trp	Gly	Ala	Gly	Thr	Thr	Val	Thr
	106	Asp	Tyr	Trp	Gly	Gln	Gly	Thr	Thr	Leu	Thr
	106	Asx	Val	Trp	Gly	Gln	Gly	Ser	Leu	Val	Thr
	116	Val	Ser	Ser							
	116	Val	Ser	Ser							
	116	Val	Ser	Ser							

[a] McPC 603 sequence from Rudikoff and Potter (1974).
[b] MOPC 315 sequence from Francis *et al.* (1974); numbering according to Rudikoff and Potter (1974) and Givol (private communication).
[c] New sequence as reported in Poljak *et al.* (1973), and Poljak (1976).

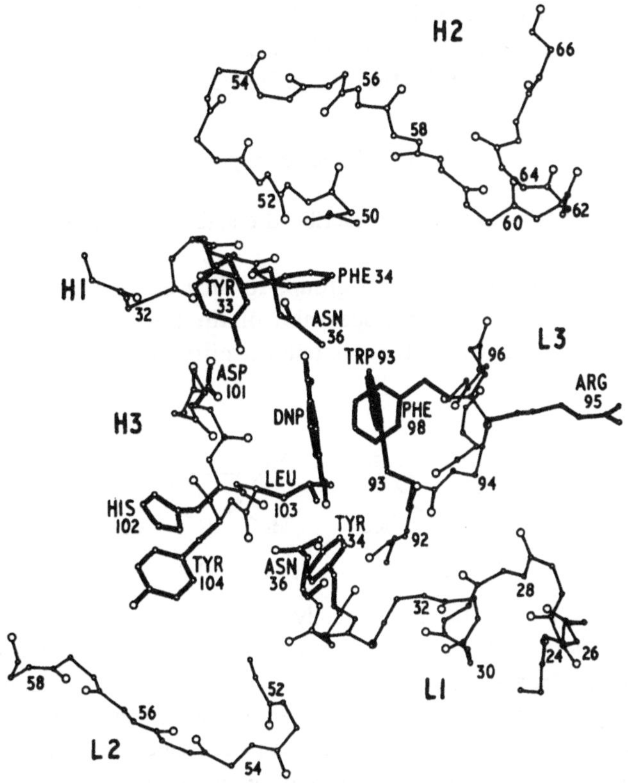

Figure 4. Predicted binding site of MOPC 315 based on the model-building studies of Padlan *et al.* (1976).

available three-dimensional data from the immunoglobulin structures. The predicted binding site of this hypothetical model is shown in Fig. 4. Both predicted models are in accordance with the results of affinity labeling studies (see Givol, 1974, for a review), but this agreement derives from coarse rather than from fine details of the model.

It is the aim of this chapter to illustrate how NMR studies in conjunction with such structure predictions can allow a picture of the site at very high resolution to be obtained so that detailed conclusions may be drawn about the reasons for specificity.

The studies involve using the predicted structure as a first approximation and then refining it by making it compatible with the physical data, mainly from the NMR studies, although other bulk properties, such as the dimensions of the site, will also suggest whether the coarser details of the model must be altered. The first section is therefore concerned with defining the dimensions and rigidity of the site using electron spin resonance (ESR) studies on a series of structurally related Dnp-nitroxide spin-labeled haptens.

II. SPIN-LABELED HAPTENS AS PROBES FOR THE DIMENSIONS AND RIGIDITY OF THE ANTIBODY COMBINING SITE

A. Spin-Labeled Haptens

The term *spin label* is used to describe the stable free radicals that are used as reporter groups.

The sensitivity of these reporter groups to their environment can be monitored by observation of the ESR spectrum of the free radical. Spin labels are molecules such as the following that contain the nitroxide moiety

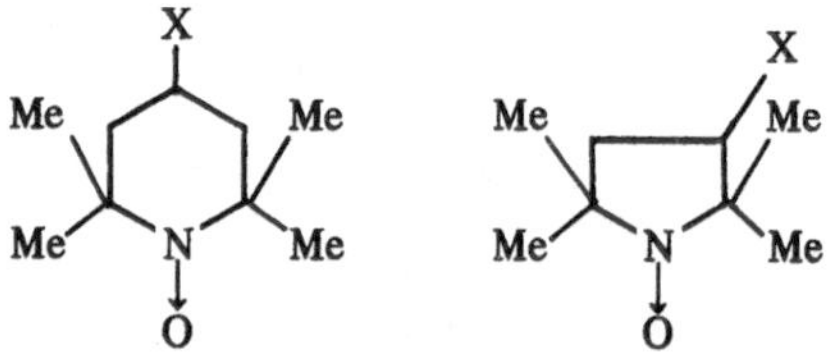

with an unpaired electron localized mainly on the nitrogen atom. By a suitable choice of X, it is possible to meet the specific requirements of many different biological systems. For instance, in antibody studies, X is the hapten group.

The ESR spectrum of a spin-label hapten consists of three lines arising from the hyperfine interaction of the spin-label unpaired electron with the nitroxide nitrogen nucleus. The mechanism by which the unpaired electron communicates with the nitrogen nucleus involves orbitals on the nitrogen that are not spherical, and therefore the hyperfine interaction is anisotropic. This means that in the extreme case of a spin label rigidly fixed in a single crystal, different hyperfine splittings would be measured when the magnetic field was directed along each of the three principal axes of the nitroxide group.

If we consider a completely random orientation of *immobilized* spin labels in the magnetic field, then the spectrum obtained (Fig. 5a) represents a sum of the spectra corresponding to all the possible orientations of the labels. If the label has any motion, this motion will cause averaging of the hyperfine anisotropy and the ESR spectrum changes. For instance, Figs 5b and c show what can happen to the spectrum of an immobilized sample if motion about a particular axis occurs. If the spin label can tumble isotropically, complete averaging occurs, and the characteristic three-line spectrum of the free label is observed (Fig. 5d). For haptens bound in the combining site, the amplitude of motion will be limited by the geometry of the combining site, and this forms the basis of the method for determining the dimensions of the site. The ESR spectra of the bound haptens, though, are often rather complex, but in all cases, the maximum

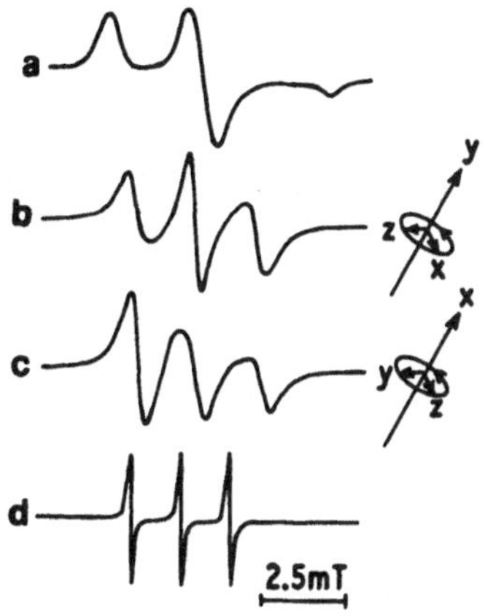

Figure 5. ESR spectrum of spin label in different motional states. (a) Completely rigid; (b) and (c) complete rotation about one axis; (d) completely isotropic.

splitting (termed $2A_{z'z'}$ or $2A_{max}$) can always be resolved, and in favorable circumstances, a minimum splitting ($2A_{x'x'}$) can sometimes be resolved.

B. Dimensions and Rigidity of the Combining Site in the Myeloma Protein MOPC 315

The geometry and flexibility of the combining site in MOPC 315 have been probed using spin-labeled haptens of different lengths and dimensions, in which the nitroxide moiety is contained in a six-membered ring. Several studies have also been reported using five-membered nitroxide spin-labeled haptens, but since these studies provide slightly different information about the site, they are best discussed as a separate group (see Section IIB2).

1. Six-Membered Nitroxide Spin Labels

The ESR spectra of various structurally differentiated dinitrophenyl hapten six-membered spin labels when bound to MOPC 315 are shown in Fig. 6. Comparison of the spectra shows that as the distance from the nitroxide to the dinitrophenyl ring increases, both the line widths and anisotropy (or extent of the spectra) decrease. The corresponds to an increased amplitude and rate of motion of the nitroxide group, which partially average out the anisotropy in the spin-label ESR spectrum. The limiting case of this is the isolated spin-label hapten rotating freely in solution, in which all the anisotropy is averaged out, giving rise to a narrow three-line spectrum as seen in Fig. 6.

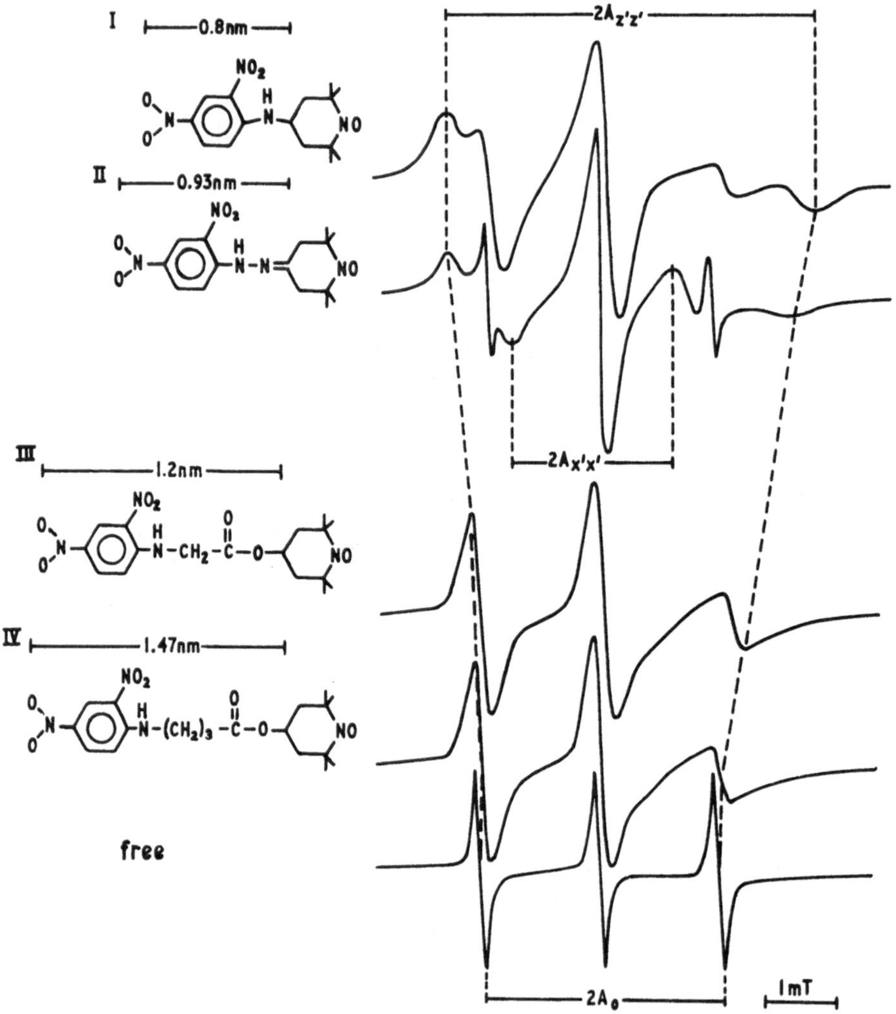

Figure 6. ESR spectra of the bound six-membered nitroxide spin labels used to probe the combining site of MOPC 315. The bottom spectrum is a free spin label in aqueous solution.

The shortest label, I, has the largest value of $2A_{z'z'}$, or 5.21 mT,* which approaches the maximum possible value of 6.4 mT expected if the spin label is completely immobilized. This value, together with the rather broad lines in the ESR spectrum, show that label I is rigidly held in the combining site. However, the reduction in the value of $2A_{z'z'}$ from 6.4 mT indicates that the spin label has a small degree of motion in the site. Calculations (Dwek *et al.*, 1975b) show

*Readers unfamiliar with these SI units should note that 1 mT ≡ 10 G.

that this motion can arise from transitions among the stable conformations of the six-membered nitroxide ring. These conformers are the "twisted," the chair, and the boat forms, of which the "twisted" conformers are likely to be the most favored on intramolecular steric considerations. The *minimum* lateral dimensions of the site that will allow interconversion (or flexing) between the twisted conformations are 0.9 × 0.6 nm (Dwek *et al.*, 1975a).

The slightly longer spin-label hapten, II, has a somewhat smaller value of $2A_{z'z'}$, 4.76 mT, indicating that it is more mobile, and since a minimum splitting ($2A_{x'x'}$) may also be measured (2.26 mT), in this case, it is possible to use an analysis of the motional averaging (Dwek *et al.*, 1975b) to show that this label has an additional motion corresponding to rotation about the N-N bond in the dinitrophenyl-nitroxide linkage. The longest hapten spin labels, III and IV, are undergoing motion of almost unlimited amplitude, since $A_{z'z'} = A_{x'x'}$, indicating that nitroxide ring is clear of the combining site. Their motion is still somewhat hindered, however, since the spectral lines are considerably broader than those obtained for the free spin label.

In summary, the different motional characteristics of haptens I-IV can be explained by assuming that (1) the hapten spin label I is accommodated wholly within the combining site; (2) the length of hapten spin label II is such that the nitroxide ring just protrudes from the combining site; and (3) hapten labels III and IV are of such a length that the nitroxide ring is sufficiently clear of the combining site for the protruding section to be able to perform almost complete, angularly isotropic motion. All these considerations would define the length of the combining site as being 1.1-1.2 nm (Dwek *et al.*, 1975a), with lateral dimensions of 0.6 × 0.9 nm around the entrance to the site. The approach used here, of considering the likely anisotropic motions of the label within the site, shows how it is possible to extend the "molecular dipstick" approach originally suggested by Hsia and Piette (1969) to obtain additional information on the transverse dimensions of the site.

2. *Five-Membered Nitroxide Spin Labels*

The spin-label haptens in this group are shown in Table III. Two have chiral centers (marked with asterisks), and so there are two pairs of enantiomers (Wong *et al.*, 1974). This feature enables certain information to be deduced about the site that cannot be provided by the six-membered spin labels. All five of the haptens give a highly immobilized "bound" signal in the ESR spectrum; haptens V and VI, consisting of a mixture of the two enantiomers, show two distinct bound signals with the IgA or Fab and Fv fragments. This is illustrated in Fig. 7 for the IgA. That two distinct signals should be obtained means that the site is asymmetric, and values of the hyperfine splitting constants (Table III) show that for both haptens V and VI, one enantiomer is completely immobilized,

Table III. Maximum Hyperfine Splittings ($2A_{max}$) of Five-Membered Nitroxide Spin Labels Bound to Myeloma Protein MOPC 315 IgA and Fragments Fab′ and Fv

Hapten	d[a] (nm)	$2A_{max}$ (mT) IgA	Fab′	Fv
V. DNP—NH—CH_2—[b] 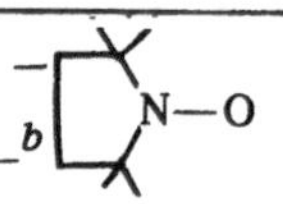	1.1	6.55 ± 0.05 5.70 ± 0.05	6.40 ± 0.05 5.70 ± 0.05	6.15 ± 0.05 5.55 ± 0.05
VI. 5—F—DNP—NH—[b] 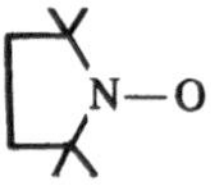	0.9	6.15 ± 0.05 5.30 ± 0.05	6.00 ± 0.05 5.25 ± 0.05	5.70 ± 0.05 5.30 ± 0.05
VII. [c]DNP—NH—N= 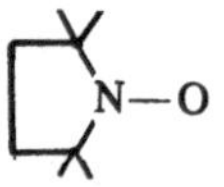	1.1	6.24 ± 0.05	–	–

[a]Measured from oxygen of the 4-nitro group to the oxygen of the nitroxide, based on results of conformational analyses (Sutton *et al.*, 1976).
[b]Denotes chiral center. In the following row of data, the two sets of figures refer to the two enantiomers.
[c]From Hsia and Little (1973).

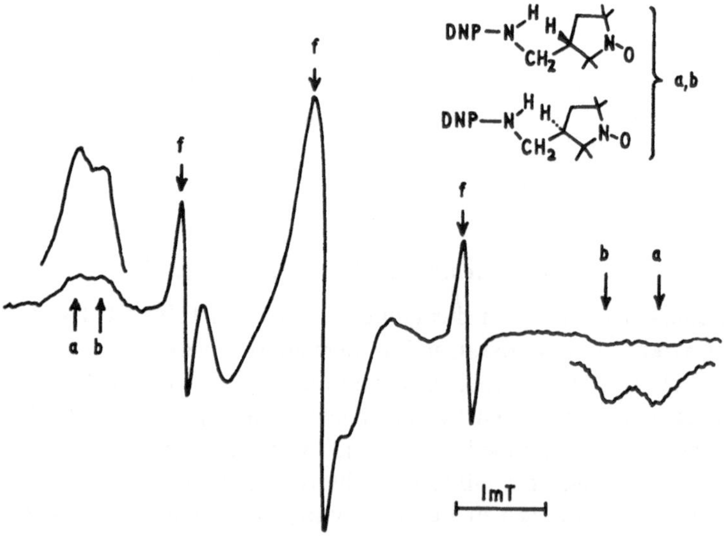

Figure 7. ESR spectrum of hapten V bound to MOPC 315 IgA, showing the bound signals (a, b) corresponding to the two enantiomers and the signal from free spin label (f).

while the nitroxide moiety of the other has some degree of mobility. The observed value of $A_{z'z'}$ for the "mobile" enantiomer must be due to motion of the label within the site (since these haptens are not long enough to have the nitroxide group clear of the site), from which it follows that the lateral dimensions around the spin label moiety can be probed. Moreover, since haptens V and VI are of different length, they will probe different parts of the site, the dimensions of which must be sufficient to allow the motion necessary to give the observed hyperfine splitting constants. For the analysis of the possible motions of the five-membered spin labels, it is necessary to know the structures of these haptens. Our analysis assumes that the N$\underline{H}$ proton is coplanar with, and hydrogen-bonds to, the 2—NO_2 group on the Dnp ring. It is possible, however, that the combining site may impose restrictions on the hapten so as to make this interaction unfavorable. In this connection, it is interesting to note that resonance Raman studies of Dnp haptens binding to MOPC 315 (Carey *et al.*, personal communication) have indicated that the N$\underline{H}$ proton is not bonded to the 2—NO_2 group of Dnp-lysine when this hapten is bound. We have therefore also considered this possibility for the five-membered spin labels used here, and find that this does not alter the overall conclusions about the dimensions of the site. A detailed picture of the dimensions of the site based on an analysis of all the spin-labeled haptens is shown in Fig. 8.

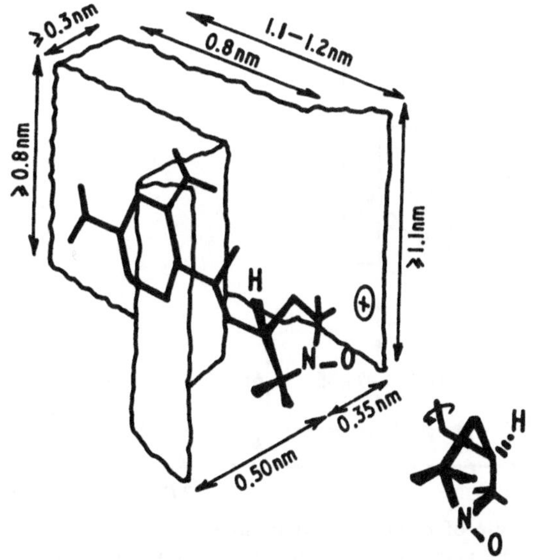

Figure 8. Combining site of myeloma protein MOPC 315 with the two enantiomers of hapten V, determined by spin-label mobility mapping.

C. Polarity of the Antibody Combining Site

The $\rangle N \rightarrow O$ bond can be considered as a hybrid of two canonical forms: $\rangle N{-}O^{\bullet} \leftrightarrow \rangle N^{\oplus}{-}O^{\ominus}$. The hyperfine splitting arises from the interaction between the unpaired electron on the nitrogen atom and the nitrogen nucleus. In the ionic form in which the unpaired electron is entirely located on the nitrogen atom, the magnitude of the interaction will be greater. The presence of a hydrogen-bonding solvent or of a positive charge near the oxygen atom that will favor the ionic form will therefore result in an increase in the hyperfine splitting constants. A convenient index of environmental polarity is the isotropic hyperfine splitting constant, A_0 (Smith *et al.*, 1975; Griffith *et al.*, 1974):

$$A_0 = {}^1\!/_3\,(A_{z'z'} + A_{x'x'} + A_{y'y'})$$

This relationship has been used to calculate the values of A_0 for some haptens (Dwek *et al.*, 1975b), and the results have been correlated with the subsites of interaction in the combining site proposed by Haselkorn *et al.* (1974) on the basis of temperature jump studies with a series of Dnp ligands. This correlation is illustrated in Fig. 9. The size of the nitroxide ring means that the spatial resolution of the spin-label data will not be as good as that from kinetic mapping. It turns out, however, that the polarity index (value of A_0) for the shortest

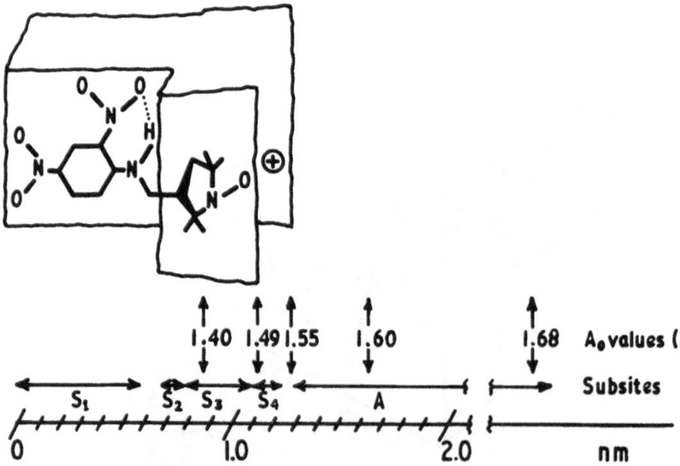

Figure 9. Combining site of myeloma protein MOPC 315 with hapten V, illustrating the correlation between the parameter A_0 (polarity index) derived from ESR studies (see the text) and the subsites of interaction deduced from binding kinetics (Haselkorn *et al.*, 1974). (S_1) Dnp-binding subsite; (S_2) first hydrophobic subsite; (S_3) second hydrophobic subsite; (S_4) positive subsite; (A) free aqueous environment.

spin-label hapten is comparable with that found in a hydrocarbon solvent, and corresponds to the second hydrophobic subsite as defined by Haselkorn *et al.* (1974). As the nitroxide grouping is further removed from the Dnp ring, the polarity index increases (Fig. 9), approaching the value found for an aqueous system. The positive subsite, S_4, of Haselkorn *et al.* (1974) corresponds to a value of A_0 in a rather polar environment, as expected. Correlation of this with the near-isotropic motion found for spin labels in this region suggests that this subsite is probably at the antibody surface.

Further information on the positive subsite can be obtained from a comparison of the values of $A_{z'z'}$, since the value of a spin-label hapten rigidly immobilized in an IgA molecule is 6.15 mT (Sutton *et al.*, 1976). While hapten V does have this value (Table III), hapten VI has a higher value of 6.65 mT. This suggests for hapten VI that a nearby positive charge is stabilizing the ionic $\rangle N^{\oplus}{-}O^{\ominus}$ form of the nitroxide bond. Calculations show (Sutton *et al.*, 1976) that the presence of a positive charge within 0.3 nm of the nitroxide bond will account for this higher value, and the position of this charge in the site has been included in Fig. 9.

In general however, polarity effects are small, and differences in $A_{z'z'}$ values between haptens will mainly arise from different degrees of motional averaging available to the haptens.

D. Comparison of the Dimensions of the Combining Sites in the DnP-Binding IgA Myeloma Proteins MOPC 315, XRPC 25, and MOPC 460

The mouse IgA myeloma proteins MOPC 315, MOPC 460, and XRPC 25 constitute a set of closely related proteins whose comparative properties are of interest, since they all possess appreciable antidinitrophenyl activity. That there are differences in specificity is illustrated by their differences in affinity for various ligands (Jaffe *et al.*, 1971; Dwek *et al.*, 1976a). In particular, it is interesting that MOPC 460 has a much higher affinity for 2,4-dinitronaphthol than MOPC 315, while no binding to XRPC 25 can be detected.

A comparison of the dimensions of the combining sites of these three myeloma proteins has been made by also applying the spin-label mapping method to MOPC 460 and XRPC 25. The experimental results are summarized in Table IV, and for completeness, those for MOPC 315 are included. The dimensions of the different sites are shown in Fig. 10.

Inspection of Table IV reveals the main features of the combining sites. Thus, the low values of $2A_{max}$ of haptens III and IV indicate that the nitroxide ring is rotating with few constraints, unlike haptens I and II, which have high

Table IV. Maximum Hyperfine Splittings ($2A_{max}$) of Spin-Label Haptens Bound to Myeloma Proteins MOPC 315, XRPC 25, and MOPC 460

Hapten	$2A_{max}$ (mT)		
	MOPC 315[a]	XRPC 25	MOPC 460
I. DNP—NH— 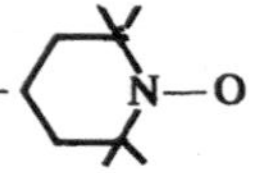	Fab′ 5.34 ± 0.02	Fab′ 6.36 ± 0.15	Fab′ 4.90 ± 0.15
II. DNP—NH—N= 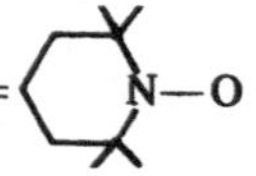	Fab′ 4.60 ± 0.10	Fab′ 5.86 ± 0.20	Fab′ 4.78 ± 0.15
III. DNP—NH—CH_2—CO—O— 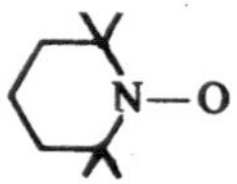	Fv 3.18 ± 0.20	Fab′ 3.18 ± 0.20	Fab′ 3.20 ± 0.02
IV. DNP—NH—$(CH_2)_3$—CO—O— 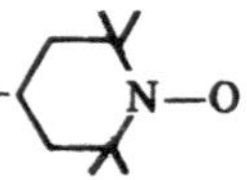	IgA 3.20 ± 0.04	Fab′ 3.18 ± 0.20	Fab′ 3.20 ± 0.02
V. DNP—NH—CH_2—[b] 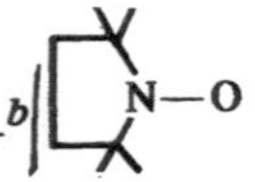	Fab′ 6.40 ± 0.05 5.70 ± 0.05	Fab′ 6.70 ± 0.05 6.40 ± 0.05	Fab′ 4.00
VI. 5—F—DNP—NH—[b] 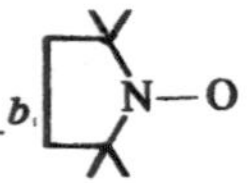	Fab′ 6.00 ± 0.05 5.26 ± 0.05	Fab′ 6.00 ± 0.05 5.46 ± 0.05	Fab′ 5.10 ± 0.05 4.86 ± 0.05
VII. DNP—NH—N=[c] 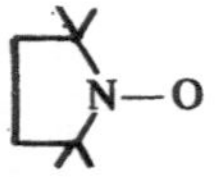	IgA 6.24 ± 0.05	—	IgA 6.24 ± 0.05

[a] Although different fragments are used in this comparison, it has been shown previously (Dwek *et al.*, 1975b) that the size of the fragment containing the combining site has only small effects on the ESR hyperfine splittings of the bound hapten.
[b] Denotes chiral center. In the following row of data, the two sets of figures refer to the two enantiomers.
[c] From Hsia and Little (1973).

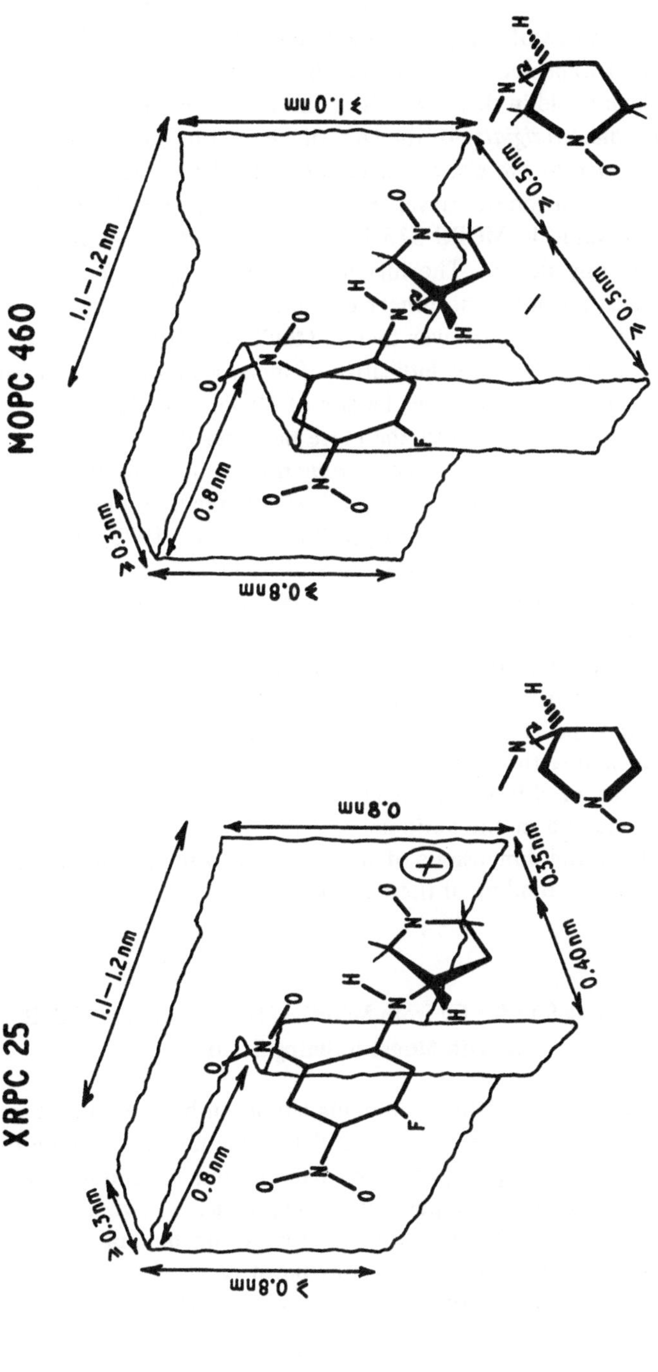

Figure 10. Combining sites of myeloma proteins XRPC 25 and MOPC 460 with the two enantiomers of hapten VI as determined by spin-label mobility mapping.

values of $2A_{max}$ indicative of constrained motion. This allows the *depth* of the combining sites of all three myeloma proteins to be estimated as 1.1-1.2 nm. Further, since the value of $2A_{max}$ for hapten VII in either MOPC 460 or MOPC 315 is about that expected if the hapten is completely immobilized, the Dnp ring must be rigidly held in these two sites. Similarly, the $2A_{max}$ value of hapten I in XRPC 25 indicates *rigidity* of the Dnp ring here too. That the *lateral dimensions of the entrance to the site* are different in the three cases, however, is well illustrated by a comparison of the values of $2A_{max}$ for hapten I. As we have seen (Section B1) the value in MOPC 315 is consistent with the dimensions being such as to allow ring flexing. The higher value of $2A_{max}$ in XRPC 25 shows, however, that such motion is no longer possible in this combining site, and that the site must therefore be narrower than in MOPC 315. By contrast, the smaller value of $2A_{max}$ in MOPC 460 is indicative of increased motion of the nitroxide ring compared with that possible in the site of MOPC 315. The entrance to the combining site in MOPC 460 must therefore be wider than in MOPC 315. *The asymmetry of the entrances to the combining sites* is shown by the observations of two ESR signals (two values of $2A_{max}$) with haptens V and VI. Further, a detailed analysis of these values of $2A_{max}$ (Sutton *et al.*, 1976) shows that the site is more symmetrical in MOPC 460 than in XRPC 25 (Fig. 10). Finally, the high $2A_{max}$ values for hapten V in MOPC 315 (6.4 mT) and XRPC 25 (6.70 mT) can be interpreted in terms of a contribution from a *positively charged residue*, which must be similarly positioned in both proteins (Dwek *et al.*, 1976a).

One limitation of the ESR technique is that it gives no information on the dimensions around the Dnp ring. The values given in the diagrams ($\geqslant$0.3 nm $\times$ $\geqslant$0.8 nm) are simply those required to fit the Dnp into the site. Although detailed explanations of differences in affinities of haptens such as 2,4-dinitronaphthol or menadione in the various myelomas must await further structural details of the sites, the dimensions of the entrance to the site in XRPC 25 are such as to preclude the binding of these particular haptens.

E. Combining Site for Fv from MOPC 315—Comparison of ESR Data with Model-Building Studies

In deciding the depth of the combining site given by the molecular model (Padlan *et al.*, 1976), it is essential to postulate some mode of hapten binding, to provide a limit to the region probed by haptens and, thus, dimensions comparable to those calculated by experiment. The presence of two nitro groups on the hapten, which appear to be necessary for strong binding, suggest some H-bonding to amino acid side chains (Haselkorn *et al.*, 1974). For instance, positioning of the Dnp ring so that it can H-bond to either or both Asn 36_L and

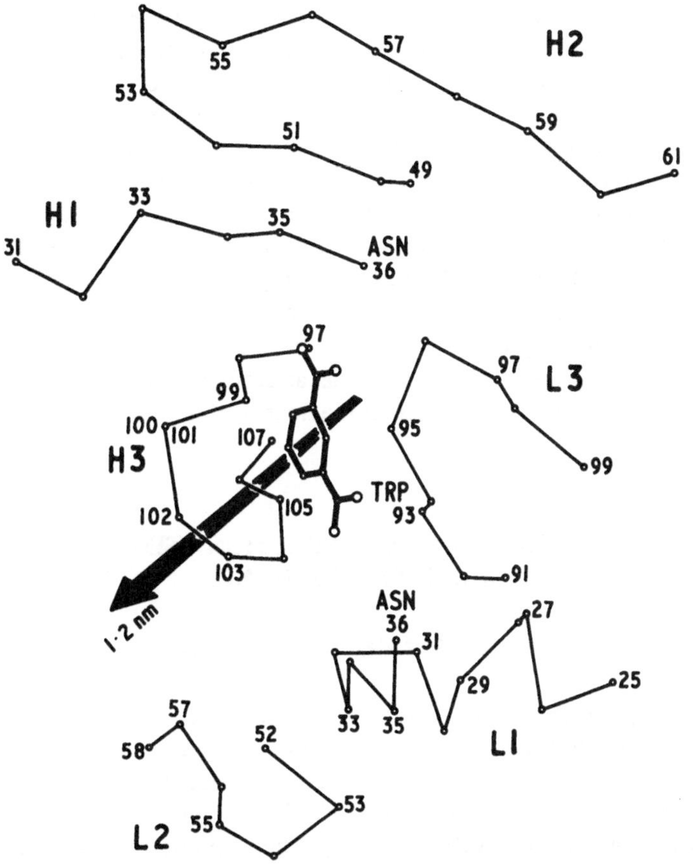

Figure 11. Predicted combining site of MOPC 315 showing the hypervariable loops of the heavy (H) and light (L) chains (Padlan *et al.*, 1976) and the hapten position relative to the two chains. The view shown is looking into the site at 35° to the plane of the Dnp ring. The heavy arrow illustrates the depth of the combining site, which is 1.2 nm.

Asn 36_H places Trp 93_L parallel to the hypervariable 3-loop of the light chain (L3), so that it "stacks" with the Dnp ring (Fig. 11). This also puts the Dnp at the back of the pocket, defined by phenylalanine side chains 98_L and 105_H, so that measurements from here should provide the desired comparability of results. A depth of 1.2 nm then results when measured from this starting point to a point entirely clear of all combining-site side chains. Significant variations in the orientations of the tryptophan can be excluded, since they result in a considerably shorter combining site.

The width and height vary greatly along the length of the hapten, being smallest around the Dnp moiety, where dimensions of 0.8 × 0.45 nm provide a tight fit for the ring. Because of the asymmetry at the entrance of the combining site and the relative freedom of motion of side chains there, which project into solution, it is more difficult to define precisely the dimensions expected from the model. Rather, it is possible to use the experimental results to define the position of the amino side chains that make up the combining site. Thus, the location of the positive charge fixes the position of the side chain of Arg 95_L. (This adjustment is incorporated into Fig. 11.) The other restrictions on the model imposed from the ESR mapping studies are all relatively small, and it should be emphasized that the ESR mapping only determines the structure at low resolution, probing such properties of the site as rigidity and overall dimensions. In solution, the actual details at atomic resolution can come only from NMR studies. This is dealt with in the next section.

III. STRUCTURAL STUDIES IN SOLUTION USING NUCLEAR MAGNETIC RESONANCE

A. Nuclear Magnetic Resonance

In this method, the nuclear orientation effects of those nuclei that possess a spin are studied. Among the biologically important nuclei that are accessible to the method are ^{1}H, ^{13}C, ^{23}Na, and ^{31}P. In the modern NMR spectrometer, a radiofrequency pulse (in the range 4–400 MHz) is applied to a sample (~1 ml) that is in a magnetic field (10^2–10^4 mT). The response to this pulse contains information about the energy involved in a transition between nuclear orientations. This energy is reflected in a resonance position on a frequency scale measured with respect to some standard, usually in units of parts per million (ppm). This scale is known as the *chemical shift scale*.

For protons, the theory is particularly simple. In a magnetic field, the proton may exist in one of two energy states in which its magnetic moment is aligned either parallel or antiparallel to the direction of the applied field. The radiofrequency pulse then causes transitions between these two energy states.

For further details of the theory and also of the applications for NMR to biochemical problems, readers are referred to the text *NMR in Biochemistry* (Dwek, 1973).

B. General Features of an NMR Spectrum

The shape of an NMR spectrum is usually governed by three factors: the chemical shifts of the various nuclei, the width of the resonances, and the hyperfine (or spin–spin) interactions between nuclei.

The Chemical Shift gives information on the environment of a nucleus. Thus, aromatic amino acids occur in regions of the spectrum quite distinct from aliphatic amino acids. In a random coil protein, all the resonances from one type of chemical grouping usually coincide, but in a globular protein with a preferred conformation in solution, this is not so because there are variations in local environment. The range of chemical shifts depends on the nucleus, but for protons it is small (~10 ppm). In a globular protein, this means that there will be an overlap of many proton resonances. The chemical shift, however, is proportional to the applied magnetic field. As the field is raised, the separation of chemically shifted resonances is increased, with corresponding simplification of the spectrum. This fact has mainly provided the impetus for the use of spectrometers operating with superconducting magnetic fields.

The Line Width of a nuclear resonance is mainly dominated by dipolar interactions with neighboring nuclei. Any motion that can cause averaging of the dipolar interactions will result in line narrowing. In a protein, the slow tumbling times will not cause much effective averaging, and the lines will be broad. However, there will be some resonances that exhibit relatively sharp lines. These resonances will arise from amino acid residues that have significant local motional freedom, such as those on the surface of a protein or on parts of the polypeptide chain having some segmental motion. The dipolar interaction is obviously reduced, too, if the number of neighboring nuclei is reduced. This and the possibility of independent motions often accounts for the sharper resonances associated with amino acids on the surface of a protein. It is also necessary to note that in addition to any dipolar broadening, the line width of a nuclear resonance may be broadened if the nucleus is involved in some sort of "exchange" process between different chemical environments. Analysis of the exchange broadening then gives information on the dynamics of these processes.

Spin–spin interactions arise from interaction of neighboring nuclei with magnetic moments, and are manifest in the spectrum as hyperfine interactions. The magnitude of these interactions depends on the nature of the chemical bonds between the nuclei and their relative geometries. In many proteins, the line widths are greater than the spin–spin couplings, and so these couplings are often unresolved.

C. 270 MHz Proton NMR Spectra of IgA, Fab, and Fv from MOPC 315

The 270 MHz NMR spectra of the IgA, Fab, and Fv from MOPC 315 are shown in Fig. 12. Even at this high frequency, there is still considerable overlap of proton resonances. This, and the broad resonance lines resulting from slow motions of proteins of this size, together with the unresolved hyperfine interactions, produce the broad envelopes for the NMR spectra. As expected, however, we note that the resolution in the spectra increases from IgA through Fab to the Fv.

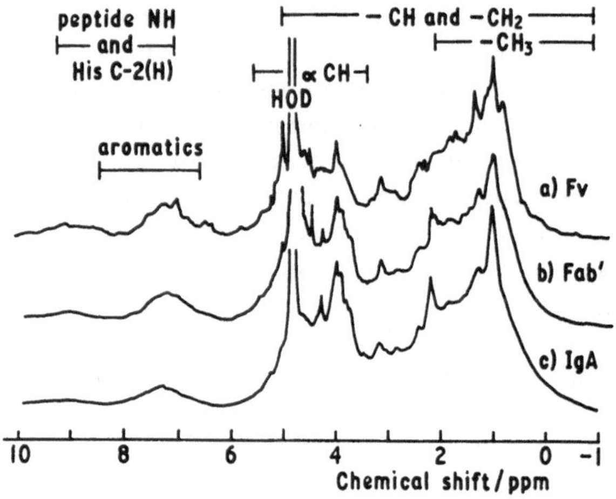

Figure 12. 270 MHz proton spectra of IgA, Fab, and Fv from MOPC 315. From Dwek *et al.* (1975b).

The main regions in which the resonances from different amino acids generally occur are also indicated in Fig. 12. The simplest *class* of proton resonances to identify are those in the range 6.5–8.5 ppm, which are from *aromatic* side chains. Of the four amino acids with aromatic side chains, the C-2 proton resonances of *histidines* are usually resolved from the aromatic envelope. Since their exact position varies with the ionization state of the histidine, these resonances can usually be identified by monitoring the effects of pH on the spectrum. Resonances from the *methyl groups* of the six amino acids containing them are also relatively easy to identify, since they have an area of three protons and they occur in the range −1 to 2 ppm. Overlapping slightly with these are the *—CH— and —*CH_2*— protons*—in the range −1 to 5.5 ppm. These are by far the hardest type of proton resonance to identify, since they often exhibit complex resonance patterns because of extensive hyperfine interactions. The *α-C$\underline{\underline{H}}$ proton* resonances occur in the region 3.5–5.5 ppm, and can sometimes be identified (Campbell *et al.*, 1975a). *Peptide NH* resonances, which occur in the range 7–9.5 ppm are often outside the bulk of the aromatic envelope, though these resonances are usually twice as broad as CH resonances, because of dipolar interaction with the ^{14}N nucleus.

Most of the observations of proton spectra of proteins are carried out in D_2O, rather than H_2O, in order to suppress the very strong H_2O resonance that can essentially "blot out" most of the protein resonances. If some of the NH protons are exchangeable, however, the consequent substitution by deuterium will simplify the spectrum. These exchangeable protons and those from any residual water in the system all contribute to an HOD peak, arising from exchange with deuterium in the D_2O. Recent improvements in techniques, though, allow spectra to be obtained quite easily in H_2O, and so it is possible to study the N$\underline{H}$ resonances if necessary.

D. Types of Amino Acid Residues in and near the Combining Site of Fv from MOPC 315

Even with Fv, the proton NMR spectrum contains some 1400 protons, and the problems of resolution and assignment of these protons are still major ones, but by a suitable trick, this spectrum can be further simplified so that only those resonances in or near the combining site are obtained. The method involves a form of *difference spectroscopy*, using a paramagnetic center such as a spin-label hapten. Paramagnetic centers such as these cause a broadening of the NMR line widths. This broadening is inversely proportional to the sixth power of the distance between the paramagnetic center and the nucleus. Thus, the greatest effects are on the resonances of nuclei close to the paramagnetic center. For illustrative purposes, consider a system that has an NMR spectrum of four resonances arising from four chemically distinct nuclei (Fig. 13). Suppose a paramagnetic spin label is added to this system, in such a way that it binds very close to one nucleus. The NMR line width of this nucleus is then broadened (Fig. 13). (For simplicity, we assume that the other nuclei are too far away from the spin label to have their resonance line widths significantly affected.) If we now subtract the two spectra in Fig. 13, we obtain essentially only the spectrum of the resonances of nuclei close to the spin label. The final spectrum is termed the NMR *paramagnetic difference spectrum*.

Figure 14 shows the 270 MHz proton spectra of the Fv in the presence and absence of the six-membered spin-label hapten 1. The resulting paramagnetic difference spectrum contains protons from those residues in or near the combining site, for it has previously been argued (Dwek *et al.*, 1975a) that the effective broadening range of this spin label extends over a sphere of radius 1.0-1.4 nm from the N-O bond, where the electron is localized. Since this length is slightly longer than the hapten itself, protons from residues in contact with the Dnp ring will be perturbed by the spin label. This is an advantage of this technique over many affinity labeling studies, which generally reveal only the residues

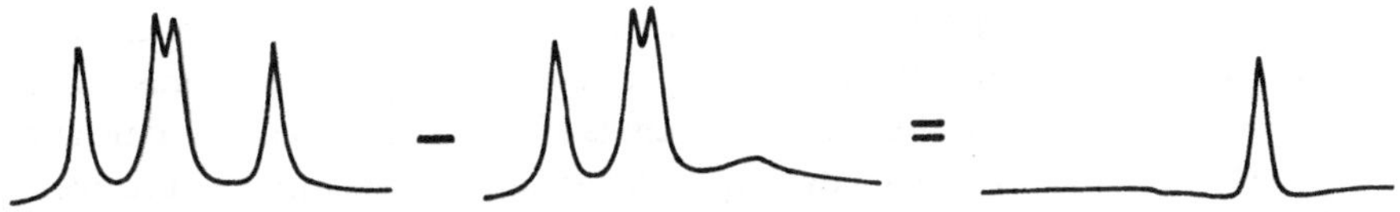

Figure 13. Schematic representation of the principle involved in obtaining a paramagnetic difference spectrum.

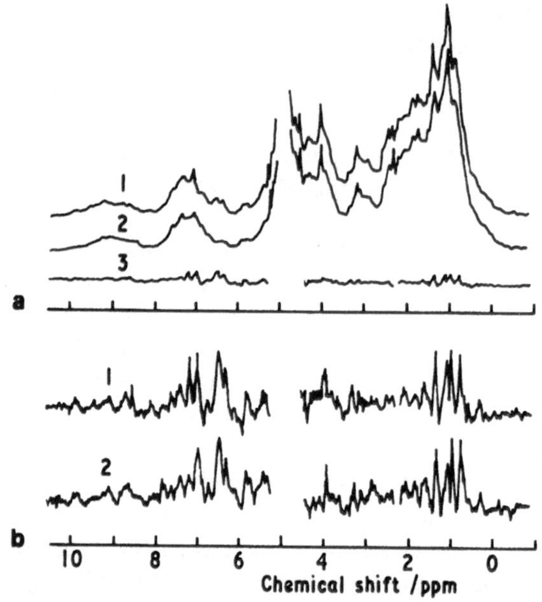

Figure 14. (a) 270 MHz proton spectrum of Fv fragment of MOPC 315 (30 mg ml^{-1}), T = 30°C, pH = 6.9, NaCl = 0.15 M, 2000 scans: (1) no addition; (2) in the presence of an equivalent amount of spin label 1; (3) paramagnetic difference spectrum (1) – (2). (b) Enlarged (×6) paramagnetic difference spectra at (1) pH 6.9, (2) pH 8.47.

in contact with the side chains of the Dnp derivatives, rather than around the Dnp itself. The difference spectrum in Fig. 14a reveals an unusually high aromatic content of residues compared with that observed in the normal Fv spectrum, suggesting that the combining site is highly aromatic. This is obviously consistent with the high affinity of MOPC 315 for Dnp derivatives. Figure 14b shows in more detail two paramagnetic difference spectra at different pHs. The slight variations with pH in the aromatic region arise from the changes in chemical shift on ionization of two histidine residues (see Section F).

E. Hapten Binding Does Not Cause Conformational Changes Outside the Combining Site

It is possible to estimate that the difference spectrum in Fig. 14 contains the equivalent of about 20 aromatic and 20 aliphatic protons. It is also interesting to note that so little (<10%) of the Fv spectrum is affected on hapten binding, and this almost certainly rules out any large conformational changes. If this were not the case, then in addition to any "broadening effects" of the spin-label hapten, the difference spectrum would also contain chemical shifts of resonances

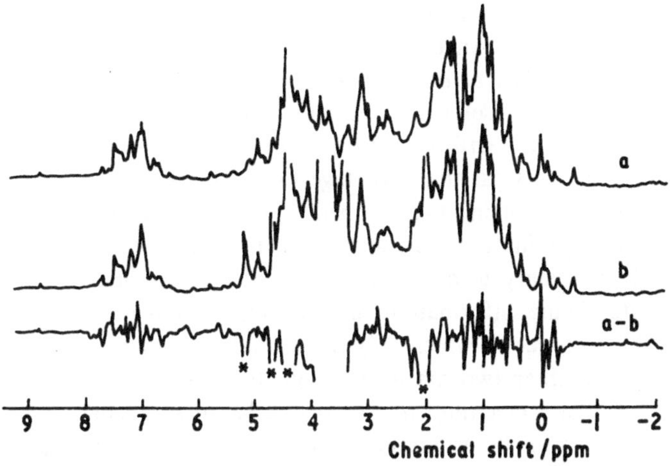

Figure 15. 270 MHz proton NMR spectra of: (a) lysozyme 5 mM, 2000 scans; (b) +*N*-acetyl glucosamine (0.2M), 2000 scans; (c) difference (a) – (b), T = 33°K, pH (nominal) = 4.0. The resonances marked with asterisks arise from *N*-acetyl glucosamine. [Note that the magnitude of the difference spectrum in (c) is of the same order as spectrum (a) or (b), in contrast to the difference spectrum in Fig. 14.]

arising from residues outside the broadening sphere. These changes in chemical shifts would result from slight changes in chemical environment of the protons caused by movements of the associated residues. An example of the sensitivity of the NMR technique in detecting such conformational changes is illustrated in Fig. 15 for the difference spectrum resulting from the addition of the inhibitor *N*-acetyl glucosamine to lysozyme. The intensity of this difference spectrum is very much greater than that in Fig. 14a, and results from many proton resonances being shifted as a result of changes in their environments. The large number of shifted resonances is also entirely consistent with the X-ray results, which indicate that there are many changes on inhibitor binding (Perkins *et al.*, to be published) that extend over almost the entire protein.

F. Assignment of Proton Resonances in the Fv

Upon obtaining some idea of the types of amino acids in and around the combining site, the next stage is to assign the resonances from these to particular amino acids. This generally involves a variety of intrinsic and extrinsic perturbations. For instance, changing the pH is often used to help identify histidine residues, since the chemical shifts of the histidine resonance varies with the degree of ionization of the residue. The changes in the NMR spectrum are most easily followed by the use of *difference spectroscopy*, which here involves the subtraction of spectra at different pHs. Only those resonances that alter their position with pH will appear in a difference spectrum. In the case of the Fv, sequence studies have shown that there are only three histidine residues (Hochman *et al.*, 1973; Dugan *et al.*, 1973), and it is therefore a relatively straightforward procedure to observe the resonances from all these residues using pH difference spectroscopy without any recourse to further simplication of the spectrum. Initially, this has the advantage that if these residues occur in different regions of the protein, they provide "windows" through which we may observe any changes in these regions on addition of haptens. Eventually, however, it will be necessary to determine which of the histidines, if any, are in the combining site. Some information on this comes from using the spin-labeled hapten—in the presence of which only one histidine resonance can be observed—showing that the other two are in the immediate region of the combining site (Dwek *et al.*, 1975a), since they are broadened by the spin label.

Typical changes in the aromatic resonances of the Fv resulting from altering the pH are shown in Fig. 16—in this case, in the presence of the hapten Dnp-NH—$(CH_2)_2$—O—PO_3. Some representative difference spectra, showing the C-2 and C-4 protons of the three histidine residues, are given in Fig. 16b. The results can be presented in the form of a pH titration in which the chemical shifts are plotted against the pH of the solution. Figure 17 shows the results of

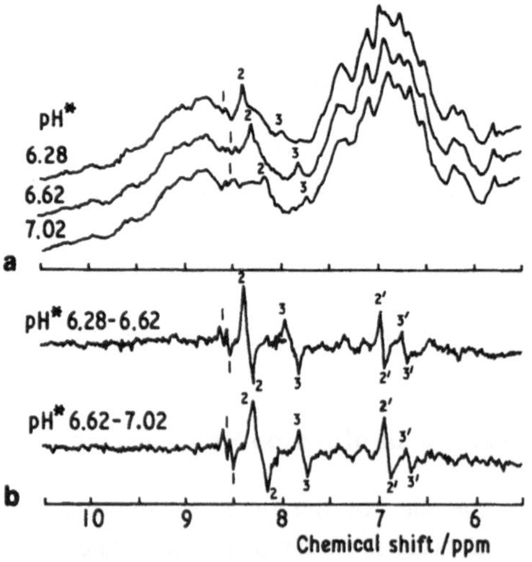

Figure 16. Effect of changing pH on the aromatic resonances of the Fv fragment. (a) 270 MHz proton spectrum of the aromatic region of fragment Fv from MOPC 315, in the presence of Dnp aminoethylphosphate at three different pH values. The numbers indicate the C-2 protons of three titrating histidines. (b) Illustration of pH difference spectroscopy showing both C-2 and C-4 protons of titrating histidine residues. The prime numerals indicate the positions of the C-4 protons. Resonance 1′ does not change over the pH range shown, and does not therefore appear in the difference spectrum.

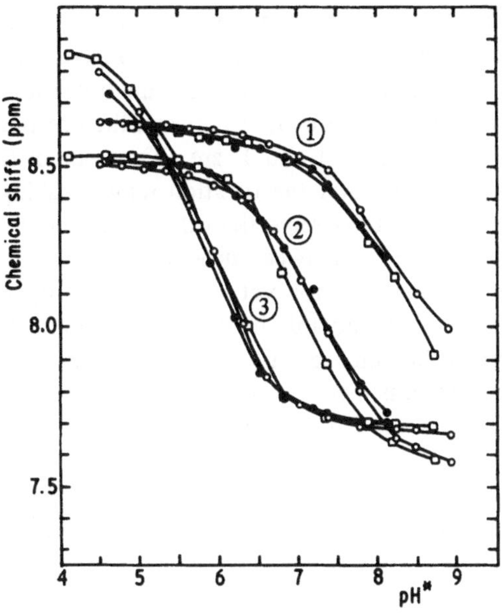

Figure 17. Titration of the histidine chemical shift vs. pH for the Fv fragment from protein MOPC 315 in the absence (□) and in the presence of Dnp aminoethylphosphate (○) and Tnp aminomethylphosphonate (●).

such titrations for the His C-2 protons of Fv alone, and also in the presence of three different haptens. The resonances 1, 2, and 3 can be assigned to the C-2 protons of the histidine ring, since the resonance positions occur in the range characteristic of C-2 protons and the chemical shifts between the protonated and unprotonated forms are approximately 1 ppm, which is also characteristic of the behavior observed for C-2 histidine protons (Dwek, 1973). Similar arguments allow the assignment of resonances 1′, 2′, and 3′ to the C-4 histidine protons. The prime numbering is assigned on the basis of the correspondence in the pK_a values, which are about 8.1 (resonances 1 and 1′), in the range 6.9–7.4 (resonances 2 and 2′), and about 5.9 (resonances 3 and 3′).

The line widths of the histidine resonances in the Fv provide further information about their environment. For example, the histidine resonances 2 and 2′ ($pK_a \sim 7.0$) are always narrower than those from the other two histidines. This and the fact that its pK_a value is almost identical with that from the imidazole grouping in model compounds such as *N*-acetyl-L-histidine (Shrager *et al.*, 1972) suggests that this particular histidine is *on the surface of the protein* and readily accessible to the solvent. Conversely, the line widths from resonances 3 and 3′ are always quite broad, and the lower pK_a value is consistent with this histidine residue being in a hydrophobic region of the protein that is not so readily accessible to solvent. Interestingly, the acid extreme of the titration curve for the C-2 proton of this histidine (resonance 3) is nearly always shifted downfield by about 0.3 ppm relative to the other two histidine C-2 protons (see, for example,

Fig. 17). It is tempting to speculate that this downfield shift is a consequence of "ring currents" (see Section IIIK1) from nearby aromatic residues. This aromatic residue could also account for the broad line width, since there would be significant dipolar interactions between the protons on it and the histidine protons.

Resonances 1 and 1′ are anomalous in that they each split into at least two components over the titration range, making it rather more difficult to observe them than to observe the other resonances. Nevertheless, the line widths of the resonances are between those of the other two histidines. The reason for the two components is not yet clear, but it might reflect some heterogeneity in the residues around this histidine. This could happen if this residue was near the region in which the Fv is cleaved from the Fab fragment. Alternatively, it may be that this histidine residue undergoes some form of restricted motion. The different components would then reflect different chemical environments for the C-2 and C-4 protons. Certainly this pK_a value of 8.2 is unusually high and suggests an extremely acidic environment for this histidine. It is to be hoped that pH titrations of the histidine residues in the Fab fragment will provide further insight into this problem.

The results of pH titrations of the three histidine resonances in the Fv alone and in the presence of a variety of haptens are summarized in Table V. Two of the histidine residues (pK_a values 8.2 and 5.9) are not significantly affected on addition of hapten. However, the pK_a value of the other histidine is always increased on addition of hapten, the trend being toward a slightly greater increase for charged haptens. The pK_a values for the second ionizations of the phosphate and phosphonate haptens in the appropriate Fv hapten complexes can also be measured using ^{31}P NMR (see Section IIIG1). These pK_a values are in the range 5.9–8.0 (see Table VI), so that although the formal negative charge on these particular haptens varies between 1 and 2 over the titration range of the histidine, there are only minor increases in its pK_a value, which probably arise from this histidine being in the vicinity of the negatively charged group.

In the presence of spin-labeled hapten 1, the resonances from the histidines with pK_a values of 5.9 and approximately 6.9 are "broadened," while the resonances from the third histidine (pK_a 8.2) are unaffected. Two histidines are therefore in or near the combining site. Taking into account the information from the line widths, the pK_a values, the effects of various haptens, and the dimensions of the site (from ESR mapping), a reasonable conclusion would be that the histidine in Fv with a pK_a value of approximately 6.9 is on the surface of the protein, at the edge of the combining site in proximity to the charged groupings on the haptens. In contrast, the histidine with a pK_a value of 5.9 is almost insensitive to the presence of haptens, so that it is unlikely to be in the immediate vicinity of the hapten. Its line width and chemical shift suggest, though, that it is partially buried and near an aromatic residue.

Table V. pK_a Values of the Histidine Residues in the Fv Fragment MOPC 315 in the Presence of Different Haptens

	Histidine pK_a values		
Hapten — Resonance:	3	2	1
[a]None	5.9	6.9	8.2
1. DNP · NH · CH_2 · $CH_2OPO_3^{\ominus}$	5.9	7.4	8.2
2. DNP · NH · CH($COO^{\ominus}$) · $CH_2COO^{\ominus}$	5.9	7.3	8.2
3. DNP · NH · CH_2—PO_3	5.9	7.3	8.2
4. DNP · NH · $(CH_2)_4$ · CH($NH_3^{\oplus}$) · $COO^{\ominus}$	5.9	7.1	8.2
[a]5. DNP · NH · CH_2— 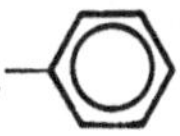	5.9	7.1	8.2
[a]6. DNP · O^-	5.9	7.1	8.2
[a]7. DNP · NH— 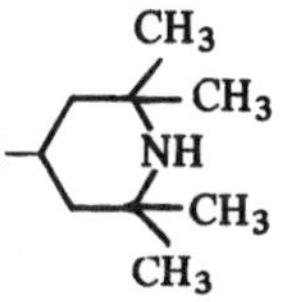	5.9	7.2	8.2
8. TNP · NH · CH_2 · PO_3	5.8	7.3	8.2
9. TNP · NH · CH_2 · CH_2 · PO_3	5.7	7.3	8.2
10. TNP · NH · $CH_2CH_2CH_2PO_3$	5.9	7.2	8.2
11. 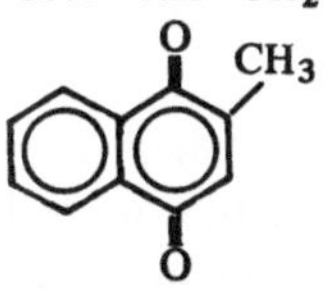	Too broad to observe	7.0	8.2

[a]From Dwek *et al.* (1975a).

G. Correlation of Histidine Data with the Hypothetical Model of Fv

The model places two histidines near the combining site and one at the back of the molecule, which would be near the C_H1 and C_L domains in the intact Fab. Correlation of the data with the model provides an unambiguous assignment of all three histidine residues, since only one (102_H) occurs on the surface of the protein, and that at the very edge of the combining site on the H3 loop. This must therefore be the residue with a pK_a value of approximately 6.9. His 97_L on

L3 is farther away (but within the spin-label broadening sphere) from the combining site in a partially hydrophobic environment, close to Phe 94_L. Assignment of this to the residue with a pK_a value of approximately 5.9 enables a positioning of His 97_L relative to the phenylalanine to be calculated by correlating its NMR chemical shift with the ring current effects (see Section IIIK1) from the benzenoid ring. The relative geometry involves a perpendicular arrangement of the rings, with center-to-center separation of 0.5 nm, i.e., the sum of the van der Waals radii. The remaining histidine residue must be the nonhypervariable His 44_L, which thus has the pK_a value of 8.2. This assignment is also consistent with its positioning 1.8 nm from the combining site (i.e., it is not within the spin-labeling broadening sphere). The model also places it adjacent to an aspartic acid, which would tend to raise its pK_a value.

H. ^{31}P Magnetic Resonance as a Probe of Electrostatic Environment

The pK_a of a phosphate or phosphonate grouping provides an extremely sensitive probe of neighboring electrostatic charges. Changes in the ionization state of ^{31}P groupings with pH can be monitored relatively easily by observing the changes in ^{31}P chemical shifts, in the same way as the histidine ionizations were monitored by following the proton chemical shifts. The phosphate or phosphonate grouping approximates a hemisphere of radius 0.3 nm, so that by using Tnp or Dnp as an anchor grouping, it is possible to choose side chains of different lengths and stereochemistries to probe different areas of the combining site for positively and negatively charged groups.

The pK_a values of several phosphate and phosphonate haptens when bound to the Fv have been measured (Wain-Hobson *et al.*, 1976) and, together with the normal pK_a values, are given in Table VI. Of the Tnp haptens, only the propyl phosphonate has its pK_a significantly affected, the decrease of approximately 1 unit suggesting the proximity of a positively charged group. The extended length of this hapten measured along the plane of the Tnp ring is 1.2 nm. From the dimensions of the site obtained from ESR mapping studies, this places the phosphonate grouping just beyond the entrance to the combining site. In contrast, Dnp ethyl phosphate is about 0.1 nm shorter, and its phosphate grouping would just be within the site. The increase in pK_a value of 0.3 unit suggests that it experiences an acidic environment. The extreme sensitivity of the pK_a values of the ^{31}P groupings is further illustrated by noting that although the extended length of the Tnp methyl phosphonate hapten is only 0.2 nm shorter than the Tnp propyl phosphonate, its pK_a value is essentially unaltered.

The intrinsic geometries of the Tnp and Dnp haptens are different, and a

Table VI. pK_a Values of Phosphonates and Phosphate Groupings of Phosphohaptens

Phosphohapten	pK_a free	pK_a bound to Fv
$TNP \cdot NH \cdot CH_2 \cdot CH_2 \cdot CH_2PO_3H^{\ominus}$	7.7	6.9 ± 0.1
$TNP \cdot NH \cdot CH_2 \cdot CH_2PO_3H^{\ominus}$	6.9	7.1 ± 0.2
$TNP \cdot NH \cdot CH_2PO_3H^{\ominus}$	5.7	5.9 ± 0.2
$DNP \cdot NH \cdot CH_2PO_3H^{\ominus}$	6.0	6.1 ± 0.2
$DNP \cdot NH \cdot CH_2 \cdot CH_2OPO_3H^{\ominus}$	6.3	6.6 ± 0.1

comparison of them can provide further information on pK_a mapping. The Dnp haptens will have the proton of the NH group coplanar (bonding to the NO_2), while in the Tnp haptens, this proton will be perpendicular to the aromatic ring. The results of this restriction mean that the phosphorous grouping is farther from the plane of the ring in the Tnp haptens than in the comparable Dnp haptens. The rotation of the phosphorous grouping in the Tnp haptens will therefore sweep out a wider area than for the Dnp haptens; thus, Tnp and Dnp haptens of essentially equal length can probe different areas of the combining site. Nevertheless, the unperturbed pK_a values of the shorter Dnp and Tnp haptens suggest that there are no positive or negative charges within a cylinder of 0.6 × 0.7 nm *from* the Dnp (or Tnp) ring (0.3 nm being the phosphonate hemisphere and 0.6 nm being the length of the animo ethyl phosphonate moiety; see Fig. 18). These dimensions are simply those obtained from considerations of van der Waals radii. They should therefore be regarded as representing minimum dimensions, since they do not take into account the range over which a pK_a value will be sensitive to a neighboring charge. It is quite clear, however, that the perturbations in pK_a values must result from charged groups at the edge of the combining site.

The ESR spin-label mapping studies (see Section IIC) have also shown that there is a positively charged group 0.1–0.3 nm beyond the entrance to the combining site. Of all the haptens considered here, only the Tnp amino-propyl phosphonate has the appropriate geometry to make contact with this charged group. The very small perturbation of the pK_a (6.9 to 7.2) of His 102_H, which is at the entrance to the site, removes this residue as a possible candidate, and examination of the amino acid sequences then leaves only Lys 52_H and Arg 95_L as positively charged groups that are expected to be in the hypervariable regions. Lysine 52_H has been shown by affinity labeling (Haimovich *et al.*, 1972) to be within the site, but it must be oriented in such a way that it does not interact with the shorter Dnp or Tnp haptens, since their pK_as are essentially unperturbed.

The increase in pK_a value of the Dnp aminoethyl phosphate grouping on

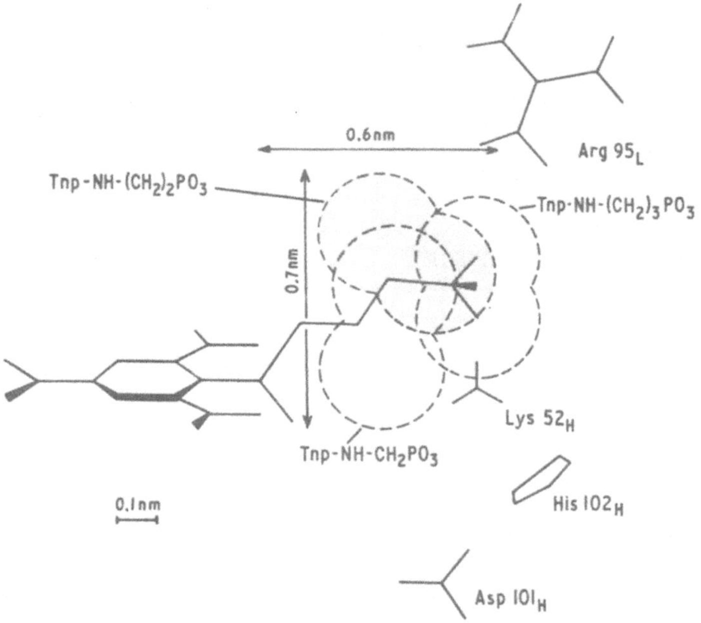

Figure 18. Mapping of pK_a, using ^{31}P magnetic resonance, of various phosphate and phosphonate haptens. The areas probed by the different Tnp haptens are shown relative to the predicted positions (Padlan *et al.*, 1976) of the charged groups at the entrance to the combining site.

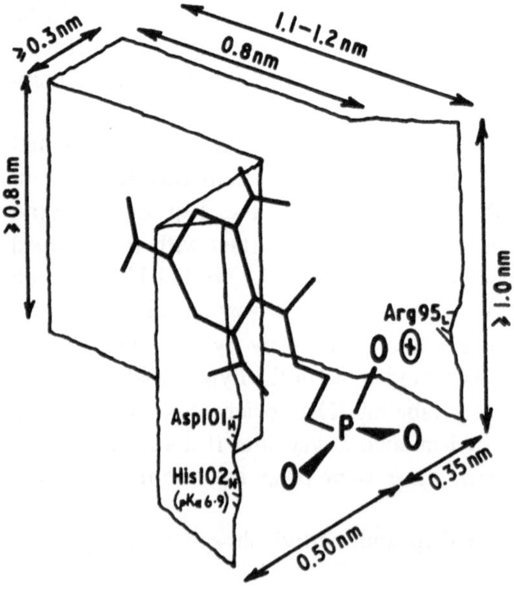

Figure 19. A picture of the combining site of MOPC 315 as deduced experimentally from NMR pH titrations and ESR studies, showing the position of the Tnp $NH(CH_2)_3PO_3$ hapten.

binding to the Fv must come from the presence of a nearby acidic grouping. From sequence studies, only three Asp groups, Asp 99_H, Asp 101_H, and Asp 106_H, are expected to be in the hypervariable regions. The increase in pK_a of one of the histidine residues, assigned as His 102_H (6.9 to 7.4), by Dnp aminoethyl phosphate suggests that the phosphate grouping has to be near both His 102_H and one of the Asp residues. Since we know His 102_H is at the edge of the combining site, Asp 101_H would also be near the entrance to the combining site and could result in the pK_a perturbation of the phosphate grouping, though this argument alone does not rule out other possibilities, since it is based on the assignment of His 102_H.

Further conclusions on the positions of the charged residues at the entrance to the combining site, responsible for the pK_a perturbations, comes from a comparison of the geometries of the haptens Dnp aminoethyl phosphate and Tnp aminopropyl phosphonate. Assuming that the Dnp or Tnp ring is rigidly held, the regions probed by the phosphate hapten will also be accessible to the phosphonate hapten, but not vice versa. The positively charged group must therefore be in a region accessible only to the phosphonate hapten, and must be some distance away from the Asp residue. A combination of these results with those from the ESR studies, which give the positioning of the positive charge, leads to the picture of the combining site shown in Fig. 19.

I. The Hypothetical Fv Model and Charged Residues

The experimental results presented above lend further support to the postulated structure. The model places Asp 101_H as the only negatively charged residue and His 102_H, Lys 52_H and Arg 95_L as the positively charged residues at the entrance to the combining site (see Fig. 18). One or more of these positively charged residues must be involved in the positive "subsite" of the combining site existing for Dnp ligands with side chains longer than four carbon atoms (Haselkorn *et al.*, 1974). The ESR and NMR studies, however, allow more detailed discussions of the actual residues likely to be involved in any particular case. Thus, on the basis of the ESR results for the dimensions of the site, we concluded that in the postulated model for Fv, the Dnp or Tnp ring must bind approximately parallel to the hypervariable L3 loop. Reference to the model then shows that the position of Arg 95_L can be such that it could be responsible for both the change in pK_a of the Tnp propyl phosphonate, possibly via H-bond interactions, and the change in the ESR spectrum of the Dnp-5 membered spin-label hapten.

J. Hapten Difference Spectra and the Aromatic Nature of the Combining Site

The 270 MHz proton magnetic resonance difference spectra resulting from the addition of a variety of haptens to the Fv are shown in Figs. 20 and 21. The intensity of these difference spectra represents only about 1-2% of the total intensity of the Fv spectrum, indicating that very few proton resonances are perturbed on hapten binding. This is again consistent with the conclusion that any conformational changes on hapten binding are very small, and are limited to the immediate vicinity of the combining site.

An important feature of these difference spectra is that the protons perturbed are almost entirely aromatic. Reference to the amino acid sequence shows that the Fv contains 29 aromatic amino acids, of which, again by analogy with human Ig variable region sequences (Kabat and Wu, 1971) and the binding sites of Fab′ New (Poljak *et al.*, 1973) and McPC 603 (Segal *et al.*, 1974), about 14 would be expected to be in the hypervariable regions. From the intensity of the histidine C-2 protons, it is possible to estimate that about 10-12 protons from aromatic residues in the Fv are perturbed on hapten binding. This means that if the perturbations in the difference spectra result from interaction of the amino acids in the Fv with the hapten, only the equivalent of about four aromatic amino acids can be in contact with the hapten.

Though there are small perturbations in the aliphatic region, the quantitative estimates of the number of protons involved are difficult because the differences ($\leqslant 1\%$ in this region, compared with $\sim 20\%$ in the aromatic region) are almost within the error limits of the technique. If, however, any of the aliphatic resonances and in particular methyl groups were shifted outside the main aliphatic envelope (e.g., above −1 ppm) in the Fv, and were perturbed on hapten binding,

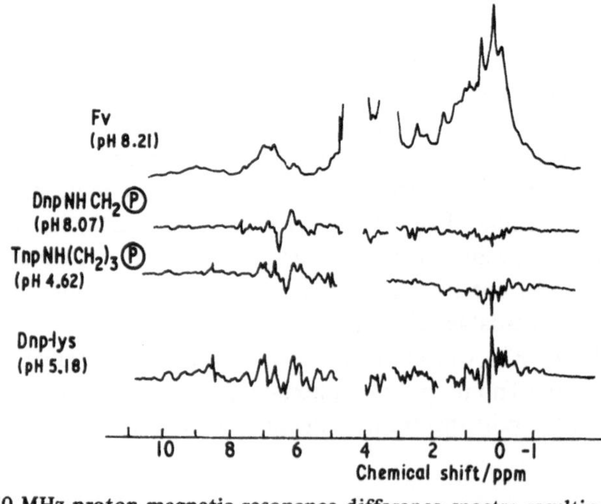

Figure 20. 270 MHz proton magnetic resonance difference spectra resulting from addition of different haptens to the Fv fragment of MOPC 315.

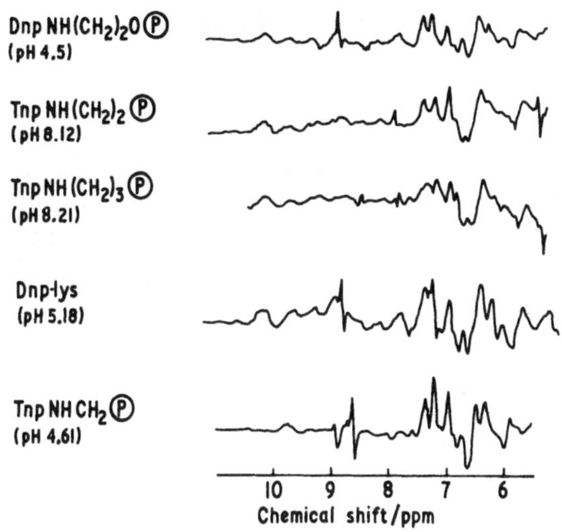

Figure 21. Aromatic region of the NMR difference spectra resulting from the addition of various haptens to the Fv fragment of MOPC 315.

differences in position ought to be detectable, since the problem of the large background no longer applies. (Such is the case, for example, for the individual histidine C-2 protons; see Section IIIF). The occurrence of upfield shifts for methyl groups is fairly common in proteins, and arises from "ring current" interactions from nearby aromatic residues. It is therefore reasonable to expect that the resonances from methyl groups of amino acid residues in or near the highly aromatic combining site of Fv would be shifted from their normal random coil positions by ring current interactions. Certainly there are no large upfield shifts of resonance (i.e., outside the aliphatic envelope) that are sensitive to hapten binding in the Fv. Even the spin-labeled difference spectrum, which contains resonances from residues within about 1.0–1.2 nm of the nitroxide, does not reveal any very unusual shifts for methyl groups. We conclude that none of the six amino acids that contain methyl groups is in the immediate vicinity of the hapten, and that any methyl groups within the spin-label broadening sphere experience only very minimal interactions with any aromatic residues. That is, they do not approach closer than about 0.4 nm; if this were not the case, significant ring current shifts would be expected (see Section IIIK1).

Comparison of the aromatic regions of the difference spectra shows that they are remarkably similar in overall pattern, indicating that the same residues are probably perturbed by all haptens. There are, however, some differences between the spectra. For instance, increasing the length of the side chains on the hapten results in larger perturbations, and in some instances, there are small but subtle differences between the Dnp and Tnp perturbations.

K. Ring Current Shifts as a Structural Intrinsic Probe of Aromatic Environment

1. Ring Current Shifts

The circulation of the delocalized π electrons of aromatic rings results in electronic currents being set up when the aromatic rings are placed in a magnetic field. Nuclei located in space on or near the sixfold axis normal to the ring plane experience a reduced total magnetic field, and the resonances of such nuclei are shifted to higher field. In contrast, nuclei located in the plane of the aromatic ring have their resonances shifted to lower fields. The extent of the shift of a given nucleus obviously depends on the magnitude of the ring current field it experiences. If we assume that these local fields (B') arise from a dipole at the center of the aromatic ring, then at a distance r from the center of the ring, we may write

$$B' = \frac{\mu}{r^3}(3 \cos^2 \theta - 1)$$

where θ is the angle between r and the applied magnetic field B_0 (see Fig. 22). The magnitude of the ring current shifts also depends on the nature of the aromatic system, being in the order Trp > Phe and Tyr > His for the amino acids.

Quantitative treatments of ring current shifts have been carried out by several authors (Johnson and Bovey, 1958; Geissner-Prettre and Pullman, 1971; Haig and Mallion, 1972), and tables have been compiled that relate the shift to the position (r and θ) of a nucleus from the center of the aromatic ring. The calculations of the tables, though, involve several approximations, so that despite considerable success in their applications, the tables must be used with caution (Mallion, 1975).

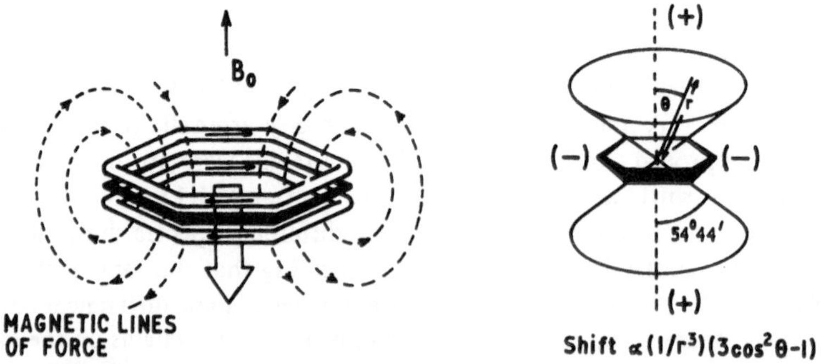

Figure 22. (a) Current and magnetic lines of force induced in benzene by an external field. (b) Dependence of the ring current shift on position: (+) represents a shift to high field, (−) represents a shift to low field.

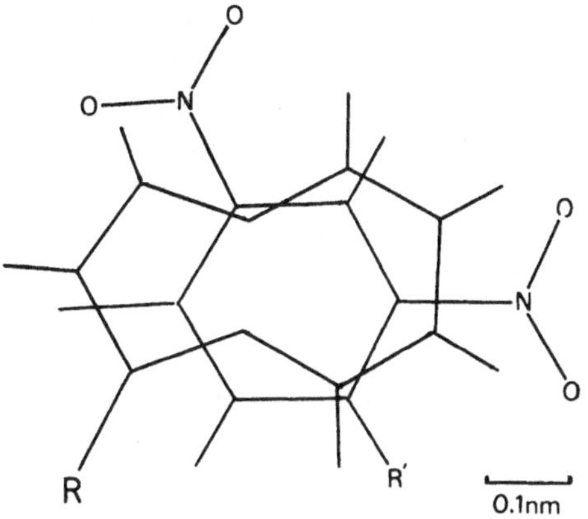

Figure 23. Structure of the Dnp-aspartate–tryptophan complex as deduced from NMR ring current interactions.

2. *Interaction of Tryptophan and Dnp Haptens*

As an illustration of the use of ring current interactions to obtain structural interactions, we may consider the interactions of Dnp-aspartate with L-tryptophan (Dower *et al.*, 1976). Complex formation results in shifts of both the Dnp and Trp protons, and by the use of suitable titrations, the fully bound shifts for each proton can be obtained. Assuming that the origins of the shifts arise from ring currents, reference to the appropriate tables allows the positions of the individual protons on one aromatic ring to be determined relative to the others. The reciprocal effects of the aromatic rings on the shifts of each others' protons allows the consistency of any structure to be tested. The structure of the Dnp–Trp complex, in solution, is shown in Fig. 23. The structure is very much that expected for a charge-transfer complex, the Dnp ring with its high affinity for electrons "stacking" approximately over the "electron-rich" tryptophan. A charge-transfer complex has also been suggested on the basis of the changes in the Dnp absorbance spectrum on interaction with tryptophan (Little and Eisen, 1967), but the NMR method now provides the structural basis for these observations.

Incidentally, only extremely weak complexes of this sort could be detected using NMR with Dnp and the other aromatic amino acids. The specificity for tryptophan by Dnp and Tnp ligands (Dower *et al.*, 1976), particularly in a hydrophobic environment (Johnston *et al.*, 1974), could well be a major factor in the very tight binding of these ligands to anti-Dnp and anti-Tnp antibodies, and also to MOPC 315.

In proteins, ring current effects from aromatic residues are a major cause of chemical shifts of resonances from their random coil positions. Thus, in lysozyme, ring current shifts account qualitatively for the observed differences between the native and random coil chemical shift values for many of the methyl group resonances (Campbell *et al.*, 1975b). In principle, therefore, it ought to be possible to use the magnitude of the bound shifts of a hapten in an antibody combining site as an intrinsic probe of the relative geometries of neighboring aromatic residue. This, of course, would be particularly relevant to the detection of interactions of Dnp and Tnp ligands with tryptophan residues in the appropriate antibody combining sites.

L. Aromatic Combining Site of MOPC 315

The addition of Dnp-aspartate to the Fv results in changes in the chemical shifts of the proton resonances of both hapten and protein. These changes are indicated in Fig. 24, which shows the 270 MHz proton difference spectra resulting from successive additions of hapten. The serial difference spectra (shown in Fig. 25) illustrate that after the ratio of hapten Fv exceeds 1 : 1, only the hapten resonances continue to shift; the actual position of each of these resonances then represents the "weighted" mean of that in the free hapten and that when bound to the Fv. Using the histidine resonances as internal markers, it is possible to estimate the number of protons associated with each perturbed resonance (Table VII).

The most notable feature of Table VII is the extremely large upfield chemi-

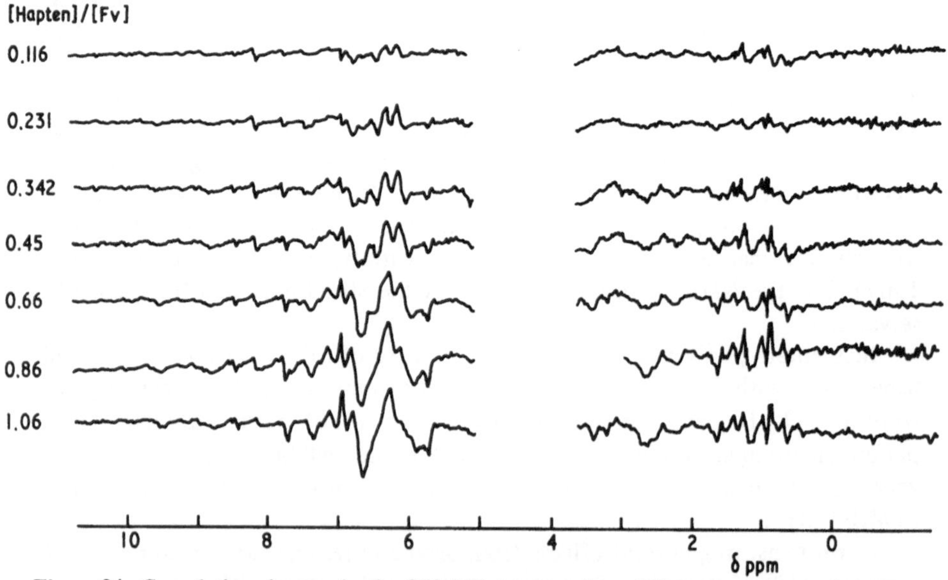

Figure 24. Cumulative changes in the 270 MHz spectra (i.e., difference spectra) of the Fv fragment of MOPC 315 resulting from the addition of Dnp-aspartate.

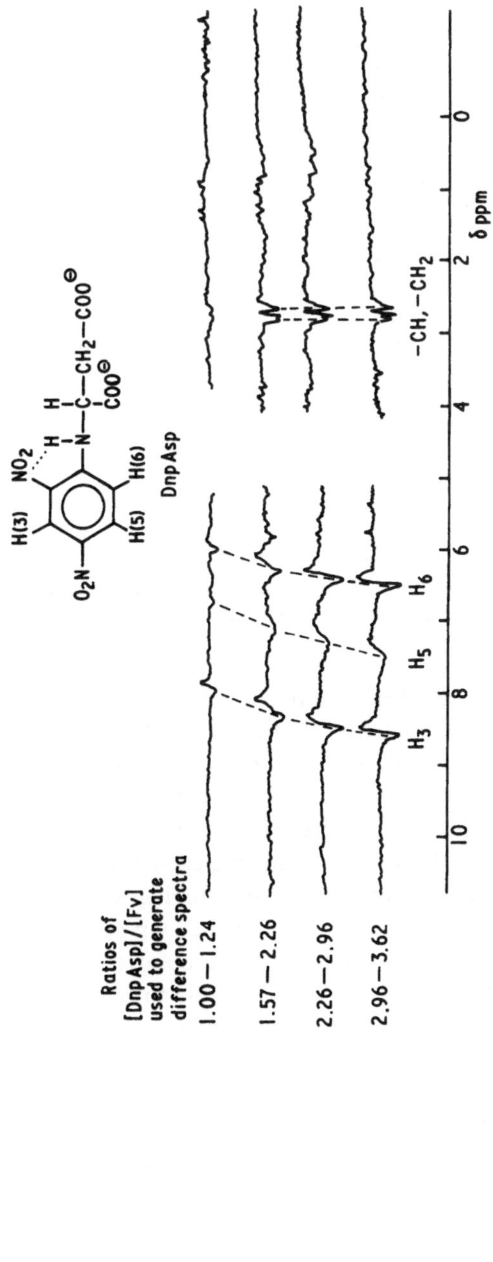

Figure 25. Difference spectra resulting from the addition of Dnp-aspartate illustrating the titration behavior of the hapten resonances. (Differences are between successive additions of hapten, and the ratios of Dnp-Asp: Fv are indicated each time.)

Table VII. Chemical Shifts (δ_0) and the Change in Chemical Shift ($\Delta\delta$) of Resonances Perturbed on Binding of DNP-Aspartate to the Fv from MOPC 315 at pH 6.9

Resonances	δ_0(ppm)	$\Delta\delta$ (ppm)[a]	Number of protons
Hapten			
H_3	9.18	−1.68	1
H_5	8.36	~−2.3	1
H_6	7.04	−1.31	1
$—CH_2—$	2.76	−0.1	
(complex pattern with	2.91	−0.2	2
3 main peaks)	2.99	−0.26	
—CH—		Not observable	
Protein			
5.9 His C2	7.82	−0.06	1
–	7	Broadens out	~2
5.9 His C4	6.95	−0.07	1
–	6.9	−0.19	1
–	6.62	0.08	1
–	6.37	0.296	2
	6.33	−0.175	2
	6.16	−0.256	2
Peak decreases as hapten is added.	7.2		~2
Peak increases as hapten is added.	7.42	Poss. 0.22	2

[a]Positive sign is downfield, negative upfield, shift change.

cal shifts experienced by the Dnp protons. These shifts are on the order of that found in lysozyme for the resonances of methione 105 (Campbell *et al.*, 1975b), which sits at the center of an "aromatic box" of amino acid residues (Imoto *et al.*, 1972). On the protein, apart from the resonances of His 97_L ($pK_a = 5.9$), only five protons have their resonances shifted upfield. The magnitudes of these shifts are very similar to the Dnp-induced ring current shifts of the five tryptophan protons in the model Dnp-aspartate–tryptophan complex (Dower *et al.*, 1976). When it is noted that the changes in the Dnp absorbance spectrum on interaction with the Fv are also similar to those observed in the Dnp-aspartate–tryptophan complex (Fig. 26), it seems reasonable to conclude that some if not all of the resonances in the protein shifted upfield on addition of the hapten belong to a tryptophan residue, and that the Dnp ring when bound in the Fv interacts with this tryptophan in an almost identical manner to that shown in the model system in Fig. 23. This would be expected if the interaction between Dnp and tryptophan is of the charge-transfer type, since the steric requirements for such complexes are fairly stringent to allow efficient electron transfer to

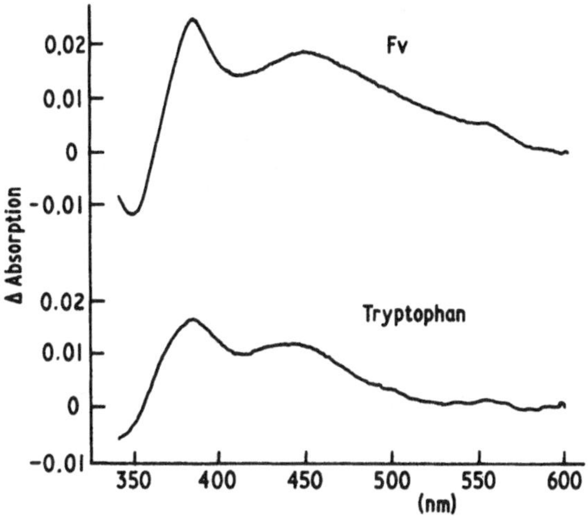

Figure 26. A comparison of the changes in the absorbance spectrum of Dnp-aspartate on interaction with either Fv or tryptophan. Dnp-Asp: 70 μM; Fv: 40 μM; Trp: 20 mM; pH 6.8; PIPES buffer: 40 mM; NaCl: 0.15M; T: 20°C.

occur (Foster, 1969). Thus, if the Dnp and tryptophan do form a charge-transfer pair in the Fv, the relative orientation of the two residues should be very similar to that in the model compounds. An interaction of this nature may help to explain the extremely large quenching of the tryptophan fluorescence of the Fv on binding Dnp (or Tnp) haptens.

The upfield shifts of the Dnp protons when bound to the Fv are far greater than those in the Dnp-aspartate–tryptophan complex, and indicate interaction with a *minimum* of two additional aromatic residues. By using tables of ring currents, it is possible to work out the relative geometries of the Dnp-aspartate and the three aromatic residues surrounding it. A picture of the resulting "aromatic box" is shown in Fig. 27. This picture also accounts for some of the resonances on the protein that move downfield on addition of hapten, since they could result from the ring current shifts of the Dnp ring on the aromatic residues above and below it. It should be noted that the ring current interactions are sensitive to changes in average positions as small as 0.05 nm. Thus, we know that while His 97_L (pK_a 5.9) is near but not in the combining site, it is close to an aromatic residue. A relative movement on hapten binding between this aromatic residue and His 97_L of approximately 0.05 nm would be sufficient to cause the observed shifts of the His proton resonances.

Further information on the aromatic nature of the combining site is obtained by comparing the resonance positions and intensities of the aromatic protons *of the Fv* that are perturbed on hapten binding (Table VII) with the resonance positions and intensities expected for the aromatic protons in random

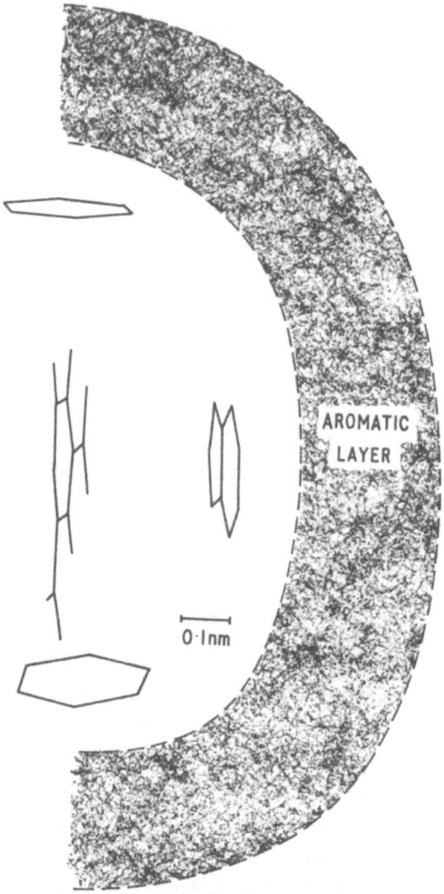

Figure 27. A picture of the combining site of the Fv fragment of MOPC 315 showing the "aromatic box" deduced from ring current interactions, which also indicate the presence of a second layer of aromatic residues.

coil positions (Table VIII). Thus, the resonances (two protons each) at 6.33 and 6.16 ppm (Table VII) are significantly ring current-shifted upfield irrespective of whether they originate from Trp, Phr, or Tyr residues. The magnitude of these shifts, approximately 1 ppm, is such that these protons must be approximately 0.3 nm above the plane of the neighboring aromatic residues giving rise to these ring interactions. A minimum of two aromatic rings are necessary to account for these shifts, even if all the four perturbed proton resonances come from one tryptophan residue. A further two aromatic residues would also be

Table VIII. Random Coil Positions of Aromatic Protons in Protein High-Resolution NMR Spectra

Amino acid	Number of carbon-bound protons	Expected multiplet structure[a]	Number of protons	ppm
Histidine	2	2 singlets	1, 1	6.5–9[b]
Tyrosine	4	2 doublets	2. 2	6.9, 7.2
Phenylalanine	5	1 triplet 1 doublet 1 triplet	1 2 2	7.4
Tryptophan	5	1 singlet 2 doublets 2 triplets	1 1, 1 1, 1	7.3 7.7, 7.5 7.2, 7.3

[a]The multiplet structure will in general not be resolved for any of the resonances in proteins the size of Fv.
[b]The C2 and C4 resonances of histidine move upfield with increasing pH.

required to account for the shifts at 6.37 ppm (two protons) and 6.62 ppm (one proton). All this leads to the concept of a "second layer" of aromatic residues around the combining site (see Fig. 27). With this high density of aromatic residues in and around the combining site and the extreme sensitivity of ring current shifts to small relative movements, the very few protons perturbed on hapten binding provide confirmation, once again, that any conformational changes on hapten binding are extremely localized. Indeed, these results suggest that the hapten just "slots" into the combining site.

An important aspect of NMR is the monitoring of interactions among nuclei that are very close in space. Thus, we have seen how ring current interactions can lead to shifts of nuclear resonances. Such shifts have an approximate $1/r^3$ dependence (where r is the distance between the ring and a given nucleus), and can therefore be significant even at distances of approximately 0.5 nm. A much shorter-range effect, proportional to $1/r^6$, arises from the dipolar interactions among nuclei. Such interactions will affect the populations of their energy levels, and it turns out that if these populations are sufficiently disturbed by the application of an additional radiofrequency field, dramatic changes in intensities of the nuclear resonances can occur (Noggle and Schirmer, 1971). If, for instance, we consider two resonances A and B from nuclei that are very close in space, then applying a radiofrequency field to resonance A will result in a change in the integrated intensity of B. This phenomenon is termed the *Overhauser effect*. In practice, such effects are only observed if the two nuclei are approximately 0.3

nm or less apart. For example, they will be detectable between adjacent protons on a benzene ring, but not between protons on opposite sides of the ring. The effects are obviously not limited simply to protons in the same amino acid residue. The main criterion is only whether a neighboring proton is sufficiently near a second proton to alter significantly the dipolar field experienced by that proton. Thus, Overhauser effects on the H_3 proton of Dnp–aspartate have been observed when Fv resonances at approximately 6.6 ppm are irradiated. More extensive experiments using Dnp-$O^{\ominus}$ showed that the effect arises from a proton (or protons) associated with the resonance at 6.37 ppm in the Fv that move downfield on hapten binding. Irradiation of a further resonance in the Fv at 7.6 ppm also resulted in an Overhauser effect, even though no resonance at this position occurred in the difference spectrum. The ring current shifts on the ring protons of Dnp-$O^{\ominus}$ indicated that the Dnp orientation in the site is very similar to that of Dnp-aspartate.

The situation is thus: the H_3 of the Dnp ring sits below the plane of an aromatic ring, and experiences a substantial ring current shift. This fixes, quite accurately, the relative geometry of the H_3 proton and the aromatic ring, and also places at least one proton on this ring within 0.3 nm of the H_3 proton. The Overhauser effect is then used to identify the resonance positions of protons on the Fv within 0.3 nm of the H_3 proton. One such proton has a resonance position at approximately 6.6 ppm, and the sensitivity of this proton resonance to hapten binding suggests that it actually comes from a proton *on* the aromatic ring above the H_3 proton.

As we have already discussed, the aromatic proton at 6.6 ppm responsible for the Overhauser effects is itself within 0.3 nm of a further aromatic ring. This allows some additional deductions to be made about the nature of the second aromatic proton on the Fv (resonance 7.6 ppm) within 0.3 nm of the H_3 proton. If the protons with resonances at 7.6 ppm and 6.6 ppm both come from the same aromatic residue, they would have to be adjacent to be within 0.3 nm of the H_3. We would then have a situation in which one proton resonance (6.6 ppm) is substantially shifted upfield, while the adjacent proton resonance is shifted downfield. This would put considerable restraints on the geometry on any neighboring aromatic residue. Alternatively, the proton resonance at 7.6 ppm may be associated with a different aromatic residue from the proton with the resonance at 6.6 ppm. Both explanations involve at least two more aromatic residues around the H_3, and thus support the concept of a large concentration of aromatic residues around the combining site. Nevertheless, the Overhauser results illustrate the type of sophistication that NMR can give. Any model of the combining site will have to be consistent with the Overhauser results, and these results can provide an extremely sensitive filter among different possible models.

M. Combining Site for Fv—Comparison of NMR Data with Model-Building Studies

To a first approximation, there is excellent agreement between the predicted combining site (see Fig. 4) based on the model-building studies of Padlan *et al.* (1976) and the observed experimental results. The outstanding feature of the model is a double layer of aromatic residues that would surround the Dnp ring. Because of the proximity of these rings to one another and the sensitivity of ring current shifts to the position of nearby aromatic residues, NMR provides the means of positioning at least the first layer accurately to within 0.1 nm at most, something that model-building does not and could not hope to achieve. Thus, the orientation of the indole side chain of Trp 93_L is pointing back into the site, where its protons can be upfield shifted by Phe 98_L and where it forms the side of the aromatic box required to account for the chemical shift positions of bound Dnp aromatic protons. Location of the Dnp ring to overlap with Trp 93_L in this position also gives a binding site depth of 1.1-1.2 nm, in agreement with ESR and other determinations. Since the second layer of aromatic residues is less perturbed by hapten binding, accurate positioning will probably involve unambiguous identification of individual proton resonances, something that may well require the higher resolution of a larger NMR spectrometer for a molecule as large as Fv. Nevertheless, NMR is able to provide some information about other nonaromatic side chains. Thus, Leu 103_H is placed inside the combining site on the model postulated by Padlan *et al.* (1976), and yet the NMR results are entirely contrary to this view. If it were in the site before hapten binding, it would obscure Tyr 34_L, a residue required (from ring current effects) to be in contact with the Dnp ring. If Leu 103_H moves out of the site on addition of hapten, this would give large shifts of the methyl resonances, which are not observed. [In fact, with the hapten Tnp-$NHCH_2PO_3H^-$, *no* methyl resonances at all are perturbed (Dower *et al.*, 1976).] Another possibility is that if the light and the heavy chains moved apart on hapten binding, Leu 103_H could still be in the site. Such a movement is ruled out, however, since it would destroy the "aromatic box" by separating the "top" (Phe 34_L) from the "bottom" of the box (Tyr 34_L). We thus conclude that Leu 103_H has to be repositioned so that its side chain projects away from the binding site. This also allows closer approach of Tyr 104_H and Tyr 34_L, enabling them to ring current-shift each other's aromatic resonances, perhaps accounting for the unusual chemical shifts of some of the aromatic protons perturbed on hapten binding. It is interesting to note that in the model postulated by Poljak (1975) and based on Fab′ New, Leu 103_H would in fact be on the outside of the site, as suggested by the NMR studies. This again illustrates how NMR can help to differentiate among various hypothetical models, and indicates how model-building studies in conjunction with magnetic resonance experiments afford a most attractive possibility for the future.

N. NMR Can Give Both Dynamic and Structural Information

The binding of a hapten to an antibody generally results in chemical shifts of the hapten resonances. These shifts reflect the changes in chemical environment of the hapten. If there is an excess of hapten and the rate of chemical exchange (denoted $1/\tau$, where τ is the lifetime of the hapten antibody complex) between the two environments (free and bound) is *slower* than the corresponding differences in chemical shift (denoted $\Delta\omega$), then, in principle, two separate sets of resonances for the hapten will be observable.

At the other extreme, if the hapten exchanges much more rapidly between its two environments (free and bound) than the difference in chemical shift, i.e., $1/\tau \gg \Delta\omega$, one set of resonances is observed that occurs in the "average" positions of those in the two environments. In the intermediate case, the resonances are broadened and the observed exchange broadening can be related to the lifetime of the complex. It is the possibility of obtaining both dynamic and structural information from NMR experiments that makes the technique so attractive for studying proteins (Dwek, 1973).

In situations in which fast exchange conditions (defined as above) are satisfied, the "average" positions of the hapten resonances will be weighted according to the hapten populations in the two environments. This means that it is possible, by titrating the antibody with the hapten, to follow the shifts in the hapten resonances. At concentrations of hapten in excess of the antibody, the hapten resonances will be clearly visible over those from the antibody, and by suitable extrapolations, the values of the bound chemical shifts can be obtained (see Fig. 25). As with the chemical shift, the line width, under fast exchange conditions, is again the weighted average of those in the two environments.

The introduction of a hapten into the antibody combining site may also cause the environment of several amino acids to alter, with consequent chemical shift in the corresponding antibody nuclear resonances. As before, the lifetime of the antibody-hapten complex, and the magnitude of each protein chemical shift, will be the important factors in determining whether slow or fast exchange conditions apply. The situation may even be quite complex, with fast exchange conditions applying to some resonances and slow exchange to others, the critical factor being the magnitude of the shift.

The advantage of fast exchange conditions being applicable to the protein resonances is that as discussed for the hapten, titrations can be performed in which the resonances can be followed into their new positions. This is a valuable aid to the assignment of the perturbed resonances, for it enables the effects of the hapten on each resonance to be accurately determined, as we have seen in the case of Dnp-aspartate. Under slow exchange conditions, this is not possible, for the addition of hapten will then cause the perturbed protein resonances to "grow in" at their new positions, and it is difficult to know where each resonance originated.

O. The Antibody-Hapten Reaction Is a Single Association Step

In NMR, the exchange rate ($1/\tau$) is usually identified with the dissociation rate constant k_{off} in the relationship

$$A + B \underset{k_{off}}{\overset{k_{on}}{\rightleftharpoons}} AB$$

Thus, one may define fast exchange conditions as $1/\tau > \Delta\omega$ or as $k_{off} > \Delta\omega$. Conversely, the definition of slow exchange is then $k_{off} < \Delta\omega$.

With hindsight, we note that the majority of resonances perturbed on binding Dnp-aspartate to the Fv exhibit fast exchange conditions. The magnitudes of the shifts depend on the fractions of the hapten bound, and in most cases, no line broadenings were observed. This is also the case for the H_3 and H_6 protein resonances of the Dnp ring and the shift of approximately 1.7 ppm ($\equiv 3000\ s^{-1}$) on the H_3 gives a lower limit for k_{off}. On the other hand, the H_5 resonance of the Dnp ring does show some broadening. The effect is at a maximum when about 50% of the Fv is bound, and indicates an exchange contribution to the line width. A simple relationship for maximum broadening is $k_{off} \approx \Delta\omega$. The shift of 2.3 ppm ($\equiv 3900\ s^{-1}$) for the H_5 resonance thus gives an approximate value for k_{off}.

This value of k_{off}, together with the measured binding constant, allows k_{on} to be calculated as approximately $2 \times 10^8\ s^{-1}$. This is of the same order as the values obtained by Haselkorn *et al.* (1974) for a variety of Dnp haptens, and is fairly typical for bimolecular diffusion controlled reactions. The NMR results thus support the idea of Haselkorn *et al.* (1974) that the antibody hapten reaction can be visualized as a single *association step* in which the Dnp enters the site and immediately senses the aromatic environment as manifested by the ring current shifts on the hapten protons.

Further support for the single-step mechanism comes from the results for the binding of Dnp-lysine to the Fv. The resonances that are perturbed simply grow into their new position, exhibiting chemical slow exchange conditions. Using the results of the Dnp-aspartate titration, the smallest shift on a protein resonance is approximately 0.07 ppm ($\equiv 120\ s^{-1}$), and this gives an upper limit for k_{off} in the Dnp-lysine system. A value of k_{on} can then be calculated as equal to or greater than 3×10^8 s^{-1}, in good agreement with that from the temperature jump method (Pecht *et al.*, 1972).

Careful inspection of the difference spectra in Fig. 25 reveals that there are more resonances in the positive than in the negative in the aromatic region. As we noted in Table VII, certain aromatic resonances in the Fv are broadened on addition of hapten. In the light of Section IIIL, a possible mechanism for such broadening is "exchange," in which resonances experience a variety of environments with different chemical shifts. The resulting "uncertainty" in the chemical shift can result in broad resonances. As we have seen, though, the broadening will also depend on the rate at which these environments are sampled. The most likely source of line-broadening in proteins comes from alterations in the environments of either phenylalanine or tyrosine residues. The work of Campbell *et al.* (1975c) has shown that both these residues can flip rapidly about their axes of symmetry. This makes the two *ortho* (and the two *meta*) proton resonances equivalent. The rates of flipping are approximately 10^3-10^4 s^{-1}, and if the motion becomes less rapid, or if the inequivalence between the *ortho* (or *meta*) environments is increased, severe broadening could result. In the case of the Fv, the small shifts on the protein resulting from hapten binding suggest that the environment of the protein protons are not much altered so that the broadening of the protein resonances arises most probably from the hapten altering the rate of flipping of a nearby tyrosine or phenylalanine.

P. Orientation of the Dnp Ring in the Combining Site of MOPC 315

A major question that remains unsolved is the orientation of the Dnp ring in the combining site, and thus the possible H-bonding scheme. Only four amino acid residues in the model shown in Fig. 4 are suitably disposed for H-bonding to the two nitro groups of the hapten. These are Asn 36_L, Asn 36_H, Tyr 34_L, and Tyr 33_H. Tyr 33_H can be eliminated, since nitration of this residue causes no reduction in the affinity of normal Fv for Dnp lysine (Dwek *et al.*, 1976b), even at pH values at which the NO_2 Tyr is ionized (so that there is no H atom available for bonding). Further support that this residue is not involved comes from the fact that the NMR difference spectra in the nitrated Fv resulting from addition of Dnp-aspartate are almost identical with those obtained for the unmodified Fv.

The remaining possibilities can be distinguished only if the orientation of the Dnp ring is known. If the H(3) proton of the Dnp ring points toward Tyr 34_L (part of the aromatic box), the NO_2 groups could bond both to the —OH of this residue and to Asn 36_L. If the hapten is the other way up, only one H bond (from Asn 36_H) can form to a NO_2 group. The NMR studies reported here do not distinguish, thus far, between these two schemes, although other schemes

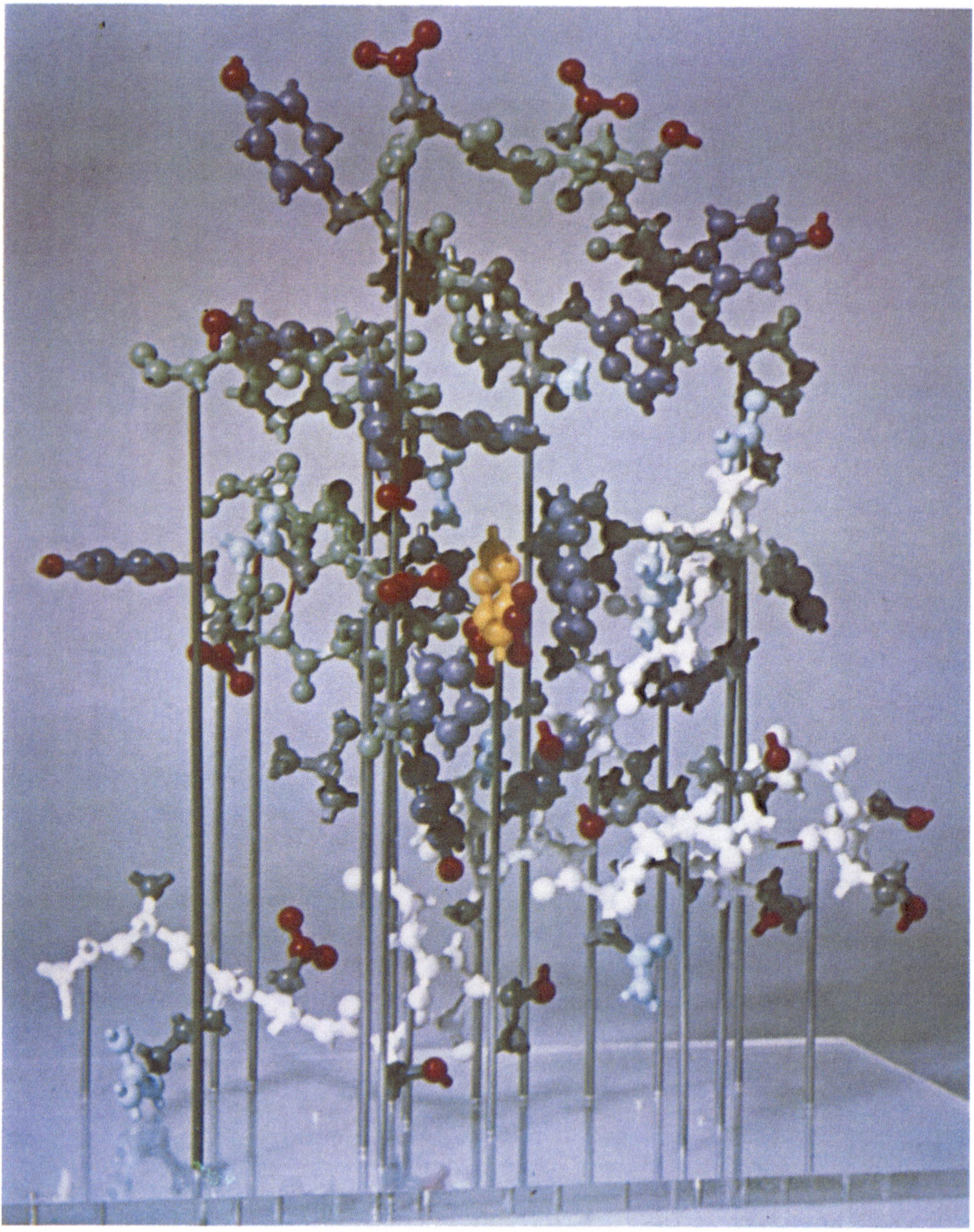

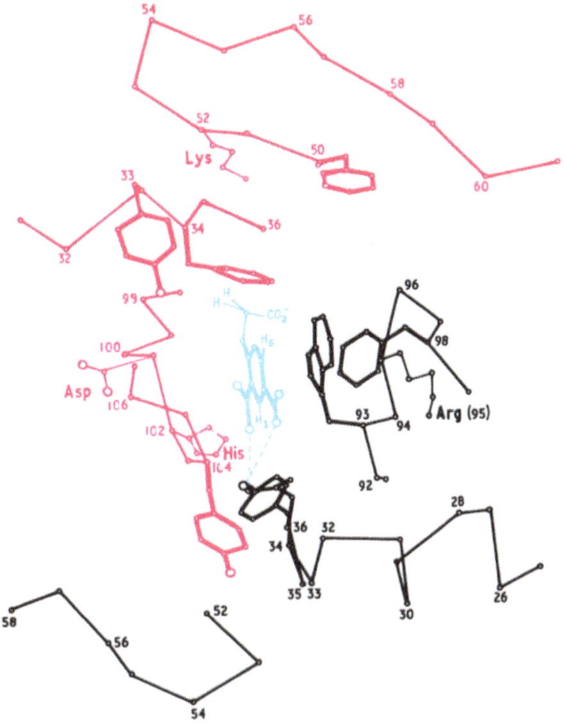

Figure 28. Combining site of MOPC 315. The site is shown with just the Dnp ring present. The heavy chain is colored green, the light chain white. The Dnp ring is shown in yellow (the hole indicates where the side chain is attached), and the two NO_2 groups are in red. (For the picture in general, red groupings represent acidic, and light blue, basic, groups.) The Dnp ring is parallel to a Trp residue (93_L); on the immediate right, the H(5) proton of the Dnp ring is perpendicular to and directly beneath Phe 34_H, while the H(3) proton (between the two NO_2 groups) is perpendicular to Tyr $34_{(L)}$ (on the lower right). The OH of this Tyr (34_L) – in red – is conveniently placed to form an H-bond to one of the NO_2 groups of the Dnp; the other NO_2 group can bond to Asn 36_L (light blue), which is just visible at the back of the site. The side chains involved in the specificity are His 102_H, which is at the front (left) of the site; Asp 101_H, which is just above it; and Arg 95_L (on the right in light blue), which is positioned just in front of Trp 93_L. Lys 52_H (which has been affinity labeled) is at the top of the site (light blue), and is included for completeness. The computer drawing highlights these features, and is shown with Dnp glycine in the site. The heavy chain is in red, the light chain in black. Note that each of the residues forming the "aromatic box" (Phe 34_H, Tyr 34_L, and Trp 93_L) is interacting with a further aromatic residue (Phe 50_H, Phe 98_L, and Tyr 104_H) – the second layer of aromatic residues referred to in the text. The H-bonding scheme of the two NO_2 groups of the Dnp ring (blue) is also indicated. The CH_2 group of the glycine (which projects outward toward the reader) is parallel to Tyr 33_H (in the photo, Tyr 33_H is just above Asp 101_H, and the plane of the ring is perpendicular to the reader). His 102_H, Asp 101_H, Arg 95_L, and Lys 52_H are also indicated.

can be ruled out, since they would destroy the very exact geometrical requirements of the "aromatic box." On energetic grounds, it would be expected that the scheme involving two hydrogen bonds to the Dnp would be preferred. Experiments using Dnp glycine indicate that this is indeed the case (Dwek *et al.*, 1976b).

IV. CONCLUDING REMARKS–SPECIFICITY OF MOPC 315 FOR Dnp LIGANDS

The results of the studies summarized in this article support the use of model building as a basis for structural analysis in immunoglobulins. The predicted properties of the binding site of MOPC 315 based on this assumption are in good agreement overall with the experimental results. With the predicted structure of the binding site as a first approximation, the use of different physical techniques, but in particular NMR, leads to this structure being refined (see Figure 28). These refinements then allow detailed conclusions to be made about the structural reasons for the specificity of MOPC 315 for Dnp ligands. The Dnp ring forms a charge-transfer complex with Trp 93_L, and this interaction, when carried out in an "aromatic box" (essentially Phe 34_H and Tyr 34_L), results in highly favorable contributions to the free energy of binding. There is also an enthalpy contribution from at least one hydrogen bond involving one of the NO_2 groups on the Dnp ring. The binding-energy contributions from the Dnp side chains appear to be essentially entropic, again reflecting their transfer into the nonpolar site.

This is well illustrated by comparing the affinity of Dnp-$O^{\ominus}$ (~1 mM) with Dnp-aspartate for MOPC 315 (~10 μM). The NMR studies show that in each case, the Dnp ring binds in the "aromatic box" of the combining site in an *identical* manner (Dower *et al.*, 1976). The difference in affinity reflects mainly the substitution by the NH in Dnp-aspartate for the $O^{\ominus}$ of Dnp-$O^{\ominus}$. Additionally, in the case of haptens carrying charged tail groups, there is also the possibility of electrostatic interactions with the charged groups at the entrance to the site (Asp 101_H, Lys 52_H, Arg 95_L, and His 102_H), which can give some contribution to the binding energy.

The NMR studies are currently being extended to other aromatic haptens such as menandione and 2,4-dinitronaphthol. The NMR method provides an extremely powerful and relatively rapid structural readout for comparative binding studies. Thus, the initial results show quite clearly that both these fused ring systems bind in the rigid combining site, but, as expected, in a slightly different manner from the Dnp haptens discussed here. A more general application of NMR should also be able to put concepts such as strange cross-reactions

(Michaelides and Eisen, 1974) and multispecificity (Richards *et al.*, 1975) on a firmer structural basis.

Finally, the NMR evidence shows that any conformational changes on hapten binding are essentially limited to the combining site. Secondary immunological functions such as complement fixation may involve subtle changes in the flexibility of certain groupings that only experiments in solution will reveal. In this respect, NMR studies may also be able to make a contribution, for such studies can give both structural and dynamic information.

ACKNOWLEDGMENTS

The studies in this article are very much a group effort, and I hope that I have done justice to my colleagues in giving a taste of the exciting possibilities of their research. In particular, I wish to acknowledge the experimental contributions of S. Wain-Hobson, S. K. Dower, K. Willan, P. Gettins, B. Sutton, and C. Sunderland. Throughout this project, we have all benefited from the interest and encouragement of Professor R. R. Porter and members of his M.R.C. Unit, in particular Miss E. M. Press, who was involved in the initial studies, and also from Professors D. Givol, D. C. Phillips, and R. J. P. Williams.

V. REFERENCES

Amzel, L.M., Chen, B.L., Phizackerley, R.P., Poljak, R.J., and Saul, F., 1974, *Prog. Immunol. II* **1**:85–92.

Campbell, I.D., Dobson, C.M., and Williams, R.J.P., 1975a, *Proc. R. Soc. London Ser. A* **345**:23.

Campbell, I.D., Dobson, C.M., and Williams, R.J.P., 1975b, *Proc. R. Soc. London Ser. A* **345**:41.

Campbell, I.D., Dobson, C.M., and Williams, R.J.P., 1975c, *Proc. R. Soc. London Ser. B* **189**:503.

Davies, D.R., Padlan, E.A., and Segal, D.M., 1975a, *Ann. Rev. Biochemistry* **44**:639.

Davies, D.R., Padlan, E.A., and Segal, D.M., 1975b, in: *Contemporary Topics in Molecular Immunology*, Vol. 4 (F.P. Inman, ed.), Plenum Press, New York, p. 127.

Dower, S.K., Wain-Hobson, S., Gettins, P., Givol, D., Jackson, W.R.C., Perkins, S.J., Sunderland, C., and Dwek, R.A., 1976, *Biochem. J.*, submitted for publication.

Dugan, E.S., Bradshaw, R.A., Simms, E.S. and Eisen, H.N., 1973, *Biochemistry* **12**:5400.

Dwek, R.A., 1973, *NMR in Biochemistry*, Clarendon Press, Oxford.

Dwek, R.A., Knott, J.C.A., Marsh, D., McLaughlin, A.C., Press, E.M., Price, N.C., and White, A.I., 1975a, *Eur. J. Biochem.* **53**:25.

Dwek, R.A., Jones, R., Marsh, D., McLaughlin, A.C., Press, E.M., Price, N.C., and White, A.I., 1975b, *Philos. Trans. R. Soc. London Ser. B.* **272**:53.

Dwek, R.A., Marsh, D.M., Sunderland, C., Sutton, B., Willan, K., Wain-Hobson, S., and Givol, D., 1976a, *Biochem. J.*, submitted for publication.
Dwek, R.A., Wain-Hobson, S., Dower, S.K., Gettins, P., Perkins, S.J., and Givol, D., 1976b, *Nature*, submitted for publication.
Epp, O., Colman, P., Fehlhammer, H., Bode, W., Schiffer, M., Huber, R., and Palm, W., 1974, *Eur. J. Biochem.* **45**:513.
Foster, R., 1969, *Organic Charge Transfer Complexes,* Academic Press, London.
Francis, S.H., Leslie, R.G., Hood, L., and Eisen, H.N., 1974, *Proc. Natl. Acad. Sci. U.S.A.* **71**:1123.
Geissner-Prettre, G., and Pullman, B., 1971, *J. Theor. Biol.* **31**:287.
Gettins, P., 1976, Part II thesis, Oxford.
Givol, D., 1974, *Essays Biochem.* **10**:73.
Griffith, O.H., Dehlinger, P.J., and Van, S.P., 1974, *J. Membr. Biol.* **15**:159.
Haigh, C.W., and Mallion, R.B., 1972, *Org. Magn. Reson.* **4**:203.
Haimovich, J., Eisen, H.N., Hurwitz, E., and Givol, D., 1972, *Biochemistry* **11**:766.
Haselkorn, D., Friedman, S., Givol, D., and Pecht, I., 1974, *Biochemistry* **13**:2210.
Hochman, J., Inbar, D., and Givol, D., 1973, *Biochemistry* **12**:1130.
Hsia, J.C., and Little, J.R., 1973, *FEBS Lett.* **31**:80.
Hsia, J.C., and Piette, L.H., 1969, *Arch. Biochem. Biophys.* **129**:296.
Imoto, T., Johnson, L.N., North, A.C.T., Phillips, D.C., and Rupley, J.A., 1972, in: *The Enzymes* (P.D. Boyer, ed.), Vol. VII, Academic Press, New York.
Inbar, D., Hochman, J., and Givol, D., 1972, *Proc. Nat. Acad. Sci. U.S.A.* **69**:2659.
Jaffe, B.M., Simms, E.S., and Eisen, H.N., 1971, *Biochemistry* **10**:1693.
Johnson, C.E., and Bovey, F.A., 1958, *J. Chem. Phys.* **29**:1012.
Johnston, M.F.M., Barisas, B.G., and Sturtevant, J.M., 1975, *Biochemistry* **13**:390.
Kabat, E., and Wu, T.T., 1971, *Ann. N.Y. Acad. Sci.* **190**:382.
Little, J.R., and Eisen, H.N., 1967, *Biochemistry* **6**:3119.
Mallion, R., 1975, *Chem. Soc. (London), Specialist Per. Reports* (R.K. Harris, ed.), vol. 4, p. 1.
Michaelides, M.C., and Eisen, H.N., 1974, *J. Exp. Med.* **140**:687.
Noggle, J.H., and Schirmer, R.E., 1971, *The Nuclear Overhauser Effect,* Academic Press, New York.
Padlan, E.A., Davies, D.R., Pecht, I., Givol, D., and Wright, C.E., 1976, *Cold Spring Harbor Symp. Quant. Biol.*, in press.
Pecht, I., Givol, D., and Sela, M., 1972, *J. Mol. Biol.* **68**:241.
Perkins, S., Johnson, L.N., Phillips, D.C., and Dwek, R.A., 1976, to be published.
Poljak, R.J., 1975, *Adv. Immunol.* **21**:1.
Poljak, R.J., 1976, private communication.
Poljak, R.J., Amzel, L.M., Avery, H.P., Chen, B.L., Phizackerley, R.P., and Saul, F., 1973, *Proc. Nat. Acad. Sci. U.S.A.* **70**:3305.
Porter, R.R., 1959, *Biochem J.* **73**:119.
Richards, F.F., Konigsberg, W.H., Rosenstein, R.W., and Varga, J.M., 1975, *Science* **187**:130.
Rudikoff, S., and Potter, M., 1974, *Biochemistry* **13**:4033.
Schiffer, M., Girling, R.L., Ely, K.R., and Edmundson, A.B., 1973, *Biochemistry* **12**:4620.
Segal, D.M., Padlan, E.A., Cohen, G.H., Rudikoff, S., Potter, M., and Davies, D.R., 1974, *Proc. Nat. Acad. Sci. U.S.A.* **71**:4298.
Shrager, R.I., Cohen, J.S., Heller, S.R., Sachs, D.H., and Schecter, A.N., 1972, *Biochemistry* **11**:541.

Smith, I.C.P., Marsh, D., and Schrier-Mucillo, S., 1975, *Free Radicals in Molecular Biology and Pathology*, Vol. 1, Academic Press, New York.

Sutton B., Dwek, R.A., Gettins, P., Marsh, D., Wain-Hobson, S., Willan, K.J., and Givol, D., 1976, *Biochem. J.*, submitted for publication.

Wain-Hobson, S., Dower, S.K., Gettins, P., Givol, D., McLaughlin, A.C., Pecht, I., Sunderland, C., and Dwek, R.A., 1976, *Biochem. J.*, submitted for publication.

Wong, L.T.L., Piette, L.H., Little, J.R., and Hsia, J.C., 1974, *Immunochemistry* **11**:377.

Wu, T.T., and Kabat, E., 1970, *J. Exp. Med.* **132**:211.

Isolation and Structure of Human Histocompatibility (HLA) Antigens

Michael J. Crumpton and David Snary

National Institute for Medical Research
Mill Hill, London, England

I. INTRODUCTION

Histocompatibility (transplantation) antigens were initially described as being responsible for the rejection of tumor and tissue grafts between nonsyngeneic individuals (Gorer, 1938; Snell, 1948). Genetic analyses subsequently established that the major transplantation antigens are the products of genes located at two separate, but closely linked, loci. More recent studies have indicated that these loci delineate a chromosomal region that controls a complex series of cell-mediated reactions. This region is referred to as the *major histocompatibility complex*. In mice, it is denoted as *H-2*; in humans, as *HLA*. The *H-2* complex has been more extensively studied than the analogous human region, and many of the functions of the *HLA* complex are based on analogies with the mouse data. The exact number of genes present in each complex is not known, although most workers are agreed that the number is large. Thus, for example, Klein (1975) has suggested that the *H-2* complex contains sufficient DNA to code for up to 2000 polypeptide chains, each of about 200 amino acids. The relationships among the genes have not been established, but their functions appear to be related and to be primarily concerned with the control of expression of cell-surface antigenic determinants, immune-response differences, certain complement functions, and probably other functions related to cell–cell recognition.

Genetic maps of the mouse and human major histocompatibility complexes are shown in Fig. 1. The *H-2* complex occupies 0.5 recombination units on

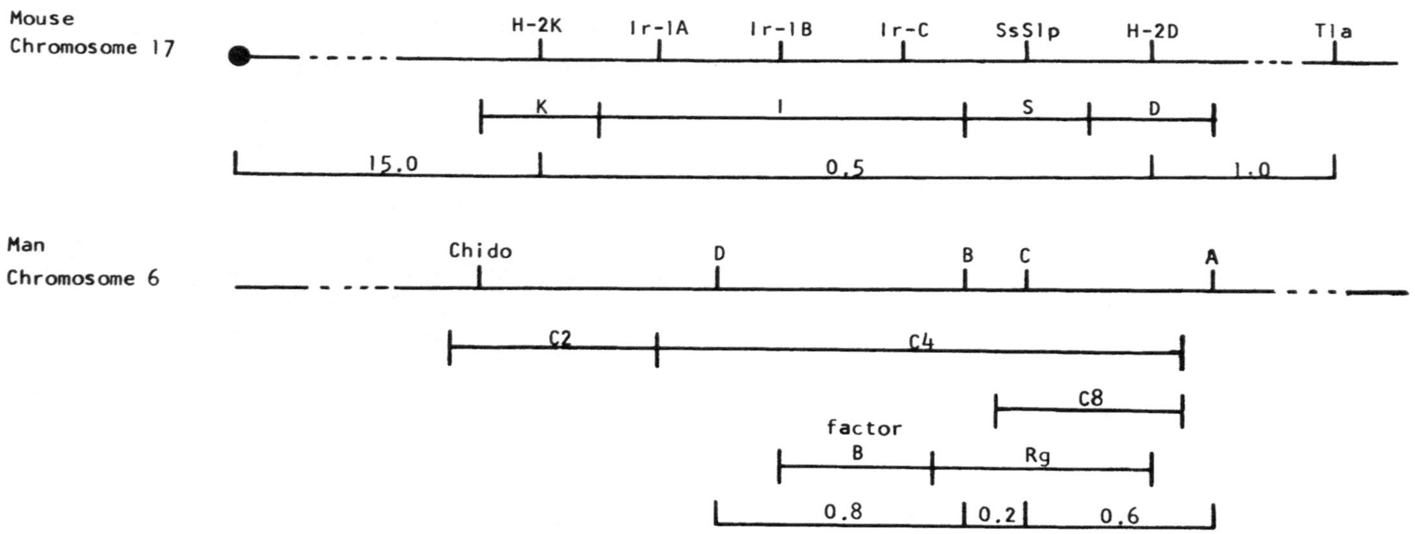

Figure 1. Major histocompatibility gene complexes of mouse (*H-2*) and man (*HLA*). Map distances are expressed in terms of percentage recombination frequencies, and are given in centiMorgans. Many of the letters apparently depict point loci, but actually denote regions. The *H-2* gene complex is taken from Klein (1975) and Shreffler and David (1975). The *HLA* gene complex is primarily based on data given in *Histocompatibility Testing 1975* (Kissmeyer-Nielsen, 1975). It is at present not known whether the complex is located on either the long or the short arm of chromosome 6. The locations of the complement components C2, C4, C8, factor B, and Rg are tentative. Factor B is a complement-activating factor; Rg is a blood-group antigen.

chromosome 17, and is divided into four major regions, *K*, *I*, *S*, and *D*. The *I* region is further subdivided into at least three subregions. The *K*, *S*, and *D* regions, and the *I* subregions, are denoted by the *H-2K*, *SsSlp*, *H-2D*, *Ir-1A*, *Ir-1B*, and *Ir-C* loci, respectively. The *HLA* complex occupies at least one to two recombination units on chromosome 6. It comprises three serologically defined loci, *A*, *B*, and *C*. It also contains two regions, *D* and another closely linked to the *C* locus, that are responsible for the mixed lymphocyte reaction.

The *K* and *D*, and the *A* and *B* (formerly *LA* and *FOUR*), loci of mouse and man are apparently analogous and, together with the *C* (formerly *AJ*) locus in humans, control the expression of the highly polymorphic series of serological specificities that comprise the classic major transplantation antigens. In man, 19, 26, and 6 alleles of the *A*, *B*, and *C* loci are currently recognized. The gene products are integral membrane glycoproteins of molecular weight about 43,000 that, *in situ*, interact specifically via noncovalent bonds with an equimolar amount of β_2-microglobulin. The gene controlling the expression of β_2-microglobulin is not included in the major histocompatibility complex, and is located on a different chromosome (No. 15 in humans; Goodfellow *et al.*, 1975). The molecular basis of the polymorphic allogeneic specificities has not been established, although various studies suggest that β_2-microglobulin does not contribute to the polymorphism, and that the specificities are determined solely by the polypeptide structure of the larger chain. β_2-Microglobulin is a nonglycosylated polypeptide of molecular weight about 12,000 (Cresswell *et al.*, 1973; Springer *et al.*, 1974; Tanigaki and Pressman, 1974), the amino acid sequence of which shows a marked homology to the C_H-3 domain of the γ-1 chain of immunoglobulin G (Cunningham *et al.*, 1973). This homology adds credibility to the proposals that histocompatibility antigens and immunoglobulins have a common evolutionary origin (Bodmer, 1972; Gally and Edelman, 1972).

The biological relevance of the extreme polymorphism of the *K*, *D*, *A*, and *B* antigens is not known, although Bodmer (1972) has proposed that the polymorphism evolved through the necessity for cell–cell recognition systems during development and morphogenesis. Some support for this proposal is provided by the striking analogies between mouse embryonic *T*/*t* antigens and adult *K* and *D* antigens (Artzt and Bennett, 1975). Thus, the *T*/*t* complex is of critical importance in the early stages of embryonic development and is located on the same chromosome as *H-2*, and it has been claimed (Vitetta *et al.*, 1975) that the gene products are also associated with a polypeptide chain of similar molecular weight to β_2-microglobulin. Direct evidence that the *H-2* and *HLA* antigens may mediate cell–cell recognition has recently been obtained at the level of cell-mediated lymphocytolysis. Thus, *H-2D* and/or *H-2K* antigen compatibility has proved to be essential for T-lymphocyte killing of virus-infected cells (Doherty and Zinkernagel, 1975) and of cells incompatible at minor histocompatibility loci (Bevan, 1975), including *H-Y* (Gordon *et al.*, 1975). The way in which the apparent requirement for common *H-2D* and/or *H-2K* genes between the cytotoxic and target cells is expressed at the molecular level is not understood, although it has been proposed that altered *H-2D* and/or *H-2K* antigens are recognized as "nonself" by the responding T cells (Blanden *et al.*, 1976).

The *I* region of the mouse is concerned primarily with determining the level of immune responses to T-cell-dependent antigens (Benacerraf and McDevitt, 1972; Katz and Benacerraf, 1975). Although the nature of the region has not been clearly established, various results can be accounted for if it contains two types of genes (Munro and Taussig, 1975). First, *Ir* (immune-response) genes. As all the responses regulated by *Ir* genes are T-cell-dependent, it seems logical to equate the *Ir* gene product with T cells, where it may serve as the antigen receptor (regulator) (Katz and Benacerraf, 1975). Interaction with antigen appears to induce release of the receptor, which then functions as either the activator (Munro and Taussig, 1975) or the suppressor (Tada *et al.*, 1975) of B-lymphocytes. Second, the *I* region also regulates the expression of a set of serological specificities called *Ia* (immune-associated) antigens that are expressed on B lymphocytes, but only in trace amounts or not at all on T cells (Shreffler and David, 1975). In man, these antigens probably represent the products of several loci (Mann *et al.*, 1976), some of which show a close association with the *D* locus that controls the expression of the major antigenic determinants involved in mixed lymphocyte responses (Thorsby and Piazza, 1975).

The *I* region probably also plays a crucial role in determining an individual's susceptibility to disease. Following the initial observation in mice of an association between virus-induced leukemogenesis and the *H-2* antigenic type, striking correlations have been reported between the *HLA-A* or *-B* type and susceptibility to a number of diseases including especially ankylosing spondylitis (McDevitt and Bodmer, 1974; Möller, 1975). Disease susceptibility has been directly correlated with the *A* and *B* loci. Due to nonrandom segregation, however, it is possible that the genes mediating disease susceptibility are actually closely linked with *A* and *B*, but are not the *A* and *B* genes *per se* (Winchester *et al.*, 1975b). The most attractive candidates are the *Ir* genes, although these genes have not as yet been clearly identified in man.

The *S* region of mice controls the expression of a serum α-globulin and includes the structural/control gene for the C4 component of complement. This region has not been identified in humans, but the demonstrations of genetic linkage between *HLA* antigens and the serum levels of the C2 (Fu *et al.*, 1975), C3 proactivator (Albert *et al.*, 1975), C4 (Rittner *et al.*, 1975), and C8 (Merritt *et al.*, 1976) components of complement imply strongly that the *HLA* region controls complement function. The recent finding of genetic independence between antigen type and serum levels of C1 and C6 (Mittal *et al.*, 1976) indicates, however, that not all components of the human complement system are controlled by the major histocompatibility region.

A clear understanding of the biological relevance of the gene products of the *HLA* region and of the interrelationships among the gene products relies ultimately on their isolation and the determination of their structure. Purified antigens will also permit the raising of antisera that should prove invaluable in tissue typing and disease diagnosis. The isolation and molecular structures of the mouse *H-2* antigens have been extensively studied (reviewed by Nathenson and Cullen, 1974). The results are complementary to and frequently precede those of the studies of the *HLA* antigens, so that, in many cases, interpretations of the human data are based on analogies with the mouse results.

II. ISOLATION OF ANTIGENS

The isolation of *HLA* antigens presents a number of problems due primarily to their polymorphic nature, their low level of expression on the cell surface, and their insolubility in conventional aqueous solvents. These problems can be circumvented in various ways.

A. Source of Material

The choice of tissue for the isolation of the *A*, *B*, *C* and *Ia* antigens is dictated by several considerations. *A*, *B*, and *C* antigens are expressed on the surface of almost all tissues except erythrocytes and placenta. *Ia* antigens, however, show a much more restricted distribution, being found on B lymphocytes, monocytes, and possibly some endothelial and epithelial cells, but not on T lymphocytes and fibroblasts (Jones *et al.*, 1975; Winchester *et al.*, 1975a). As a result, B lymphocytes represent the only reasonably convenient source of *Ia* and *A*, *B*, and *C* antigens, whereas platelets and human cultured lymphoblastoid T-cell lines provide relatively easily accessible sources of *A*, *B*, and *C* antigens devoid of *Ia* antigens.

Estimates of the amount of *A* and *B* antigens on normal T and B cells indicate about 20,000 molecules of each antigen per cell (Sanderson and Welsh, 1974). Assuming that the lymphocyte surface membrane has 10^7 protein molecules per cell, and that the membrane protein represents about 4% of the total cell protein (Crumpton and Snary, 1974), then the *A* and *B* antigens correspond to 0.5% of the plasma membrane protein, or 0.02% of the cell protein. Despite these low levels, amounts of antigen suitable for structural studies have been obtained from various natural sources, including especially spleen, and leukemic cells and platelets separated by plasmaphoresis. Serum and urine may also represent a useful source, particularly of the A9 antigen, although the solubility characteristics and molecular size of the purified antigen indicate that it has been degraded (Oh *et al.*, 1975; Bernier *et al.*, 1976). Natural tissues have the notable advantage of low cost. They suffer, however, from the major disadvantage that due to the extreme polymorphism of the *A* and *B* antigens, it is difficult to obtain reproducible sources of particular specificities, apart from those such as A2, A9, and B7 that occur at high frequency (50, 22, and 21%, respectively, in North European Caucasians, Bodmer, 1973, 1975).

The ideal source of *A*, *B*, *C*, and *Ia* antigens is the human cultured lymphoblastoid B-cell lines, although their high cost is somewhat restrictive. Thus, they circumvent the problem of polymorphism by providing reproducible antigenic types, and given mass-culture facilities are available in unlimited amounts. They also offer the opportunity of choosing particular *A* and *B* specificities and of developing cell lines homozygous at the *A*, *B*, and *C* loci to promote the separation of different specificities (see Fig. 5, for example), as well as doubling the antigen yield. Although lymphocytes transformed by Epstein-Barr virus have been claimed to possess 36-fold as much *A* and *B* antigens as normal cells (McCune *et al.*, 1975), in our experience, the increased content of a number of lymphoblastoid cell lines, including BRI 8, can be completely accounted for in terms of their increase in cell size (P. Goodfellow and W.F. Bodmer, personal communication).

The cell surface membrane, as either a crude or a highly purified preparation, is usually employed as the starting material for antigen isolation. Crude preparations have the disadvantage that they may promote degradation due to

Table I. Purification of *HLA* Antigens from BRI 8 cells[a]

		A2 activity		*Ia* activity	
Fraction	Protein (% recovery)	Recovery (%)	Degree of purification	Recovery (%)	Degree of purification
BRI 8 cells	100	100	1	100	1
Plasma membrane	1.0	46	45	46	45
Na deoxycholate-soluble	0.95	39	41	48	51
Gel-filtration	0.26	36	136	41	158
Glycoprotein	0.026	33	1240	32	1390

[a]Experimental details are given in Bridgen *et al.* (1976). BRI 8 cells were disrupted using the Stansted cell disruptor, and the plasma membrane fraction was separated as previously de-described (Crumpton and Snary, 1974). The membrane was solubilized in 2% (wt/vol) sodium deoxycholate and immediately centrifuged at 100,000*g* for 1 hr. The supernatant was fractionated by gel-filtration on Ultragel AcA 34 in 0.5% deoxycholate (see Fig. 2). Fractions containing *A*, *B*, *C*, and *Ia* antigens were pooled and added to *Lens culinaris* lectin-Sepharose in 0.5% deoxycholate, and the bound glycoproteins were subsequently eluted with 2% (wt/vol) methyl-α-D-mannopyranoside (see Fig. 3). Antigen activities were monitored by inhibition of cytotoxicity (Snary *et al.*, 1974). The purification of the A1, B8, and B13 antigens was similar to that illustrated for A2. The distribution of CW2 activity paralleled that of A2 up to the glycoprotein step, but differed from A2 in its behavior on *L. culinaris* lectin-Sepharose (see the text). *Ia* antigen activity was determined using allogeneic antisera (Jones *et al.*, 1975). An identical distribution was obtained using xenogeneic (rabbit) antisera (Snary *et al.*, 1977).

protease (lysosomal) contamination and the generation of structural artifacts such as dimerization through disulfide interchange (endoplasmic reticulum). Such alterations can be greatly reduced by using purified plasma membrane, which has the added advantage of providing a considerable increase in specific antigenic activity (about 46-fold; Table I). Methods of preparing the plasma membrane in good yield are, however, an essential prerequisite to their use for antigen isolation. The preparation of lymphocyte plasma membrane has been reviewed previously (Crumpton and Snary, 1974).

B. Solubilization

Two basic approaches have been used to overcome the problem of the insolubility of the *A*, *B*, *C*, and *Ia* antigens in conventional aqueous solvents (Strominger *et al.*, 1975). First, the intact membrane-associated molecules have been solubilized with detergents; second, the whole molecules have been cleaved, thereby releasing a water-soluble, antigenically active fragment from a nonpolar domain inserted in the lipid bilayer of the membrane (see Fig 9.)

1. Detergents

Detergents are extremely effective solubilizing agents for cell membranes (Helenius and Simons, 1975). The strongly cationic and anionic detergents such as sodium dodecylsulfate are the most effective, but have the disadvantage of also inducing protein denaturation and loss of biological activity. On the other hand, nonionic detergents such as Nonidet P40, Triton X100, and Ammonyx Lo combine good solubilization with a negligible effect on antigenicity. *A* and *B* antigens have been extracted from whole cells using Nonidet P40 and Triton X100, which fail to solubilize the nucleus, whereas Springer *et al.* (1974) used Brij 99 to extract the antigens selectively from crude membranes. Alternatively, purified plasma membrane has been solubilized using sodium deoxycholate (Snary *et al.*, 1974). This detergent has proved especially efficient at solubilizing lymphocyte plasma membrane (Allan and Crumpton, 1971), extracting about 95% of the membrane protein together with about 90% of the antigenic activity (see Table I). It has also proved superior as a solubilizing agent to Nonidet P40, Triton X100, and Ammonyx Lo. Thus, 1% Triton X100 solubilized only 40% of the antigens of the purified membrane. Sodium deoxycholate has the added advantage of having a much smaller micelle size (about 6000 mol. wt.) than the nonionic detergents (about 100,000 mol. wt. for Nonidet P40). As a result, it is the detergent of choice for the fractionation of membrane proteins by gel-filtration, since it gives a better resolution of low-molecular-weight proteins due to its smaller relative contribution to the protein's apparent molecular size (see Section IIIA and Helenius and Simons, 1975). The major disadvantage of deoxycholate arises from its charge and precipitation (gelation) at pHs less than about 7.5, which preclude its use as a solvent in isoelectric focusing and certain other charge separations. This problem can be avoided, however, by replacing the deoxycholate with a nonionic detergent. This has been achieved by adding Triton X100 to deoxycholate-solubilized membrane and then removing the deoxycholate by ion-exchange on a column of Zeolit FFIP.

2. *Cleavage*

Water-soluble antigenically active fragments of *A* and *B* antigens have been obtained by digestion with papain, extraction with 3 M KCl (Reisfeld *et al.*, 1971), and sonication (Kahan and Reisfeld, 1971). Papain digestion has proved especially effective, releasing up to about 40% of the *A* and *B* activities from crude membranes together with B lymphocyte specific polypeptides that most probably represent *Ia*-antigen fragments (Strominger *et al.*, 1975). Although 3 M KCl extraction and sonication were initially claimed to solubilize the whole molecule, a comparison of the properties of the purified products with those of the detergent-solubilized materials indicates that they must have been degraded (Snary *et al.*, 1974).

C. Fractionation of Solubilized Antigens

Papain-solubilized *A* and *B* antigens have proved very amenable to purification in good yield with the use of traditional fractionation methods such as gel-filtration and ion-exchange chromatography. For example, Turner *et al.* (1975) reported a yield of about 1 mg of purified antigen per 100 g packed, frozen, lymphoblastoid cells (cell line RPMI 4265), with a degree of purification of about 70-fold relative to the purified membrane preparation. Incidentally, the latter value indicates that the *A* and *B* antigens comprised about 1 to 2% of the protein of the cell surface membrane, which is 2- to 4-fold greater than that calculated for normal lymphocytes (see Section IIA). An important feature of the fractionation procedure was the relative ease of separation of the A2 antigenic activity from the mixed B7 and B12 activities by chromatography on DEAE-cellulose.

The fractionation of the detergent-solubilized antigens has not been explored as extensively as the papain-solubilized material. A simple efficient scheme that gives extensive purification of the *A*, *B*, *C*, and *Ia* antigens in good yield is outlined in Table I. BRI 8 cells, a lymphoblastoid B cell line, were used as the source of antigens (HLA-A1, A2, B8, B13, and CW2). The scheme comprises essentially four steps. First, the cells were broken by using a commercial model of the cell-disrupting pump (Crumpton and Snary, 1974). The plasma membrane was separated from the cell homogenate by differential centrifugation followed by discontinuous sucrose density-gradient centrifugation, and was washed by homogenizing under hypotonic conditions. Under the conditions described above, yields of plasma membrane in excess of 50% were often achieved, and the purified membrane was not contaminated by significant amounts of other subcellular organelles as judged by various morphological, biochemical, and immunological criteria. Second, solubilization of the purified membrane in 2% sodium deoxycholate and centrifugation at 100,000*g* for 1 hr gave 95% of the membrane protein and about 90% of the *A*, *B*, *C*, and *Ia* antigen activities in the supernatant. Third, fractionation of the supernatant on a column of Ultragel AcA 34 in 0.5% sodium deoxycholate gave about a 40% recovery and a 150-fold purification of *A*, *B*, *C*, and *Ia* antigens relative to whole cells. Ultragel AcA 34 was used in preference to Sephadex G200 and Bio-gel P150 due to its superior column stability and flow rate in deoxycholate. Antigen A2 was eluted as a single peak (Fig. 2a) that was coincident with the *Ia* antigenic activity (Fig. 2b). The distribution of A1, B8, B13, and CW2 antigenic activities was identical with that shown for the A2 and *Ia* antigens. Fourth, the glycoproteins, including the *A*, *B*, and *Ia* antigens, of the gel-filtration fraction were next separated from the nonglycosylated proteins by selective adsorption to *Lens culinaris* lectin-Sepharose in sodium deoxycholate and subsequent elution with methyl-α-D-mannopyranoside (Fig. 3). In contrast to the previous steps, the distribution of CW2 antigenic activity did not parallel that of the *A*, *B*, and *Ia* antigens. Thus, about half the CW2 antigen was bound reversibly by *L. culinaris* lectin-Sepharose and emerged from the column just subsequent to the initial protein peak, whereas the rest remained attached to the column and was eluted with sugar. A similar behavior has been described previously for the Thy-1 antigen of rat thymocytes (Letarte-Muirhead *et al.*, 1975). As shown in Table I, the overall purification procedure gave about a 1300-fold increase in the specific activities of A2 and *Ia* antigens relative to BRI 8 cells, with a recovery of about 32%.

Since *A*, *B*, and *C* antigens contain β_2-microglobulin, they can be selectively separated from other components, including *Ia* antigens, that lack the β_2-microglobulin chain (Jones *et al.*, 1975) by using immunoadsorbents against β_2-microglobulin. The glycoprotein fraction in 0.5% sodium deoxycholate was further fractionated by passage down a column containing the immunoglobulin fraction of a rabbit antiserum to human β_2-microglobulin attached to Sepharose. Under these conditions, the *A* and *B* antigens were specifically adsorbed, and were subsequently eluted using 3 M potassium thiocyanate in 0.5% deoxycholate as the dissociating solvent. A similar procedure has been used by Strominger *et al.* (1975), except that the adsorbed protein was specifically eluted using free β_2-microglobulin. Incidentally, this procedure should be applicable to the direct purification of the *A*, *B*, and *C* antigens from the deoxycholate-solubilized membrane, although in this case the purified *Ia* antigens would not be obtained as a by-product (see below).

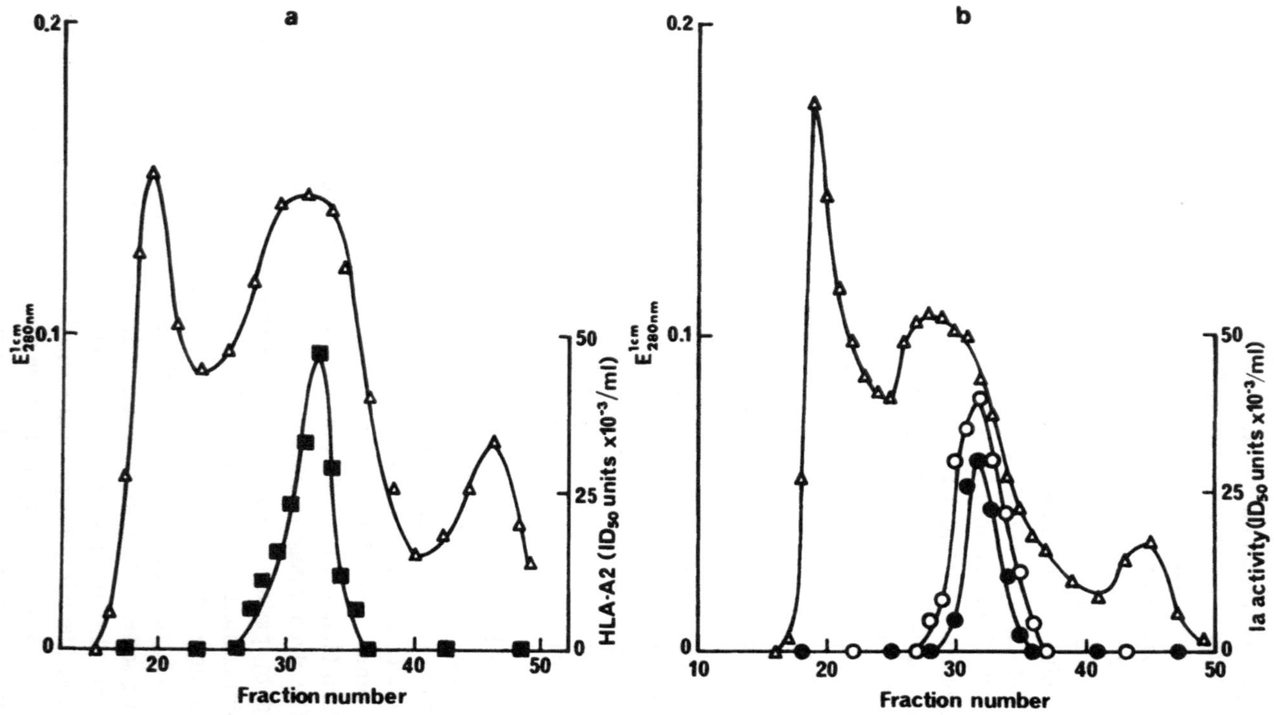

Figure 2. Gel-filtration of deoxycholate-solubilized BRI 8 plasma membrane. Membrane (4 mg protein/ml) was solubilized in 2% (wt/vol) sodium deoxycholate at 0°C and immediately centrifuged at 100,000*g* for 1 hr. The supernatant (1 ml) was eluted from a column (91 × 1.6 cm) of Ultragel AcA 34 with 0.5% sodium deoxycholate. Fractions (2.45 ml) were assayed for protein at 280 nm (△). (a) Distribution of A2 activity (■). The A1, B8, B13, and CW2 antigenic activities occupied an identical position with A2. (b) Distribution of *Ia* antigenic activity assayed using allogeneic (●) and xenogeneic (○) antisera. ID_{50} represents the amount of antigen giving 50% inhibition of cytotoxicity (Snary *et al.*, 1974).

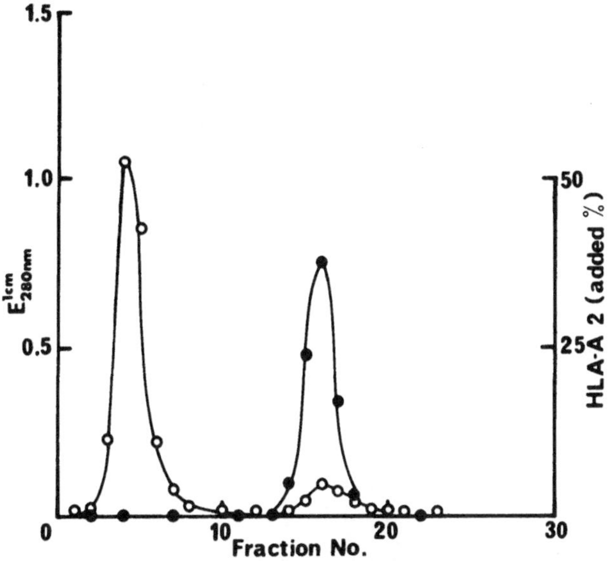

Figure 3. Fractionation of deoxycholate-solubilized BRI 8 plasma membrane using *Lens culinaris* lectin–Sepharose. Membrane solubilized in sodium deoxycholate (7.5 mg protein in 2 ml) was eluted from a column of *L. culinaris* lectin–Sepharose (10 ml containing about 10 mg lectin) with 1% sodium deoxycholate. The adsorbed glycoproteins were released by washing with 2% (wt/vol) methyl-α-D-mannopyranoside in 1% sodium deoxycholate. Fractions were assayed for protein (○) and for A2 activity (●). A1, B8, B13, and *Ia* antigenic activities were distributed similarly to A2.

The various fractions were recovered by precipitation at -20°C for 48 hr with 66% (vol/vol) ethanol, and were analyzed by polyacrylamide gel electrophoresis in sodium dodecylsulfate. Figure 4 shows that the glycoprotein fraction has a very restricted polypeptide composition compared with that of the original plasma membrane preparation. Only five bands with positions corresponding to molecular weights of 43,000, 39,000, 33,000, 28,000, and 12,000 were detected. Analysis of the fraction that was adsorbed and eluted from the β_2-microglobulin immunoadsorbent (Fig. 4C) revealed two polypeptides of molecular weights 43,000 and 12,000 together with bands of molecular weight 50,000 and 25,000 that most probably represent the H and L chains of immunoglobulin that was eluted from the immunoadsorbent. The 43,000-molecular-weight chain corresponds to the glycosylated polypeptide of the *A* and *B* antigens that carries the polymorphic allogeneic specificities, whereas the 12,000-molecular-weight chain represents β_2-microglobulin (see Section IIIB). The 39,000-molecular-weight polypeptide of the glycoprotein fraction is of unknown function, but various results indicate that those of molecular weight 33,000 and 28,000 represent the human counterparts of the mouse *Ia* antigens. This conclusion is based on three

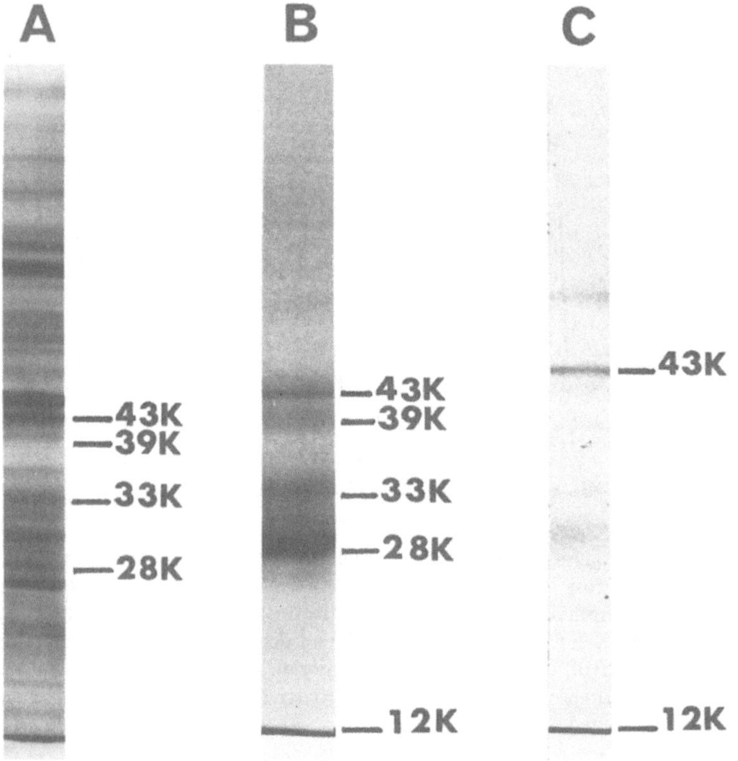

Figure 4. Polyacrylamide gel electrophoresis in sodium dodecylsulfate. (A) BRI 8 plasma membrane; (B) glycoprotein fraction (see Table I); (C) fraction adsorbed by antibody to β_2-microglobulin: the glycoprotein fraction was added to a column of the immunoglobulin fraction of an anti-β_2-microglobulin serum attached to Sepharose, and the adsorbed protein was eluted with 3 M potassium thiocyanate in 0.5% sodium deoxycholate. Electrophoresis was performed in 10% (wt/vol) polyacrylamide slab gels using the discontinuous buffer system of Laemmli (1970). Samples were dissolved by heating at 100°C in 2% (wt/vol) sodium dodecylsulfate, 0.1 M dithiothreitol, and 0.02% bromophenol blue. Gels were stained with Coomassie blue, and molecular weights were calculated by reference to the mobilities of standard proteins. Under these conditions, β_2-microglobulin was coincident with the bromophenol blue band at the gel front. The presence in gels B and C of a band with a molecular weight of 12,000 was revealed by using 12% (wt/vol) polyacrylamide gels. The unlabeled bands of gel C represent H and L chains due to contaminating immunoglobulin eluted from the anti-β_2-microglobulin–Sepharose column.

arguments. First, Table I shows that the antigens detected using antisera against human "*Ia*-type" antigens (Jones *et al.*, 1975) were concentrated in the glycoprotein fraction. Second, mouse *Ia* antigens are made up of two polypeptide chains with molecular weights of about 30,000 (Sachs *et al.*, 1975). Third, the most compelling evidence is based on the observation that antisera raised in rabbits and mice by immunizing with the glycoprotein fraction reacted exclusively with the 33,000- and 28,000-molecular-weight polypeptides and had many of the properties expected for heterologous anti-*Ia* sera (Snary *et al.*, 1977). Thus, they reacted preferentially with human B lymphoblastoid cell lines, purified peripheral blood B lymphocytes, and monocytes, but not T cell lines, peripheral T cells, fibroblasts, or erythrocytes. The immunoglobulin fraction of the antisera and its Fab fragments blocked mixed lymphocyte reactions, and the Fab fragments also blocked the cytotoxicity of the allogeneic antisera. Similar

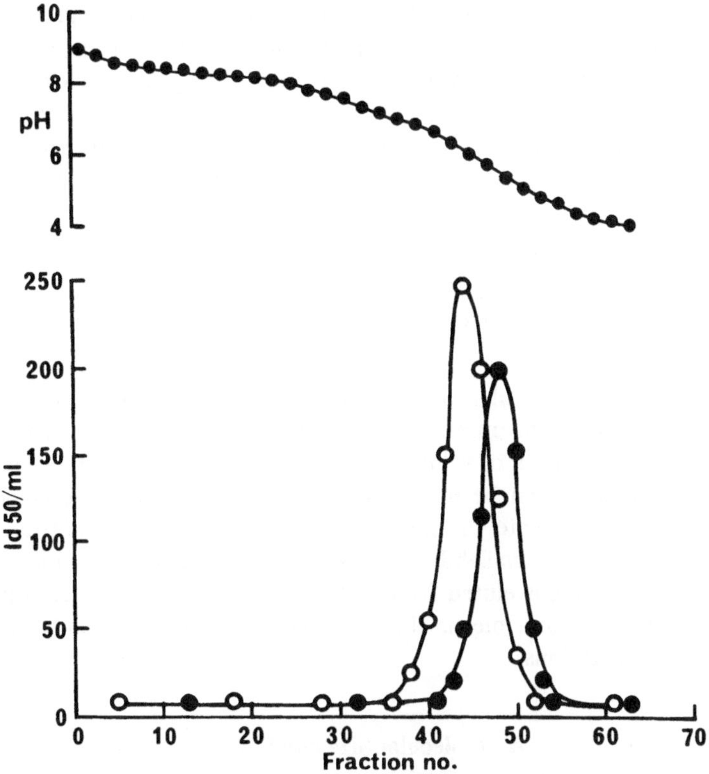

Figure 5. Isoelectric focusing of Triton X100–solubilized BRI 8 plasma membrane. Membrane (20 mg protein) was solubilized in 20 ml 1% Triton X100 and centrifuged at 100,000*g* for 1 hr. The supernatant, which contained about 40% of the *A* and *B* antigenic activities of the membrane, was incorporated into a continuous sucrose density-gradient [50 ml 5–50% (wt/vol) sucrose] containing 1% ampholine (pH range 3–10) and 1% Triton X100. The electrode solutions were 1% ethanolamine and 1% ascorbic acid. After electrophoresis for 72 hr at 750 V, the column was displaced with 60% (wt/vol) sucrose, and fractions of about 0.8 ml were collected. The upper curve illustrates the pH gradient. The fractions were assayed for the A2 (○) and A1 (●) alloantigenic activities. The B8, B13, and *Ia* activities coincided with the A1 peak.

B-lymphocyte-specific antisera have been described by Cresswell and Geier (1975) and Strominger *et al.* (1975).

The fractionation scheme outlined above provides purified mixtures of *A* and *B* antigens with different allogeneic specificities. Separations of different alloantigens have been achieved by utilizing the charge differences between the water-soluble fragments of some *A* and *B* antigens. For example, papain-solubilized antigen A2 was separated from mixed B7 and B12 by Strominger *et al.* (1975), and urinary antigen A9 from B12 by Bernier *et al.* (1976). Charge fractionation methods have also been assessed for the separation of the whole, detergent-solubilized antigens. Figure 5 illustrates the fractionation of BRI 8 plasma membrane solubilized in Triton X100 by isoelectric focusing. Antigen A2 was partly separated from the A1, B8, B13, CW2, and *Ia* antigens, all of which apparently occupied an identical position. It seems likely that a more complete separation of the A2 antigen would be achieved by using a shallower pH gradient.

The fractionation scheme described commends itself for the separation of highly purified *A*, *B*, and *Ia* antigens in good yield by using simple, traditional procedures.

III. STRUCTURE OF ANTIGENS

Information on molecular structure is conventionally obtained using pure materials. The isolation of pure *HLA* antigens is not, however, an essential prerequisite to the acquisition of valuable information on their structure. Thus, molecular size and shape can be derived from hydrodynamic data obtained using biological activity to locate the positions of the antigens on gel-filtration and centrifugation. Also, the availability of amino acid sequencing techniques, which are applicable to proteins eluted from polyacrylamide gels after electrophoresis in sodium dodecylsulfate, means that sequencing information can be obtained using impure preparations.

A. Molecular Size and Shape

The molecular size and shape of the deoxycholate-solubilized antigens can be adduced from measurements of their Stokes radii and $s_{20,w}$ determined by gel-filtration and sucrose density-gradient centrifugation, respectively, in the presence of sodium deoxycholate. The values obtained are summarized in Table II, which also includes the results for papain-solubilized *A* and *B* antigens measured under identical conditions.

Gel-filtration of deoxycholate-solubilized BRI 8 plasma membrane on Ultragel AcA 34 gave a single slightly asymmetric peak for each antigen. The peaks

Table II. Molecular Size and Shape of *HLA* Antigens[a]

	HLA antigen	$s_{20,w}$	Stokes radius (Å)	Molecular weight	f/f_0
Na deoxycholate-solubilized	*A*	5.15[b]	44.0	88,000	1.49
	B	4.55[b]	44.0	78,000	1.55
	C	5.15	44.0	88,000	1.49
	Ia[c]	4.48	44.0	77,000	1.57
Papain-solubilized[d]	A, B	3.68	29.8	46,000	1.26

[a] $s_{20,w}$ values were determined by sucrose density-gradient centrifugation in 1% sodium deoxycholate (see Fig. 6) relative to the sedimentation of aldolase (7.5 S), bovine serum albumin (4.41 S), ovalbumin (3.55 S), and myoglobin (2.08 S). The Stokes radii were measured by gel-filtration in 0.5% sodium deoxycholate (see Fig. 2) relative to the elution of standard proteins of known Stokes radii: aldolase (45 Å), bovine serum albumin (35.5 Å), ovalbumin (27.3 Å), and soybean trypsin inhibitor (23.9 Å). Molecular weights and frictional ratios (f/f_0) were calculated according to Siegel and Monty (1966), as described by Snary *et al.* (1975, 1977).
[b] Membrane that had been solubilized in deoxycholate under reducing conditions (2 mM 2-mercaptoethanol) gave similar $S_{20,w}$ values for the *A* and *B* antigens (5.24 and 4.35 S, respectively).
[c] Assayed using allogeneic and xenogeneic antisera.
[d] Mixture of A1, A2, B7, and B12 activities donated by Dr. A. R. Sanderson.

due to the *A*, *B*, *C*, and *Ia* antigens occupied identical positions (see Fig. 2). Similar elution patterns were obtained with a variety of gel filtration media and with purified plasma membranes from spleen and various lymphoblastoid cell lines. In each case, no evidence was obtained for the presence of aggregates or for gross polydispersity. The absence of aggregates contrasts with the results of a similar experiment reported by Cresswell and Dawson (1975), in which about 40% of the *A* and *B* antigenic activity of a crude membrane preparation was eluted from Sephadex G200 in deoxycholate in the position of dimers and larger oligomers. The origin of this difference in behavior is not clear, but it seems possible that Cresswell and Dawson's pattern reflects aggregation through disulfide interchange, which would be expected to be promoted in crude membrane preparations by the presence in the contaminating endoplasmic reticulum of an enzyme catalyzing sulfhydryl–disulfide interchange. This interpretation is supported by the demonstration that no oligomeric *A* and *B* antigens were detected when the cells were pretreated prior to breakage with iodoacetamide to block free sulfhydryl groups (Strominger *et al.*, 1975). If this explanation is correct, then the lack of aggregates in the present experiments emphasizes one of the advantages to be gained from using purified vs. crude plasma membrane preparations.

Sedimentation of the solubilized BRI 8 membrane on sucrose density gradients in deoxycholate gave an essentially symmetrical peak for each antigen

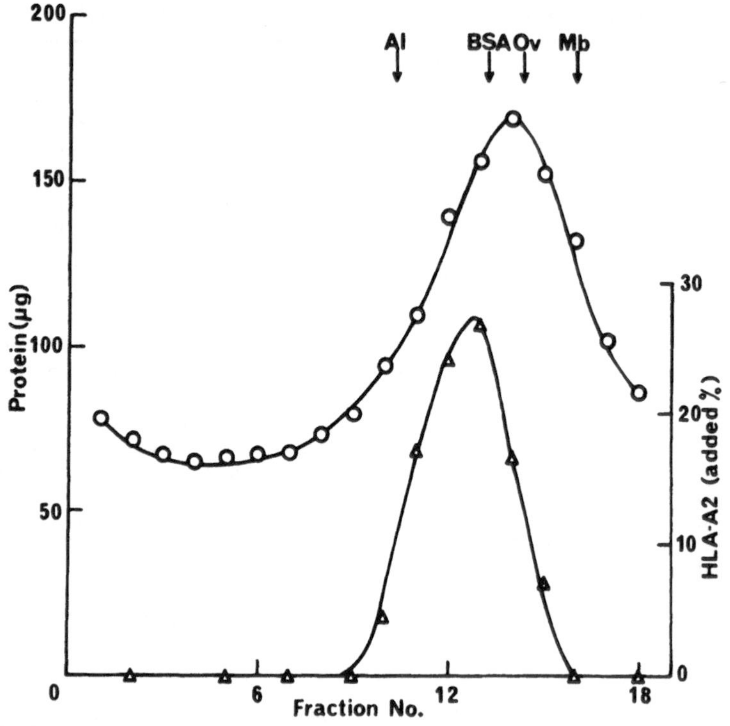

Figure 6. Sucrose density-gradient centrifugation of BRI 8 plasma membrane solubilized in sodium deoxycholate. Distribution of protein (○) and of A2 activity (△) across the gradient. A1 and CW2 antigens occupied identical positions with that shown for A2, but the B8, B13, and *Ia* antigens sedimented slightly more slowly (see Table II). The arrows indicate the positions of marker proteins run under identical conditions: (Al) aldolase; (BSA) bovine serum albumin; (Ov) ovalbumin; (Mb) myoglobin. Experimental details are given in Snary *et al.* (1974).

(Fig. 6). A comparison of the widths of the antigen peaks with those of the marker proteins suggested that the antigens were slightly polydisperse. Solubilization of the antigens under reducing conditions failed to cause any significant reduction in either the widths of the peaks or their sedimentation rates. The *A* and *C*, and the *B* and *Ia* antigens occupied identical positions, but the *B* and *Ia* antigens sedimented a little more slowly than the *A* and *C* antigens.

Calculation of molecular weights gave about 88,000 for the *A* and *C* antigens and a slightly lower value of about 78,000 for the *B* and *Ia* antigens (see Table II). The values for the *A*, *B*, and *C* antigens were larger than those predicted for a monomer comprising one each of the 43,000- and 12,000-molecular-weight polypeptides, but were too small to accommodate a four-chain dimer of molecular weight 110,000. Similarily, the value for the *Ia* antigen was greater than that for two chains of 28,000 and/or 33,000 molecular weight. The most likely explanation for the difference between the molecular weights determined for the deoxycholate-solubilized antigens and those estimated from their polypeptide chain compositions is that the *A*, *B*, *C*, and *Ia* antigens resemble other integral membrane proteins (e.g., cytochrome b_5 and rat Thy-1 antigen; Spatz and Strittmatter, 1973, and Letarte-Muirhead *et al.*, 1974, respectively) in that they incorporate a hydrophobic domain that binds detergent (Helenius and Simons, 1975). As a result, the deoxycholate-solubilized *HLA* antigens will be of anomalously high molecular weight when assessed relative to water-soluble globular proteins that fail to bind detergent. If it is assumed that the true molecular weight of the *A*, *B*, and *C* antigens is 55,000 and that of the *Ia* antigen is 61,000 (see Section IIIB), and that the difference between these molecular weights and those reported for the deoxycholate–antigen complexes in Table II is entirely due to bound detergent, then the *A*, *B*, *C*, and *Ia* antigens bind 0.57, 0.39, 0.57, and 0.28 g of deoxycholate per gram of protein, respectively. These values are in accord with those reported for various membrane proteins (0.29–0.64 g per gram of protein; Helenius and Simons, 1975). The apparent differences in the amounts of deoxycholate bound by the *A* and *C* vs. the *B* and *Ia* antigens most probably reflect differences in their hydrophobicities, in which case they may indicate that *A* and *C* antigens are inserted more deeply into the membrane lipid bilayer than *B* antigens. The very much larger molecular weights estimated for *A* and *B* antigens solubilized in Brij 99 (460,000; Springer *et al.*, 1974) can be explained in terms of the larger micelle size of Brij 99 compared with deoxycholate.

Estimates of the frictional ratios of the *A*, *B*, *C*, and *Ia* antigens gave values within the range 1.49–1.57 (see Table II). These values indicate that the deoxycholate–antigen complexes are moderately asymmetrical. The decreased asymmetry of the papain-solubilized *A* and *B* antigens suggests that either the hydrophobic domain and/or the bound detergent is responsible for the apparent asymmetry of the intact molecules.

In contradistinction to the deoxycholate-solubilized *A* and *B* antigens, the molecular weights of the papain-solubilized antigens in deoxycholate (46,000; Table II) agreed closely with those calculated from polyacrylamide gel electrophoresis for one each of the 12,000- and 34,000-molecular-weight chains (Turner *et al.*, 1975). This result, together with the water solubility of the papain fragments, implies that the hydrophobic domain, which presumably binds detergent and is inserted into the membrane, is cleaved by papain. It is also apparent that the region extrinsic to the membrane lipid that carries the allotypic antigenic determinant binds little or no detergent. Although the hydrophobic domain may correspond to the difference in size between the complete and the papain-solubilized *A* and *B* gene products (10,000 mol. wt.), studies of another human integral membrane glycoprotein, glycophorin, indicate that it need be no larger than approximately 32 amino acid residues (Tomita and Marchesi, 1975). Thus, it is possible that the *A* and *B* gene products have a terminal hydrophilic domain that may be exposed on either the external or the cytoplasmic surface of the membrane (see Section IVC and Fig. 9).

B. Gross Structure

Analyses of the purified *A* and *B* antigens indicate that the whole antigens comprise two noncovalently bonded polypeptide chains of 43,000 and 12,000 molecular weight (Cresswell *et al.*, 1973; Springer *et al.*, 1974; Tanigaki and Pressman, 1974), and that in the papain-solubilized antigens, the larger polypeptide chain has a decreased molecular weight of 34,000 (Turner *et al.*, 1975; Henriksen *et al.*, 1976). As far as can be judged, the 12,000-molecular-weight chain is identical to human urinary β_2-microglobulin (see also Section IIID). According to some recent data, *C* antigens are analogous in structure to the *A* and *B* antigens (Rask *et al.*, 1976). The structure of the membrane-associated *A* and *B* antigens has not been defined, but it has been suggested that it resembles immunoglobulin in having two basic units of one each of the larger and smaller polypeptide chains linked either noncovalently or by a disulfide bridge to give a four-chain dimer of molecular weight 110,000 (Strominger *et al.*, 1974; Peterson *et al.*, 1975). This proposal was largely based on the presence of dimers and larger oligomers in detergent-solubilized preparations. Our experiments, however, have failed to reveal any dimers. These results have led to the suggestion that dimers are an experimental artifact, rather than a naturally occurring structure (see Section IIIA and Snary *et al.*, 1975), and that the immunoglobulinlike model for the membrane-associated *A* and *B* antigens described above is unlikely to be correct.

The gross structure of the *Ia* antigens is less certain than that of the *A* and *B* antigens, although some preliminary results are consistent with the suggestion that they comprise two noncovalently bonded polypeptide chains of molecular weights 33,000 and 28,000 (Snary *et al.*, 1977). This suggestion is based on the results of the following experiments: First, rabbit antisera, which according to various criteria recognized the human counterparts of the mouse *Ia* antigens, selectively precipitated the 28,000- and 33,000-molecular-weight chains from ^{125}I-labeled, deoxycholate-solubilized BRI 8 plasma membrane. Second, treatment of the glycoprotein fraction of Table I with dimethyl-3,3′-dithiobispropionimidate dihydrochloride, which cross-links adjacent polypeptide chains with an efficiency of about 30% (Wang and Richards, 1974), gave only one new polypeptide chain of molecular weight 61,000 (Fig. 7). Cleavage of the cross-linked species using dithiothreitol caused the disappearance of this chain. Obviously, a single species of molecular weight 61,000 readily accommodates one each of the 33,000- and 28,000-molecular weight chains, but argues strongly against other possible combinations. The 33,000- and 28,000-molecular-weight chains were not linked by disulfide bridges prior to cross-linkage, since no 61,000-molecular-weight chain was detected in the untreated glycoprotein fraction that had not been reduced with dithiothreitol prior to polyacrylamide gel electrophoresis.

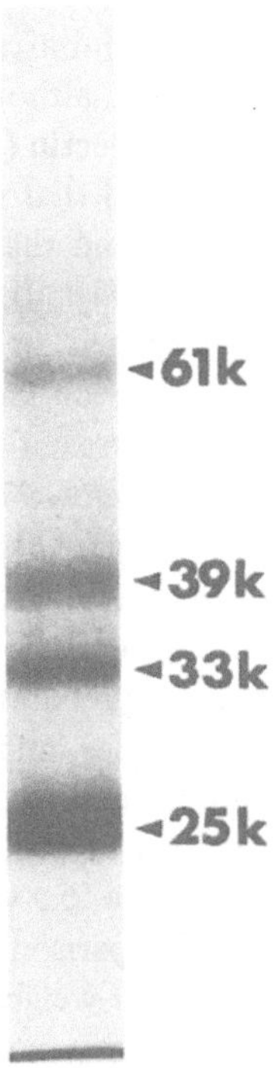

Figure 7. Polyacrylamide gel electrophoresis in sodium dodecylsulfate of the BRI 8 glycoprotein fraction that had been cross-linked with dimethyl-3,3′-dithiobispropionimidate dihydrochloride. The glycoprotein fraction (see Table I) in sodium deoxycholate was treated with the reagent as described by Wang and Richards (1974). Electrophoresis was performed as described in the Fig. 4 caption, except that the sample was not reduced with dithiothreitol. The polypeptide pattern should be compared with Fig. 4B. The 43,000- and 28,000-mol. wt. chains of Fig. 4B have mobilities equivalent to molecular weights of 39,000 and 25,000, respectively, when not reduced prior to electrophoresis.

Third, the molecular weight of the deoxycholate–antigen complex is contrary to a single polypeptide chain of molecular weight about 30,000 (see Section IIIA).

If, as seems likely, the B lymphocyte-specific antisera described by Strominger *et al.* 1975) are in fact anti-*Ia* reagents, then it is apparent that the polypeptides comprising *Ia* antigens can be cleaved by papain to give a water-soluble fragment composed of 30,000- and 23,000-molecular-weight chains.

C. Composition

The *A*, *B*, and *Ia* antigens are glycoproteins. This conclusion is based on direct analyses of the papain fragments of the *A* and *B* antigens (Henriksen *et al.*, 1976, Terhorst *et al.*, 1976), and on the adsorption of the deoxycholate-solubilized *A*, *B*, and *Ia* antigens by *L. culinaris* lectin and their specific elution with α-methyl mannoside (see Table I). Although water-soluble preparations of

A and B antigens that lack carbohydrate (less than 1%) have been described (Reisfeld and Kahan, 1972), it now appears likely that the carbohydrate had been cleaved from the portion of the molecule bearing the allotypic determinant during solubilization. The situation with respect to the *C* antigen is at present confused, although since the antigen was either retarded or adsorbed by *L. culinaris* lectin (see Section IIC), it is probably also a glycoprotein. Most workers are agreed that the β_2-microglobulin chain of the *A* and *B* antigens is nonglycosylated, and that all the carbohydrate is associated with the *A* and *B* gene products. In *Ia* antigens, both the 28,000- and 33,000-molecular-weight chains are glycosylated, as judged by their capacities to bind ^{125}I-labeled *L. culinaris* lectin after polyacrylamide gel electrophoresis (Snary *et al.*, 1977).

Analyses of the papain fragments of the A2 and A7 polypeptide chains (Henriksen *et al.*, 1976; Terhorst *et al.*, 1976) revealed about 13% by weight of carbohydrate per 34,000 molecular weight. The carbohydrate comprised sialic acid, mannose, galactose, glucosamine (presumably *N*-acetylglucosamine), and possibly fucose. Variations in the relative amounts of the sugars reported for different antigen preparations were apparently unrelated to differences in their allogenic specificities, and were most probably due to artifacts, to variations in technique, and, at least in the case of sialic acid, to microheterogeneity. Thus, on isoelectric focusing, a purified preparation of the papain-solubilized A2 antigen gave four bands due to a variable number of sialic acid residues (Parham *et al.*, 1974).

Comparison of the polypeptide structures of the A2 and A7 34,000-molecular-weight chains has revealed some differences superimposed on an overall similarity in structure. For example, Henriksen *et al.* (1976) detected no more than 15 amino acid differences between the amino acid compositions of the A2 and A7 polypeptides, whereas peptide mapping revealed that 5 of the 6 half-cystine tryptic peptides of the A7 chain were shared by the A2 chain.

D. Amino Acid Sequence

Some information is available on the *N*-terminal sequences of the papain-solubilized A2, and mixed B7 and B12 antigen fragments (Terhorst *et al.*, 1976), and of the whole 43,000-molecular-weight polypeptide chain from a mixed A1, A2, B8, and B13 antigen preparation (Bridgen *et al.*, 1976). Very different approaches were used to collect the data. Thus, Terhorst *et al.* (1976) applied conventional sequencing techniques to extensively purified preparations of the water-soluble A2 and mixed B7 and B12 antigens. Alternatively, Bridgen *et al.* (1976) exploited a solid-phase, microsequencing method by applying it directly to the 43,000- and 12,000-molecular-weight chains eluted after polyacrylamide gel electrophoresis of a partly purified preparation of the intact *A* and *B* antigens of mixed allotypic specificities. The latter approach has the advantage that it is applicable to much smaller amounts of protein (less than 1 nmol) than the conventional methods, and that it exploits the considerable resolving power of sodium dodecylsulfate–polyacrylamide gel electrophoresis as an aid to purification. The applicability of the method was evident from the analysis of the 12,000-molecular-weight chain of the glycoprotein fraction (see Fig. 4), the *N*-terminal amino acid sequence of which was clearly the same as the *N*-terminus of human urinary β_2-microglobulin (Bridgen *et al.*, 1976).

The *N*-terminal sequences of the whole *A* and *B* antigens and their papain fragments are summarized in Table III. Clearly, the sequence of the whole 43,000-molecular-weight polypeptide chain represents the sum of the sequences of the papain-solubilized *A* and *B* antigens, apart from some slight variation at residues 6, 8, 10, and 13. This marked similarity in *N*-terminal sequences indicates that papain must cleave the polypeptide chain toward the *C*-terminus, and that the *N*-terminus is exposed on the cell surface. In other words, the hydrophobic portion of the polypeptide chain that is inserted into the membrane lipid bilayer must be located close to the *C*-terminus, although it is still possible that the *C*-terminus is exposed on the inner or outer face of the membrane.

If, as seems likely, the *C* gene product was not present to a significant extent in the 43,000-molecular-weight polypeptide used for analysis, then several interesting points emerge from the data shown in Table III. First, at least 10 of the *N*-terminal 16 residues were constant for both the *A* and *B* antigens, and all the amino acid changes could be accounted for as single nucleotide base changes. This marked restriction in heterogeneity is consistent with the antigenic cross-reactivity observed between *A* and *B* antigens with xenogeneic antisera (Cresswell and Ayres, 1976; Rask *et al.*, 1976), and endorses the suggestion that the *A* and *B* genes arose from a common ancestral gene by duplication (Bodmer, 1972). In this context, the sequence of the *C* antigen will be particularly informative because although the strong linkage disequilibrium between the *C* and *B* loci determinants suggests that that *C* gene(s) arose from the *B* gene(s), a comparison of the molecular sizes of the deoxycholate-solubilized antigens (see Table II) indicates that the *C* antigen resembles the *A* antigen more closely than the *B* antigen. Second, the sequence differences at residues 9 and 11 can be interpreted as *A*- and *B*-locus differences but those at residues 6, 8, 10, and 13 cannot be interpreted in this way. Thus, the A1, A2, B8, and B13 antigens collectively have arginine at residue 6, whereas the B7 and B12 antigens have arginine and valine. This variation is consistent with the suggestion that the B7 or B12 antigen differs from other *A* and *B* antigens in having valine at this position. Similarly, the serine and alanine residues at positions 10 and 13, respectively, may represent changes that are directly related to the A1, B8, and/or B13 specificities. If these and other changes do contribute to the serologically defined polymorphism, then each allele may represent the sum of a number of changes at positions remote from each other in the unfolded polypeptide chain.

Table III. Comparison of *N*-Terminal Amino Acid Sequences of *A* and *B* Antigens[a]

Protein	Antigenic specificity	Residue 1	2	3	4	5	6	7	8	9	10	11	12	13	14	15	16
Papain-solubilized 34,000-molecular-weight chain[b]	A2	Gly	Ser		Ser	Met	Arg	Tyr	Phe	Phe	Thr	Ser	Val	Ser			Gly
	B7 B12	Gly	Ser		Ser	Met	Arg Val	Tyr	Phe	Tyr	Thr	Ala	Val	Ser	Arg	Pro	Gly
43,000-molecular-weight chain[c]	A1, A2								Phe	Phe	Thr	Ala		Ala			
	A1, A2, B8, B13		Ser		Ser	Met	Arg	Tyr					Val		Arg	Pro	Gly
	B8, B13								Tyr	Tyr	Ser	Ser		Ser			

[a]*N*-Terminal sequences of the larger polypeptide chains of the papain-solubilized A2, and of the mixed B7 and B12 antigens (Terhorst *et al.*, 1976), compared with the sequence of the *N*-terminal 16 residues of the 43,000-molecular-weight polypeptide chain. Blank positions indicate that no information is available on the residue at this point.

[b]Data obtained by Terhorst *et al.* (1976) using conventional sequencing techniques.

[c]Data of Bridgen *et al.* (1976). The 43,000-molecular-weight polypeptide chain was eluted from polyacrylamide gels after electrophoresis of the glycoprotein fraction (see Fig. 4), and the *N*-terminal sequence was determined using a solid-phase, high-sensitivity technique. The *A* and *B* antigenic specificities are based on the known specificities of the glycoprotein fraction and on reports that the allogeneic *A* and *B* specificities are associated exclusively with a polypeptide of molecular weight 43,000 (Tanigaki and Pressman, 1974). Its sequence begins at residue 2, since residue 1 remains attached to the resin and is not identified. Residue 3 of the 43,000-molecular-weight chain gave a detectable spot on thin-layer chromatography, but the spot could not be identified with any known phenylthiohydantoin-amino acid.

E. Antigenicity and Immunogenicity

The results of various studies suggest that β_2-microglobulin does not contribute to the activities of the *A* and *B* antigens detected using allogeneic antisera. The most compelling evidence in support of this view is provided by the demonstration that the alloantigenic activity of the papain-solubilized antigens persisted after the removal of β_2-microglobulin (Nakamuro *et al.*, 1975). The role of the carbohydrate, if any, in defining the *A* and *B* antigenic activities is more controversial. Thus, results such as the amino acid composition and sequence (see Sections IIIC and IIID), peptide maps, and effect of heating (Fig. 8) argue strongly in support of the proposal that the alloantigenic activities are determined solely by the polypeptide structure. It is difficult, however, to categorically rule out any involvement of carbohydrate, especially if, as has been proposed (Sanderson *et al.*, 1971), the antigenic site is located close to the carbohydrate moiety. Although, *a priori*, the alloantigenic differences can be accounted for in terms of single amino acid changes (Crumpton, 1974), the preliminary data on amino acid composition are more in keeping with multiple changes that may not be located within a variable region, but may be remote from one another in the unfolded polypeptide chain. Definitive answers to these questions must await the complete sequence analysis of the *A* and *B* gene products. It will also be interesting to see whether cross-reacting antigens such as A2 and A23 have some common changes that distinguish them from all other antigens, as well as additional changes that distinguish them from each other.

Few data are at present available on the molecular basis of the allogeneic activity of the *Ia* antigens. However, the similar heat labilities of the A2 alloantigenic activity and the *Ia* activities, measured using allogeneic and xenogeneic antisera (see Fig. 8), and the destruction of *Ia* activity by proteolysis argue in favor of the view that the *Ia* antigenic activity is also dependent on the polypeptide structure. This interpretation agrees with the results of similar experiments that suggest that mouse *Ia* alloantigenic activity is also determined by the protein moiety (Cullen *et al.*, 1975).

Antisera against the papain-solubilized, purified *A* and *B* antigens have been raised primarily in rabbits and monkeys by various workers (Miyakawa *et al.*, 1973; Sanderson and Welsh, 1973; Robb *et al.*, 1975; Cresswell and Ayres, 1976; Rask *et al.*, 1976). In general, rabbit antisera against *A* antigens contained precipitating antibodies directed toward antigenic determinants that were shared by all *A* antigens, irrespective of their allogeneic specificities; the rabbit anti-*B* sera behaved similarly. Anti-*A* sera also cross-reacted with *B* antigens and vice versa. As the antisera either failed to precipitate β_2-microglobulin (Cresswell and Ayres, 1976) or had been absorbed with β_2-microglobulin (Rask *et al.*, 1976), the common antigenic determinants must be associated with the *A* and *B* gene products. These results clearly demonstrate that the *A* and *B* polypeptides share a consid-

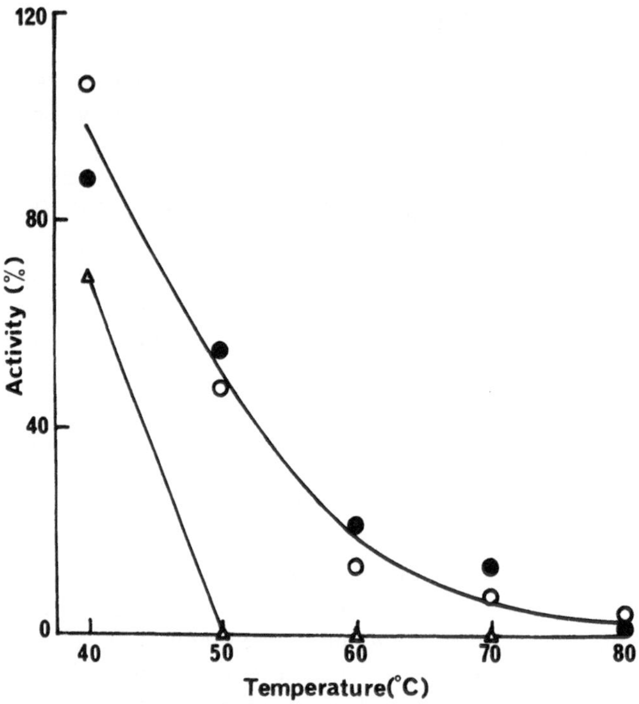

Figure 8. Effect of heating on the antigenic activities of the BRI 8 plasma membrane. Samples of the plasma membrane (see Table I) were heated for 15 min at various temperatures prior to assaying for A2 alloantigenic activity (△), and for the *Ia* antigens using allogeneic (○) and xenogeneic (●) antisera.

erable degree of structural homology (Crumpton, 1974). In some cases, the antisera also contained antibodies against the alloantigenic determinant, and could be rendered specific for the allotype of the immunizing antigen by absorption with lymphoblastoid cells that lacked the particular *A* specificity (Robb *et al.*, 1975).

Immunization of rabbits with a purified preparation of the *A*, *B*, and *Ia* antigens (the glycoprotein fraction in Table I) stimulated the preferential production of antibodies against the *Ia* antigen (Snary *et al.*, 1977). The specificity of the antibodies was assessed in terms of their reactivity with B and T lymphocytes and other cell types, as well as their capacity to inhibit mixed lymphocyte reactions. Antisera with similar properties that were prepared in a similar manner except that the antigen was derived from papain-solubilized material have been described by Strominger *et al.* (1975).

IV. DISCUSSION AND CONCLUSIONS

There seems to be little doubt that the *A*, *B*, *C*, and *Ia* antigens are integral plasma membrane glycoproteins. This conclusion is based primarily on the hydrodynamic properties of the detergent-solubilized antigens, which can be satisfactorily accounted for only in terms of the molecules incorporating a hydrophobic domain that binds detergent. It is supported by the apparent close association of the antigens with the cell membrane, which survives cell breakage, dilution, and extensive washing. Being integral membrane proteins, the antigens are insoluble in conventional aqueous buffers. This insolubility initially frustrated attempts to purify the antigens, but the problem has been solved either by using weakly anionic and nonionic detergents as solubilizing agents or by using papain to cleave the hydrophilic portion of the antigen from the membrane.

A. Papain vs. Detergent Solubilization

Papain digestion releases the *A*, *B*, *C*, and apparently the *Ia* antigens in a form that is readily amenable to purification in good yield (Strominger *et al.*, 1975). The products preserve their antigenicity, and have been used as immunogens to prepare allogeneic and xenogeneic antisera. Given the recent improvements in plasma membrane preparation (see Table I), detergent-solubilization shares all the positive features of papain-solubilization, and, as judged by these features, there seems to be little to dictate the choice between the two procedures. Detergent-solubilization has, however, one important extra advantage: it provides the complete molecule with the capacity of being incorporated into an artificial membrane, rather than just the hydrophilic portion extrinsic to the cell surface. Since the biological function of the antigens is apparently intimately associated with the cell surface, possibly as a macromolecular structure, it appears that a study of the whole antigen, rather than just a portion, will prove more valuable in unraveling the molecular basis of the function.

B. Molecular Structure of *Ia* Antigens

Preliminary results suggest that the *Ia* antigens are composed of two noncovalently linked, glycosylated polypeptides of molecular weight 33,000 and 28,000. Since both chains are apparently cleaved on papain-solubilization, it appears possible that each dips into the membrane lipid. Assuming this structure is correct, it is of considerable interest to determine whether, as in the case of the *A*, *B*, and *C* antigens, one chain carries all the polymorphism and the other is the product of a gene that is not located in the major histocompatibility complex. Other interesting questions concern the degree of structural homology between the 33,000- and 28,000-molecular-weight chains and whether one or both chains, together with the *A*, *B*, and *C* gene products, arose by duplication of one primordial gene (Bodmer, 1972).

C. Molecular Structure of *A* and *B* Antigens

Figure 9 summarizes our current knowledge of the molecular nature of the *A* and *B* antigens. The *A* and *B* gene product is a glycosylated polypeptide of molecular weight about 43,000, of which the carbohydrate contributes about 10%. Approximately three-quarters of the chain can be released in a water-soluble and alloantigenically active form by cleavage with papain. This portion carries all the carbohydrate and the *N*-terminus of the whole chain, and is presumably external to the cell surface. At least a portion of the remainder of the chain is hydrophobic, and is inserted into the membrane lipid bilayer. Although

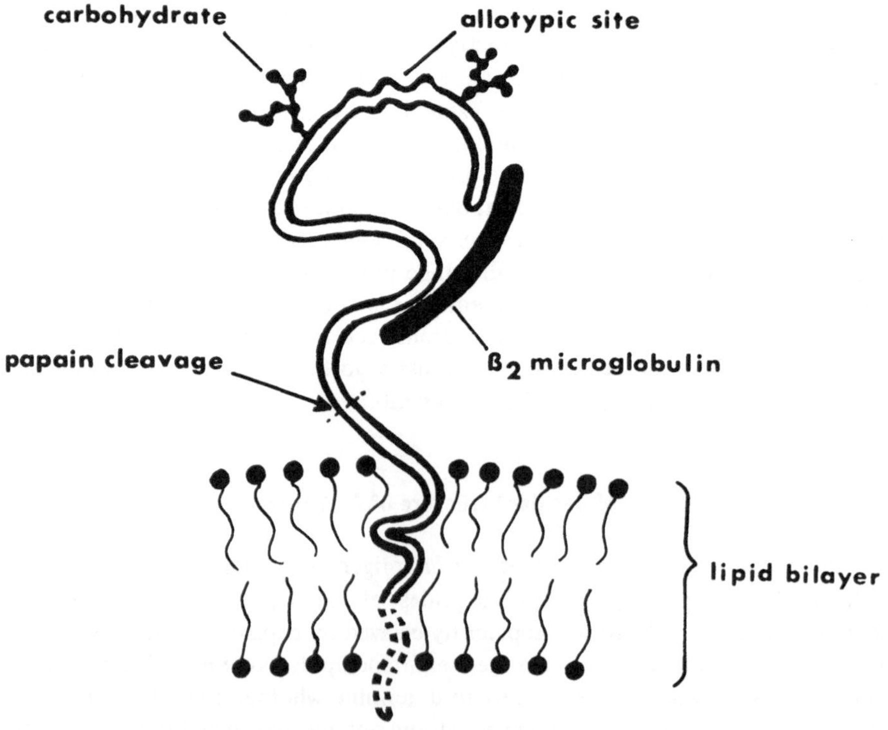

Figure 9. Model of the structure of the *A* and *B* antigens.

it is shown in Fig. 9 as spanning the membrane, this is hypothetical. Alternative arrangements are that it is located entirely within the lipid layer, or that it loops through the lipid with the *C*-terminus also exposed on the cell surface. The alloantigenic activity is most probably determined solely by the polypeptide structure, and different allotypes probably differ by a small number of amino acid residues.

The *A* and *B* gene products are noncovalently linked to a polypeptide of molecular weight 12,000 that is apparently identical with urinary β_2-microglobulin. This polypeptide does not contribute to the alloantigenic activity of the larger chain, and is most probably not glycosylated. In all probability, it does not dip into the lipid layer, and its membrane association is mediated entirely by interaction with the larger chain.

Various arguments, including the intimate association of β_2-microglobulin with the *A* and *B* gene products, have led to the proposal that the *A* and *B* antigens have an evolutionary origin in common with the immunoglobulins. Although the present data on the gross structure and *N*-terminal sequences of the *A* and *B* chains provide no evidence in support of this postulate, they are too limited to supply a definitive answer.

ACKNOWLEDGMENT

The experimental work described in this chapter was carried out in collaboration with The Genetics Laboratory, Oxford. The authors are very grateful to Colin Barnstable, Professor Walter F. Bodmer, and Dr. Peter Goodfellow for making their results freely available and for many stimulating discussions.

V. REFERENCES

Albert, E.D., Rittner, C., Grosse-Wilde, H., Netzel, B., and Scholz, S., 1975, in: *Histocompatibility Testing 1975* (F. Kissmeyer-Nielsen, ed.), Munksgaard, Copenhagen, p. 941.
Allan, D., and Crumpton, M.J., 1971, *Biochem. J.* **123**:967.
Artzt, K., and Bennett, D., 1975, *Nature (London)* **256**:545.
Benacerraf, B., and McDevitt, H.O., 1972, *Science* **175**:273.
Bernier, I., Dautigny, A., Colombani, J., and Jolles, P., 1976, *FEBS Lett.* **63**:320.
Bevan, M.J., 1975, *J. Exp. Med.* **142**:1349.
Blanden, R.V., Hapel, A.J., and Jackson, D.C., 1976, *Immunochemistry* **13**:179.
Bodmer, W.F., 1972, *Nature (London)* **237**:139.
Bodmer, W.F., 1973, in: *Defence and Recognition, MTP International Review of Science, Biochemistry, Series One*, Vol. 10 (R.R. Porter, ed.), Butterworth, London, p. 295.
Bodmer, J. (ed.), 1975, in: *Histocompatbility Testing 1975* (F. Kissmeyer-Nielsen, ed.), Munksgaard, Copenhagen, p. 21.

Bridgen, J., Snary, D., Crumpton, M.J., Barnstable, C., Goodfellow, P., and Bodmer, W.F., 1976, *Nature (London)* **261**:200.
Cresswell, P., and Ayres, J.L., 1976, *Eur. J. Immunol.* **6**:82.
Cresswell, P., and Dawson, J.R., 1975, *J. Immunol.* **114**:523.
Cresswell, P., and Geier, S.S., 1975, *Nature (London)* **257**:147.
Cresswell, P., Turner, M.J., and Strominger, J.L., 1973, *Proc. Nat. Acad. Sci. U.S.A.* **70**:1603.
Crumpton, M.J., 1974, in: *The Antigens*, Vol. 2 (M. Sela, ed.), Academic Press, New York, p. 1.
Crumpton, M.J., and Snary, D., 1974, in: *Contemporary Topics in Molecular Immunology*, Vol. 3 (G. L. Ada, ed.), Plenum Press, New York and London, p. 27.
Cullen, S.E., Freed, J.H., Atkinson, P.H., and Nathenson, S.G., 1975, *Transplant. Proc.* **7** (Suppl. 1):237.
Cunningham, B.A., Wang, J.L., Berggard, I., and Peterson, P.A., 1973, *Biochemistry* **12**:4811.
Doherty, P.C., and Zinkernagel, R.M., 1975, *Lancet* **1**:1406.
Fu, S.M., Stern, R., Kunkel, H.G., Dupont, B., Hansen, J.A., Day, N.K., Good, R.A., Jersild, C., and Fotino, M., 1975, *J. Exp. Med.* **142**:495.
Gally, J.A., and Edelman, G.M., 1972, *Annu. Rev. Genet.* **6**:1.
Goodfellow, P.N., Jones, E.A., van Heyningen, V., Solomon, E., Bobrow, M., Miggiano, V., and Bodmer, W.F., 1975, *Nature (London)* **254**:267.
Gordon, R.D., Simpson, E., and Samelson, L. E., 1975, *J. Exp. Med.* **142**:1108.
Gorer, P.A., 1938, *J. Pathol. Bateriol.* **47**:231.
Helenius, A., and Simons, K., 1975, *Biochim. Biophys. Acta* **415**:29.
Henriksen, O., Appella, E., Smith, D.F., Tanigaki, N., and Pressman, D., 1976, *J. Biol. Chem.* **251**:4214.
Jones, E.A., Goodfellow, P.N., Bodmer, J.G., and Bodmer, W.F., 1975, *Nature (London)* **256**:650.
Kahan, B.D., and Reisfeld, R.A., 1971, *Bacteriol. Rev.* **35**:59.
Katz, D.H., and Benacerraf, B., 1975, *Transplant. Rev.* **22**:175.
Kissmeyer-Nielsen, F. (ed.), 1975, *Histocompatibility Testing 1975*, Munksgaard, Copenhagen.
Klein, J., 1975, *Biology of the Mouse Histocompatibility-2 Complex*, Springer-Verlag, Berlin–Heidelberg–New York.
Laemmli, U.K., 1970, *Nature (London)* **227**:680.
Letarte-Muirhead, M., Acton, R.T., and Williams, A.F., 1974, *Biochem. J.* **143**:51.
Letarte-Muirhead, M., Barclay, A.N., and Williams, A.F., 1975, *Biochem. J.* **151**:685.
Mann, D.L., Abelson, L., Harris, S., and Amos, D.B., 1976, *Nature (London)* **259**:145.
McCune, J.M., Humphreys, R.E., Yocum, R.R., and Strominger, J.L., 1975, *Proc. Nat. Acad. Sci. U.S.A.* **72**:3206.
McDevitt, H.O., and Bodmer, W.F., 1974, *Lancet* **1**:1269.
Merritt, A.D., Petersen, B.H., Biegel, A.A., Meyers, D.A., Brooks, G.F., and Hodes, M.E., 1976, in: *Proceedings of 3rd Human Gene Mapping Conference, Cytogenetics and Cell Genetics.*
Mittal, K.K., Wolski, K.P., Lim, D., Gewurz, A., Gewurz, H., and Schmid, F.R., 1976, *Tissue Antigens* **7**:97.
Miyakawa, Y., Tanigaki, N., Yagi, Y., and Pressman, D., 1973, *Immunology* **24**:67.
Möller, G. (ed.), 1975, *Transplant. Rev.* **22**:3.
Munro, A.J., and Taussig, M.J., 1975, *Nature (London)* **256**:103.

Nakamuro, K., Tanigaki, N., and Pressman, D., 1975, *Transplantation* **19**:431.
Nathenson, S.G., and Cullen, S.E., 1974, *Biochim. Biophys. Acta* **344**:1.
Oh, S.K., Pellegrino, M.A., Ferrone, S., Sevier, E.D., and Reisfeld, R.A., 1975, *Eur. J. Immunol.* **5**:161.
Parham, P., Humphreys, R.E., Turner, M.J., and Strominger, J.L., 1974, *Proc. Nat. Acad. Sci. U.S.A.* **71**:3998.
Peterson, P.A., Rask, L., Sege, K., Klareskog, L., Anundi, H., and Ostberg, L., 1975, *Proc. Nat. Acad. Sci. U.S.A.* **72**:1612.
Rask, L., Lindblom, J.B., and Peterson, P.A., 1976, *Eur. J. Immunol.* **6**:93.
Reisfeld, R.A., and Kahan, B.D., 1972, in: *Transplantation Antigens* (B.D. Kahan and R.A. Reisfeld, eds.), Academic Press, New York, p. 489.
Reisfeld, R.A., Pellegrino, M.A., and Kahan, B.D., 1971, *Science* **172**:1134.
Rittner, C., Hauptmann, G., Gross-Wilde, H., Grosshans, E., Tongio, M.M., and Mayer, S., 1975, in: *Histocompatibility Testing 1975* (F. Kissmeyer-Nielsen, ed.), Munksgaard, Copenhagen, p. 945.
Robb, R.J., Humphreys, R.E., Strominger, J.L., Fuller, T.C., and Mann, D.L., 1975, *Transplantation* **19**:445.
Sachs, D.H., Cullen, S.E., and David, C.S., 1975, *Transplantation* **19**:388.
Sanderson, A.R., and Welsh, K.I., 1973, *Transplant. Proc.* **5**:471.
Sanderson, A.R., and Welsh, K.I., 1974, *Transplantation* **17**:281.
Sanderson, A.R., Cresswell, P., and Welsh, K.I., 1971, *Nature (London) New Biol.* **230**:8.
Shreffler, D.C., and David, C.S., 1975, *Adv. Immunol.* **20**:125.
Siegel, L.M., and Monty, K.J., 1966, *Biochim. Biophys. Acta* **112**:346.
Snary, D., Goodfellow, P., Hayman, M.J., Bodmer, W.F., and Crumpton, M.J., 1974, *Nature (London)* **247**:457.
Snary, D., Goodfellow, P., Bodmer, W.F., and Crumpton, M.J., 1975, *Nature (London)* **258**:240.
Snary, D., Barnstable, C., Bodmer, W.F., Goodfellow, P.N., and Crumpton, M.J., 1977, *Scand. J. Immunol.*, in press.
Snell, G.D., 1948, *J. Genet.* **49**:87.
Spatz, L., and Strittmatter, P., 1973, *J. Biol. Chem.* **248**:793.
Springer, T.A., Strominger, J.L., and Mann, D., 1974, *Proc. Nat. Acad. Sci. U.S.A.* **71**:1539.
Strominger, J.L., Cresswell, P., Grey, H., Humphreys, R.E., Mann, D., McCune, J., Parham, P., Robb, R., Sanderson, A.R., Springer, T.A., Terhorst, C., and Turner, M.J., 1974, *Transplant. Rev.* **21**:126.
Strominger, J.L., Chess, L., Herrmann, H.C., Humphreys, R.E., Malenka, D., Mann, D., McCune, J.M., Parham, P., Robb, R., Springer, T.A., and Terhorst, C., 1975, in: *Histocompatibility Testing 1975* (F. Kissmeyer-Nielsen, ed.), Munksgaard, Copenhagen, p. 719.
Tada, T., Taniguchi, M., and Takemori, T., 1975, *Transplant. Rev.* **26**:106.
Tanigaki, N., and Pressman, D., 1974, *Transplant. Rev.* **21**:15.
Terhorst, C., Parham, P., Mann, D.L., and Strominger, J.L., 1976, *Proc. Nat. Acad. Sci. U.S.A.* **73**:910.
Thorsby, E., and Piazza, A., 1975, in: *Histocompatibility Testing 1975* (F. Kissmeyer-Nielsen, ed.), Munksgaard, Copenhagen, p. 414.
Tomita, M., and Marchesi, V.T., 1975, *Proc. Nat. Acad. Sci. U.S.A.* **72**:2964.
Turner, M.J., Cresswell, P., Parham, P., Strominger, J.L., Mann, D.L., and Sanderson, A.R., 1975, *J. Biol. Chem.* **250**:4512.

Vitetta, E.S., Artzt, K., Bennett, D., Boyse, E.A., and Jacob, F., 1975, *Proc. Nat. Acad. Sci. U.S.A.* **72**:3215.

Wang, K., and Richards, F.M., 1974, *J. Biol. Chem.* **249**:8005.

Winchester, R.J., Fu, S.M., Wernet, P., Kunkel, H.G., Dupont, B., and Jersild, C., 1975a, *J. Exp. Med.* **141**:924.

Winchester, R.J., Ebers, G., Fu, S.M., Espinosa, L., Zabriskie, J., and Kunkel, H.G., 1975b, *Lancet* **2**:814.

Differentiation Antigens of the Lymphocyte Cell Surface

Alan F. Williams

MRC Immunochemistry Unit
Department of Biochemistry
Oxford University
South Parks Road
Oxford, OX1 3QU, England

I. INTRODUCTION

The characterization of lymphocyte membranes is a major goal of current research in immunology. Cell-surface molecules of lymphocytes are likely to be important in a number of aspects of the immune system; in particular, molecules that are unique to lymphocytes may mediate lymphocyte-specific functions.

There are considerable difficulties in analyzing cell membranes of nucleated cells, and there are advantages in approaching the analysis of membrane molecules through their antigenicity. This is particularly so if one wishes to identify lymphocyte-specific molecules of the cell surface, since these molecules may be characterized as antigens that are found on lymphoid cells, but not generally on other tissues. Such antigens are called *differentiation antigens* (see Section IA for a definition), a term introduced by Boyse and Old (1969).

This chapter is concerned with differentiation antigens of the lymphocyte cell surface, and is divided into four main parts. Section II deals with the nature and current knowledge of differentiation antigens, Section III with the problems in immunology to which these antigens are relevant. In Section IV, quantitative techniques for the identification and purification of antigens are discussed and compared with the qualitative methods in common usage. Finally, in Section V, results of studies on differentiation antigens of rat lymphocytes are given.

Throughout, the emphasis is on a quantitative, biochemical approach, in contrast to genetic analysis, which has been discussed in detail by others (Boyse *et al.*, 1971; Bennett *et al.*, 1972).

Definitions. In this chapter, antigens are defined as molecules that can stimulate an antibody response and are recognized by interaction of antibody with the antigenic determinants they carry. Differentiation antigens of the lymphocyte cell surface are membrane molecules, the antigenic determinants of which are serologically identified on lymphocytes, but not all other tissues. The dividing line between an antigen of restricted or general distribution is not clear-cut, and the term differentiation antigen is of value for its brevity, rather than its precise definition.

Additional terms defined as they are used in this chapter are *B lymphocytes*, the mammalian equivalent of bursa-derived lymphocytes in avian species, and *T lymphocytes*, thymus-derived lymphocytes.

II. NATURE AND CURRENT KNOWLEDGE OF CELL-SURFACE DIFFERENTIATION ANTIGENS

A. Nature of Molecules and Antigens at Cell Surfaces*

Cell membranes are made up of three main constituents—protein, lipid, and carbohydrate—and most of the carbohydrate is covalently associated with either protein or lipid to give glycoproteins or glycolipids, respectively. The matrix of the membrane consists of a lipid bilayer, and the proteins can be found at the inner or outer surface, and in some cases both, with part of the molecule extending through the membrane. It appears that a part of most glycoproteins and glycolipids, which includes the carbohydrate, is exposed at the cell surface, and that unglycosylated protein is found mainly at the inner surface. It is also probable that the cell-surface glycoproteins have a hydrophobic portion that allows integration into the lipid bilayer, and those surface proteins that do not show this feature are likely to be associated with other molecules that do. The hydrophobic characteristics of the membrane glycoproteins lead to technical difficulties, and it is now clear that the use of detergents will be essential for their isolation and characterization (Helenius and Simons, 1975).

Antigenic determinants are usually protein or carbohydrate in nature, and cell-surface antigens are thus likely to be mainly glycoproteins, and to a lesser extent, proteins or glycolipids. The glycoprotein nature of many antigens is useful in that affinity chromatography with plant lectins that bind carbohydrate

*General references for this section are: Singer and Nicholson (1972), Bretscher (1973), Steck (1974), Hughes (1975), and Gahmberg (1976)

can be used in their isolation (Allan *et al.*, 1972; Lis and Sharon, 1973). However, it can also create some confusion, in that the antigenic determinants may be in the carbohydrate or protein part of the molecule. For example, one could be following differences in carbohydrate attached to a protein molecule that is common to all cells, rather than determining the distribution of the polypeptide chain. This may not matter with regard to using antigens as cell markers, but it could greatly alter interpretations of their likely biological functions.

B. Antisera to Differentiation Antigens

In raising antisera to differentiation antigens, one may immunize with anything from pure molecules to whole cells. Immunization with membranes or cells may be used in the hope of finding tissue-specific molecules through their antigenic determinants, or membrane molecules could first be purified and then tested serologically for their tissue distribution. After an antiserum is produced, the distribution of specificities recognized is analyzed, and antibodies to antigens of general distribution are removed by absorption with tissues other than lymphocytes (see Section IV). The complexity of the serum and the problems in characterization vary with the type of immunization.

There are three main categories of antisera: those raised within an inbred strain–syngeneic; those raised between strains within a species–allogeneic; and those raised between species–xenogeneic. The main use of syngeneic immunization would be in the production of antisera to fetal antigens that are foreign to the adult. These sera could recognize a number of specificities that would not be polymorphic, and thus they would be more like xenoantisera than alloantisera.

Allogeneic antisera recognize alloantigens that are determined by allelic polymorphisms within the species. The importance of alloantigens that are also differentiation antigens has been clearly recognized (Boyse *et al.*, 1971; Bennett *et al.* 1972), and a great advantage of these antigens is that they can be genetically defined. Eventually, by backcrossing, congenic strains of animals can be produced such that ideally they differ only at the locus that codes for the alloantigen (Snell, 1958). The extent to which linked regions remain associated with the gene in question is difficult to determine (Flaherty and Bennett, 1973), but there is no doubt that congenic strains are invaluable in defining an antigenic specificity. Analysis of alloantisera is also aided by the fact that usually a limited number of specificities is recognized (if histocompatibility antigens are excluded). However, this also implies a major disadvantage, which is that an alloantiserum can be produced only when a genetic polymorphism exists that results in a change in antigenicity. Such polymorphisms are relatively rare, and given the limited numbers of animal strains available, and immunizations that are possible, it is likely that many important molecules will not be detected by alloantisera. For example, in the mouse, alloantigenic determinants on κ immunoglobulin chains are yet to be described (Herzenberg and Herzenberg, 1973), and it is possible that they are not present in the available strains. Thus, if one wishes to identify most tissue-specific membrane molecules, total reliance on alloantigens would be unwise.

Xenoantisera are raised by immunization between species, and the advantage here is that most proteins are antigenic in another species, since in most cases they have diverged significantly in the course of evolution. The disadvantage is that immunization with cells or membrane will result in antibodies to a large number of antigens, and the sera will thus be difficult to analyse. If the quantitative methods described in Section IV are used, however, these problems are not insurmountable (see Section VB).

A major problem with xenoantisera is the unambiguous definition of specificity. How can one know whether two antisera are specific for the same molecule or not, and how can a specificity, once obtained, be reproduced? Potentially, analysis by somatic cell genetics may allow genetic definition of differentiation antigens identified with xenoantisera, but these techniques are in their infancy (Buck and Bodmer, 1975). Some criteria for specificity can be set up in terms of tissue distribution, and the degree to which one serum blocks binding by antibody of another (Boyse *et al.*, 1968a) may indicate the identity or nonidentity of antigenic determinants. Also, the ability of antigens to move independently or otherwise in the membrane in capping studies with different sera gives information on the molecular relationship of different determinants (Neauport-Sautes *et al.*, 1973). At present, however, none of these possibilities provides a real solution, and purification is the only clear way of defining xenoantigens and ensuring that a serum specific for a particular antigen can be produced.

C. Known Differentiation Antigens

It is not the purpose of this chapter to catalogue all known differentiation antigens of all species; however, details of alloantigens and xenoantigens of mice and rats are summarized in Tables I and II to illustrate the predominance of differentiation antigens among cell-surface antigens. This is best seen for the mouse alloantigens, which can be recognized serologically (either directly or by absorption) on lymphocytes, and are shown in Table I. Twelve sets of alloantigens have been clearly defined in this way, and of these, six are found only on lymphoid cells (the Ly antigens, Tla and G_{IX}), three are found on lymphoid cells plus a limited number of other tissues (Thy-1, Ia, and Pca-1), and only three are of broad tissue distribution (H-2 antigens and Ea-2). For the rat, two

Table I. Mouse and Rat Alloantigens That Can Be Detected Serologically on Lymphocytes

Antigen	Tissue distribution
Mouse[a]	
Ly-1	Thymocytes and T lymphocytes only; marker for helper T cells
Ly-2, Ly-3 (possibly coded by same locus)	Thymocytes and T lymphocytes only; marker for cytotoxic and suppressor T cells
Ly-4	May be on B lymphocytes only, but tissue distribution poorly defined
Ly-5	Thymocytes and T lymphocytes only
Tla	Thymocytes and leukemia cells only; could be associated with a leukemia virus
G_{IX}	In normal mice on lymphoid cells, but G_{IX} is a leukemia virus product
Thy-1	Thymocytes and T lymphocytes, brain, fibroblasts, and epidermal cells
Ia	B lymphocytes, macrophages, sperm, epidermal cells; may be on T lymphocytes in small amounts
Pca-1	Plasma cells, liver, kidney, brain
Ea-2, H2-K, H2-D	Found on most tissues
Rat[b]	
Ly-1	Thymocytes and peripheral lymphocytes only
T-cell alloantigen	Probably specific for peripheral T lymphocytes
Thy-1	Thymocytes, some bone marrow and spleen cells, brain and fibroblast
Ag-F	Lymphocyte antigen; tissue distribution not defined
Ag-B	Major rat histocompatibility antigens; found in most tissues

[a] References–Pre-1975: Klein (1975), Chap. 9. Others–Ly-1 and Ly-2/3: Cantor and Boyse (1975); Feldman *et al.* (1975); Ly-5: Komuro *et al.* (1975); G_{IX}: Obata *et al.* (1975); Ia: Shreffler and David (1975); Hammerling *et al.* (1975).
[b] References–Ly-1: Fabre and Morris (1974); T-cell alloantigen: Howard and Scott (1974); Butcher and Howard (private communication); Thy-1: see Section V; Ag-F: De Witt and McCullough (1975); Ag-B: Ivanyi (1970).

alloantigens that are probably lymphocyte-specific have been defined. Thy-1 antigen can also be identified in rat with mouse alloantiserum, and is included in the alloantigen section even though the antigen has yet to be established as being allelic in the rat.

In Table II are listed the specificities of some xenogeneic sera that have been rendered specific for lymphoid cells, and in general, results are similar for rats and mice. The notable feature of this list is that a wide range of sera identifying different categories of lymphoid cells have been described. Taken together, the

Table II. Specificities of Absorbed Xenoantisera Against Cell-Surface Determinants of Lymphoid Cells

Type of lymphoid cell or other tissue recognized[a]	Tissue of immunization	References[b]
Mouse		
Thymocytes and lymphocytes in general	Thymocytes or spleen cell subfractions	1,2
Thymocytes and T lymphocytes	Thymocytes or T lymphocytes	2,3
Thymocytes, T lymphocytes, and brain	Thymocytes or brain	4-7
Large and some small thymocytes, B lymphocytes, and plasma cells	Plasmacytoma (IgM)	8,9
B lymphocytes (not recognizing immunoglobulin)	Mainly B lymphocytes or spleen cell subfractions	2,3,10,11
Plasma cells	Plasmacytoma (IgM)	12,13
Plasma cells, kidney, brain, and liver	Plasmacytoma (IgA or IgG)	14
Rat		
Lymphocytes in general	Thoracic duct lymphocytes	15,16
Thymocytes or thymocytes and some bone marrow cells (brain not tested)	Thymocytes and thymocyte subfractions	17-19
Thymocytes and brain	Brain	6,20,21
Thymocytes and T lymphocytes	Thoracic duct lymphocyte or thymocyte membrane	15,22
B lymphocytes	Mainly B lymphocytes or thoracic duct lymphocytes	23,24
Peripheral T lymphocytes and some thymocytes	Thoracic duct lymphocytes	24

[a] Unless stated, the antigens recognized are generally not on erythrocytes, liver, kidney, or brain, although this has not been carefully tested in all references.

[b] **(1)** Shigeno *et al.* (1968); **(2)** Zeiller and Pascher (1973); **(3)** Lamelin *et al.* (1972); **(4)** Golub (1971); **(5)** Bron and Sauser (1973); **(6)** Clagett *et al.* (1973); **(7)** Thiele and Stark (1974); **(8)** Yutoku *et al.* (1974b); **(9)** Stout *et al.* (1975); **(10)** Raff (1971); **(11)** von Fellenberg and Guggisberg (1972); **(12)** Watanabe *et al.* (1971); **(13)** Takahashi *et al.* (1971); **(14)** Yutoku *et al.* (1974a); **(15)** Goldschneider and McGregor (1973); **(16)** Fabre and Williams (1977); **(17)** Colley *et al.* (1970); **(18)** Bachvaroff *et al.* (1969); **(19)** Zeiller and Dolan (1972); **(20)** Thiele *et al.* (1972); **(21)** Morris and Williams (1975); **(22)** Morris and Williams (1977); **(23)** Howard and Scott (1974); **(24)** Goldschneider (1975).

data in Tables I and II strongly suggest that many molecules on the lymphocyte cell surface are lymphocyte-specific.

The genetic loci for all the mouse alloantigens in Table I have been characterized and can be considered in 2 groups. Loci involved in the expression of H-2K, H-2D, Ia, Tla, and G_{IX} antigens are all on chromosome 17, and these antigens differ from the rest in that they are highly polymorphic (H-2K, H-2D, and Ia), or in that they are (G_{IX}), or may be (Tla), associated with leukemia virus. Genetic loci for the other antigens show no linkage pattern, nor do they seem to be particularly polymorphic. The polymorphism of most of the differentiation antigens is unlikely to be associated with their biological functions (it could be for Ia and H-2 antigens), and is probably analagous to that of immunoglobulin constant regions or hemoglobulin molecules, rather than to that of the major histocompatibility antigens.

Of all the antigens in Tables I and II, only mouse H-2 antigens (Nathenson and Cullen, 1974) and rat Thy-1 antigen (see Section V) have been characterized biochemically to any appreciable extent. Some studies have also been carried out on mouse Tla and Ia antigens (Muramatsu *et al.*, 1973; Cullen *et al.*, 1974). All these antigens are glycoproteins, and all require detergents for solubilization of the intact molecules. Both these properties suggest that they are typical of molecules that penetrate the lipid bilayer at the cell surface, as discussed in Section IIA.

Details of cell-surface immunoglobulin antigens are not given in Tables I and II, even though these are the best-characterized antigens of lymphocytes. This subject has been reviewed elsewhere (Warner, 1974).

III. IMMUNOLOGICAL INTEREST OF DIFFERENTIATION ANTIGENS OF THE LYMPHOCYTE CELL SURFACE

Studies on differentiation antigens are likely to be important in many areas of immunology, and some are discussed below. In most cases, the primary interest is not in the antigenicity *per se* (in contrast to Ia and H-2 antigens), but rather in the antigen as a cellular or molecular marker. Also, the most far-reaching applications of studies on differentiation antigens require their purification.

A. Differentiation Antigens as Membrane Molecules Responsible for Lymphocyte-Specific Functions

There are a number of properties of lymphocytes that are unique to these cells in comparison with other tissues. These properties are likely to involve cell-surface interactions, and it is possible that they are mediated by molecules specific to the lymphocyte cell surface. These surface molecules could function as receptors for soluble molecules (hormones), or could interact directly with membrane effector molecules in cell–cell interactions. The following aspects, which are also summarized diagrammatically in Fig. 1, could involve cell-surface interactions:

1. Development and migration of immature lymphocytes.

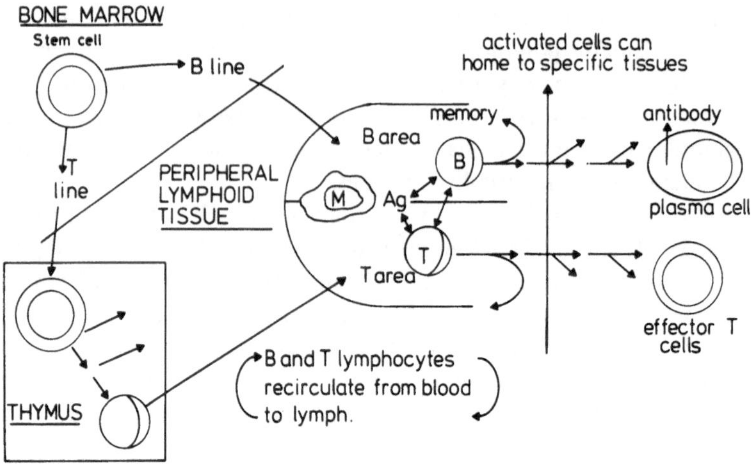

Figure 1. Stages in the differentiation of lymphocytes before and after interaction with antigen. (M) Macrophage; (Ag) antigen. After Owen (1973), and Ford (1975).

2. Interactions of B or T lymphocytes with antigen.
3. Interactions among lymphocytes and macrophages.
4. Recirculation of small lymphocytes from blood to lymph.
5. Homing of B and T lymphocytes to different parts of spleen or lymph nodes.
6. Homing of antigen-activated lymphocytes to specific target tissues.

In all these cases, the only function that can be ascribed with any confidence to a known cell-surface molecule is the specific interaction of B lymphocytes with antigen via immunoglobulin receptor (Warner, 1974). If lymphocyte-specific cell-surface molecules were identified and purified, their molecular properties could be determined, and these properties might suggest functions. Also, concentrated and specific antibodies could be prepared to investigate the role of the specific molecules in functional assays. Eventually, functions may be matched to molecules.

In characterizing lymphocyte-specific molecules, an approach via antigenicity has three great advantages: (1) By using antibody assays on intact cells that are impermeable to immunoglobulin, attention can be focused on cell-surface membrane molecules. (2) Antisera can be absorbed in such a way that only lymphocyte-specific antibodies remain; in this way, the complication of antigens common to other tissues can be removed. (3) Antibody assays can provide a rapid, quantitative technique for following antigen in purification studies, and these assays can be carried out in the presence of detergent (see Section IV).

B. Differentiation Antigens as Markers for Lymphoid Development

There are many stages in the cell lineage of lymphocytes, and a possible scheme for the development of B and T lymphocytes before and after interaction with antigen is shown in Fig. 1. The expression of cell-surface antigens changes throughout development (see Tables I and II), and this would be expected if the antigens are molecules involved in specific lymphocyte functions as suggested above. Regardless of their function, the changing expression of the antigens can be exploited to define stages in lymphocyte differentiation. This has been best used in characterizing T-cell development in the mouse, a subject recently reviewed by Cantor and Weissman (1976). It is worth noting that thus far, the genetically defined alloantisera have been much more useful than xenoantisera, mainly because of the problems in defining specificity for the latter.

Differentiation antigens as cell markers are also likely to be useful in human medicine, as well as in understanding the immune response. The monitoring of numbers of different types of lymphocytes may have diagnostic uses, and cell markers that distinguish immunocompetent lymphocytes from their precursors may facilitate advances in transplantation surgery. For example, in rodents, transplantation of allogeneic bone marrow to irradiated recipients is possible, because mature T lymphocytes that contaminate the marrow and cause graft vs. host disease can be removed by treatment with anti- (Thy-1) antibody plus complement (Tyan, 1975; von Boehmer *et al.*, 1975). In humans, transplantation of bone marrow often results in graft vs. host disease (van Bekkum and Dicke, 1972), and by analogy with the mouse, this may be alleviated if an appropriate cell-surface antigen could be defined.

Alloantisera are likely to be of minimal importance in the identification of human antigens, since experimental immunization is not possible, and the best hope for progress lies in the quantitative analysis of xenoantisera.

C. Differentiation Antigens and Immunosuppressive Anti-(Lymphocyte) Serum

For tissue transplantation in rodents, the most effective immunosuppressive agent is anti-(lymphocyte) serum. Treatment with this serum preferentially suppresses the cell-mediated (T lymphocyte) immune response, and has minimal deleterious side effects. In humans, anti-(lymphocyte) serum has given much less satisfactory results, and it is debatable whether its use in transplantation surgery is justified (Lance *et al.*, 1973).

It has been established in mice that antibody specific for lymphocytes will give immunosuppression (Shigeno *et al.*, 1968), and in an unabsorbed serum, the lymphocyte-specific antibody may give immunosuppression, while the antibody to antigens also on other tissues may lead to undesirable side effects. If this is so, the most effective anti-(lymphocyte) serum would thus have a high concentration of antibody to lymphocyte differentiation antigens, and none against antigens common to other tissues. In practice, however, one has little control over the specificity of the serum if immunization with whole cells is used. In fact, with such immunizations, there is evidence that specificity and a high concentration of antibody are incompatible, since the best immunosuppressive sera result from short immunization schedules (Lance *et al.*, 1973). The only way that the twin aims of specificity and a high concentration of antibody could be achieved is by immunization with purified cell-surface molecules. Thus, it is possible that the purification of differentiation antigens from human lymphocytes will eventually result in the production of anti-(lymphocyte) serum effective for immunosuppression. Also, serum against pure molecules could be reproducible, while by immunization with whole cells, vastly different sera may be produced in individual animals.

IV. RADIOIMMUNOASSAYS FOR THE ANALYSIS AND PURIFICATION OF CELL-SURFACE DIFFERENTIATION ANTIGENS

A. Indirect Antibody-Binding Assays

In serological studies, one ideally wants an assay that measures quantitatively the binding of antibody to antigen. This criterion is not satisfied by the serological techniques in common usage for cell-surface antigens, but is met by radioimmunoassays. Conventional radioimmunoassays, however, require purified antigen (Hunter, 1973), which is not available for most cell-surface antigens. This can be overcome by the use of indirect antibody-binding assays, the principle of which is illustrated in Fig. 2. Cells are incubated with a specific serum, or one to be analyzed, and binding is quantitated by a second incubation with purified anti-(Ig) antibody that is labeled with ^{125}I. The advantage of using the second antibody is that one well-characterized antibody can be used with a large number of different sera. Also, since the second antibody is purified, much less radioactivity need be added than would be the case if the first antibody were labeled. The indirect antibody-binding assay was used by some workers in relatively early studies on tumor (Sparks *et al.*, 1969) and lymphocyte antigens (Nossal *et al.*, 1972), but in these studies, the assays were not fully exploited. The various ways in which the assays can be used were described by Morris and

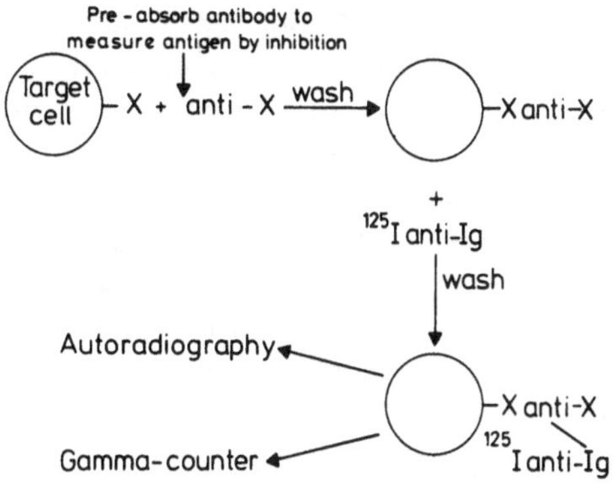

Figure 2. Indirect antibody-binding assay for cell-surface antigens.

Table III. Use of Indirect Antibody-Binding Assays in Studies on Cell-Surface Antigens

Aim of assay	Target cells	Test serum (1st incubation)	^{125}I-anti-Ig (2nd incubation)
To measure antibody concentration and quantitatively analyze specificities of a serum	In excess	Limiting	Saturating
To measure maximum antibody-binding per cell	Limiting	Saturating	Saturating
To provide a sensitive radioimmunoassay for purification studies	In excess	Limiting	At trace levels, but nonlimiting

Williams (1975), and are summarized in Table III. The number and cellular distribution of antigenic sites and antibody concentration can be measured by binding studies alone, while the analysis of antibody-specificity and measurement of antigen in different tissues is carried out by inhibition assays. These assays can be done in detergents (Williams, 1973), and can be used to measure antigenic activity in the course of biochemical purification. Details of the techniques are discussed in the following sections.

1. Assay of Cell-Bound Immunoglobulin

In the indirect binding assay, cell-bound immunoglobulin is assayed, and this can be done most rapidly by measuring the binding of ^{125}I-labeled anti-(Ig) antibody added at saturating levels. The use of a purified antibody has obvious advantages, but there are problems. In the course of eluting anti-(Ig) antibody from affinity columns, strong dissociating agents are used, and this leads to aggregation of antibody, which gives highly anomalous binding to cell-surface immunoglobulin. The simplest way to remove these aggregates is to pepsin-degrade the purified antibody to the $F(ab')_2$ fragment. When labeled with ^{125}I, $F(ab')_2$ antibody binds quantitatively to cell-surface immunoglobulin (Jensenius and Williams, 1974a). One can also remove aggregates by gel filtration, and in some studies, no anomalies were found with IgG antibody (Morris and Williams, 1975), but for routine use, $F(ab')_2$ is preferred.

The number of molecules of second antibody bound is not necessarily equal to the amount of first antibody, and the ratio between the two must be calibrated by directly measuring binding of first antibody by inhibition of a radioimmunoassay. As shown in Table IV, if anti-(Fab) or anti-(Fc) antibody was used, the ratio was usually 1–2 : 1, while when anti-(IgG) antibody was used, the ratio rose to 4 : 1. A radioimmunoassay for immunoglobulin can be set up by measuring the inhibition of binding of ^{125}I-anti-(Ig) to erythrocytes coated with immunoglobulin (Morris and Williams, 1975). If this is done, the same antibody can be used in the second step for assays as in Fig. 2, or to set up a radioimmunoassay to exactly measure immunoglobulin bound in the first step in Fig. 2.

If the amount of antibody-binding in the first step is measured with excess target cells and at a dilution at which binding is proportional to serum concentration, the weight of antibody against cell-surface antigens in a serum can be calculated.

Table IV. Ratio of Molecules of Antibody Bound at Saturation to Molecules of Antigen at a Cell Surface

Antibody	Antigen at a cell surface	Ratio	References[a]
Rabbit F(ab')2 anti-(rat Fab)	Rat IgG anti-(sheep erthyrocyte) antibody bound to sheep erythrocyte	0.7 : 1	1
Rabbit F(ab')2 anti-(rat Fc IgG_2)	Same	0.75 : 1	1
Rabbit F(ab')2 anti-(mouse Fab)	Mouse IgG anti-(Thy-1.1) antibody bound to mouse or rat thymocytes	1.1–1.5 : 1	2
Horse IgG anti-(rabbit IgG) [contained anti-(Fc) and anti-(Fab) antibody]	Rabbit anti-(rat brain) antibody bound to rat thymocytes	4 : 1	3
Horse F(ab')2 anti-(rabbit Fab)	Rabbit F(ab')2 anti-(rat Fab) antibody bound to rat lymphocytes	1.8 : 1	4
Rabbit IgG anti-(rat Thy-1)	Thy-1 on rat thymocytes	1.05 : 1	5

[a](1) Jensenius and Williams (1974a); (2) Acton *et al.* (1974); (3) Morris and Williams (1975); (4) Williams (1975); (5) Williams *et al.* (1977).

2. *Average Number of Antigenic Sites per Cell and Their Distribution Among a Cell Population*

It is desirable to measure the number of antigenic sites per cell, since this measurement may indicate whether an antigen is a major membrane component, and also give some idea as to the feasibility of purification. An estimate can be made in terms of the amount of antibody that binds per cell at saturation as described in the preceding section. Ideally, pepsin-degraded first antibody should be used, but a minimum requirement is that IgG should be prepared by gel-filtration to avoid inflated values due to the binding of IgM or aggregated IgG. The values obtained do not equal the numbers of molecules of antigen, since the binding ratio of antibody to antigen is unknown. For precipitin reactions in solution, the ratio in conditions of antibody excess is 3:1 for ribonuclease (14,000 mol. wt.), and increases to 7:1 for immunoglobulin (150,000) (Kabat and Mayer, 1968). At the cell surface, the ratio is likely to be lower than this for a given molecular weight, since part of the molecule may be buried in the membrane. Also, binding of antibody to the exposed part may be partially inhibited due to steric hindrance by the cell membrane.

The experimental values that are relevant at present are those for the binding of anti-(Ig) to antibody bound at a cell surface, and those for the binding of anti-(Thy-1) antibody to the Thy-1 glycoprotein of rat thymocytes (see Table IV). In the first case, as mentioned above, a ratio of antibody to antigen from 4:1 to 1:1 was found in various situations, while for Thy-1, the value was about 1:1. The Thy-1 value was estimated by comparing binding of antibody at saturation with the amount of cell-surface Thy-1 estimated by inhibition assays calibrated with pure Thy-1 (Williams *et al.*, 1977). Most cell-surface molecules probably present less surface area than exogenously bound antibody, and it is possible that the amount of antibody bound at saturation gives an estimate of the amount of antigen that is close to the correct value, as was the case for Thy-1.

The amount of antibody bound per cell can also be estimated by quantitative inhibition assays, and this will be discussed in the next section.

To determine the distribution of cells with antigen within a population, autoradiography can be carried out. This can be quantitated reasonably quickly by measuring grains photometrically (Rogers, 1973). Even this is time-consuming, however, and the distribution of antigen may be more rapidly measured using quantitative fluorescence techniques (see Section IVD).

3. *Use of Inhibition Assays To Define Antigenic Specificities**

The indirect antibody binding assay becomes a powerful tool when coupled with absorption analysis, which has been routinely used in association with

*General references for this section are: Morris and Williams (1975, 1977).

other assays for antigens (Reif and Allen, 1964; Boyse *et al.*, 1968b). For this purpose, target cells should be in excess so that all antibody present is bound, and cells can be fresh or glutaraldehyde-fixed. The use of fixed cells, which can be stored frozen, allows a saving of time, but these cells should be used only after specificities have been established with fresh cells. The ^{125}I-anti-(Ig) antibody used in the second step can be at saturating or trace levels, with inhibitions being 5–10 times more sensitive in the latter case for the same binding-to-background ratio in terms of counts per minute. Thus, once a specificity is established, assays using trace amounts of second antibody are preferred in purification studies.

In analyzing a complex serum against lymphocytes, one would first titrate the serum and measure binding to a fixed number of target cells with saturating second antibody. From this measurement, the greatest serum dilution consistent with a clear binding-to-background ratio would be chosen for absorption analysis. By doing this, the most concentrated antibody is examined, and complications due to the presence of minor specificities are ignored. The ability of various tissue homogenates to inhibit binding would then be measured, and compared with inhibition by lymphocytes to determine whether any lymphocyte-specific antibody is present. With the quantitative binding assays, partial absorption can be measured, and also one has a criterion for determining when absorption is completed, i.e., when further absorption fails to decrease the antibody-binding. If lymphocyte-specific antibody was identified, then bulk absorption of serum with the most appropriate tissues would be carried out and an assay for the lymphocyte specific component set up.

These principles are simply illustrated in Fig. 3, which shows binding of rabbit anti-(rat brain Thy-1) antibody to rat thymocytes and absorption by rat liver and by mouse and rat brain. Saturating amounts of the second antibody [horse anti-(rabbit IgG)] were used, and thus the amount of rabbit anti-(Thy-1) antibody binding per assay could be calculated using the ratio of second to first antibody given in Table IV. Liver homogenate gave virtually no absorption of binding, while brain homogenate from A/Jax (Thy-1.2) and A/Thy-1.1 mice (strains congenic at the *Thy-1* locus) gave partial absorption compared with complete absorption by rat brain. From this, it was calculated that 45% of the antibody was against a rat-specific determinant, 37% against a rat-mouse cross-reacting determinant, and 18% against the Thy-1.1 determinant (Barclay *et al.*, 1975). It can also be seen from Fig. 3 that amounts of tissue needed for antibody absorption can be clearly measured. Thus, absorption with 50 μg protein of A/Thy-1.1 mouse brain homogenate per 25 μl serum at 1 : 60 would be sufficient to produce a serum specific for the rat Thy-1 molecule.

For plotting data from absorption analysis, the method shown in Fig. 3 is probably the best if saturating second antibody is being used (Morris and Williams, 1977). From such a plot, the amount of tissue needed to absorb

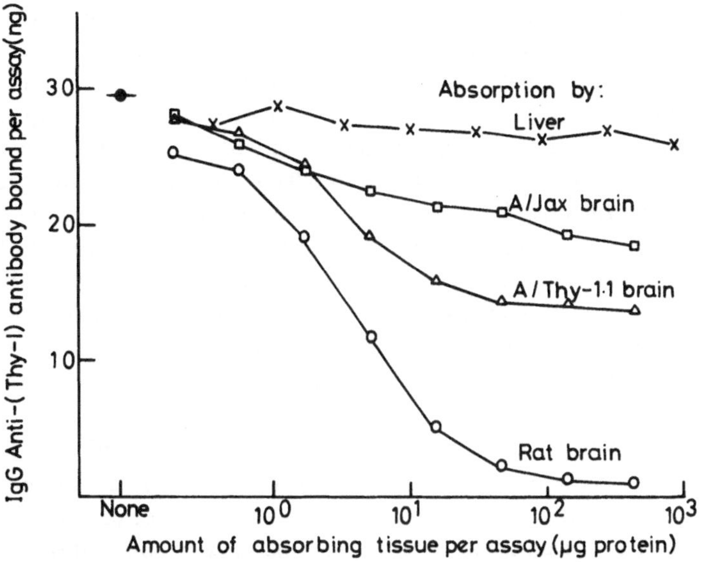

Figure 3. Absorption of anti-(rat brain Thy-1) antibody. Antiserum as in Barclay *et al.* (1975) was preabsorbed with the tissues shown, and residual binding was assayed on rat thymocyte cells using ^{125}I-horse anti-(rabbit IgG) second antibody at saturation. For each assay, 25 μl antiserum at 1:60 was used.

1 ng antibody at the point of 50% inhibition can be calculated (equals number of cells or amount of homogenate for 50% inhibition divided by nanogram of antibody bound per assay/2), and this value can be used in comparing absorption of antisera of different strength and even specificity. If absorption by cells is measured, then from the value of cells per nanogram of antibody, the amount of antibody bound per cell can be calculated. For example, in experiments on absorption of anti-(Thy-1) antibody, about 9000 thymocytes were reproducibly required for the inhibition of binding of 1 ng rabbit F(ab$'$)$_2$ anti-(rat Thy-1) antibody. This value was independent of the amount of antibody bound in the assay over a 4-fold range. From this, one can calculate that 670,000 molecules of antibody were bound per cell, which is very similar to that obtained by measuring binding of antibody at saturation (see above and Section V). This absorption method provides an alternative way of estimating the number of antigenic sites, and has the advantage that it can be carried out with antibody of very low concentration.

B. Solubilization of Antigen and Criteria for Effective Solubilization

Many cell-surface antigens are likely to be firmly embedded in the membrane, and for molecules of this type, detergents are the best agents for solubilization. The effective use of detergent on lymphocytes was initiated by Schwartz and Nathenson (1971), and it was clear from their work and others (Crumpton and Parkhouse, 1972) that nonionic and weakly ionic detergents do not affect most antigen-antibody interactions. In contrast, strongly ionic detergents, e.g., sodium dodecyl sulfate, destroy antigenic activity, although this activity is maintained to a surprising extent in moderate amounts of this detergent (Jensenius and Williams, 1974b). Indirect antibody-binding assays can be done in detergents if glutaraldehyde-fixed target cells are used (Williams, 1973), and with inhibition assays, the effect of detergent and solubilization can be monitored. Thus, one would measure inhibition by whole cells, by cells in detergent, and by supernatant from cells centrifuged at high speed to determine the effect of detergent on antigenic activity, and its power to release antigen into a high-speed supernatant.

If antigenic activity is lost in detergent, one cannot necessarily conclude that inactivation has occurred. An alternative possibility is that solubilized antigen competes poorly with the polymeric antigens of the target cell. This occurred in studies on Thy-1.1 antigenic activity, in which it was observed that with one serum, the activity was apparently lost in the presence of deoxycholate, while with another, inhibitory activity was maintained. Studies with pure Thy-1 glycoprotein in the presence and absence of deoxycholate suggested that this could be due only to differences in antibody affinity (Williams *et al.*, 1977).

With regard to the most suitable detergents for solubilization, the nonionic ones have the advantage of not releasing DNA, and thus whole cells may be extracted. Their disadvantage is that they have a low density ($\bar{v}$ = 0.9–0.96) and a large micelle size, and thus binding of detergent can have a great effect on the apparent size and hydrodynamic properties of membrane molecules. If weakly ionic detergents (e.g., deoxycholate) are to be used, membranes must be prepared prior to solubilization, since these detergents release DNA. However, deoxycholate has the advantage of a small micelle size and high density ($\bar{v}$ = 0.76 ml/g), and thus has less effect on the hydrodynamic properties of protein or glycoprotein molecules. Also, deoxycholate is a very good solubilizer of membranes (Helenius and Simons, 1975).

In solubilization studies, it is important that there should be good criteria for effective solubilization of antigens. Failure to sediment with high *g* forces is not sufficient, particularly if nonionic detergents that have low densities are used. There is much to be said for determining the hydrodynamic properties of a solubilized molecule and obtaining an estimate of the size of the antigen-detergent complex. From gel-filtration, one can measure Stoke's radius, and from zone sedimentation on sucrose gradient in H_2O and ^2H_2O, sedimentation coefficients and partial specific volumes can be measured. From these values, an estimate of molecular weight can be made (Meunier *et al.*, 1972; Letarte-Muirhead *et al.*, 1974; Clarke, 1975). This estimate will be 0–100% greater than the correct size of the antigen, since membrane molecules bind up to 100% of their own weight of nonionic and weakly ionic detergents (Helenius and Simons, 1975). If the estimated size is very large, one suspects that an aggregate or complex is present, rather than a discrete molecular form. These procedures are not an academic exercise, for in studies on Thy 1.1, it was found that Lubrol-PX and deoxycholate, both released antigen into a supernatant after centrifugation at high speed. In Lubrol-PX, however, the molecule was shown to be in a low-density aggregate, while in deoxycholate, it was in a discrete molecular form. Following this, deoxycholate was used in successful purification studies (Letarte-Muirhead *et al.*, 1974, 1975).

C. Steps in the Purification of Antigens

In the purification of membrane molecules, one faces the problem of having small amounts of material and working in detergents. To purify milligram amounts of molecules that are predominant in the membrane, a regular supply of cells in amounts of greater than 10^{11} per batch is needed. Lymphocytes from medium-sized laboratory animals can be obtained in these amounts, while for human lymphocytes, and probably also for mouse lymphocytes, tissue culture cell lines will be needed.

Most conventional techniques for purification of proteins are likely to be applicable to the purification of molecules in detergents, although ion-exchange chromatography and electrophoresis are probably not feasible in deoxycholate. Gel-filtration in deoxycholate seems particularly useful, since with rat thymocytes, for example, the main glycoproteins (see Fig. 4) chromatograph in gel-filtration in the same order as they electrophorese on polyacrylamide gels in sodium dodecyl sulfate. They all behave as asymmetrical molecules, but move in proportion to their apparent size on gels, and can thus be separated (Williams, unpublished observations).

While techniques such as these are valuable, affinity chromatography will undoubtedly be vital in most purifications, and in particular, the ability to separate glycoproteins from proteins and lipids by affinity chromotography with plant lectins is of great use (Allan *et al.*, 1972). The different specifities of lectins may also be exploited to separate within a glycoprotein fraction (Lis and Sharon, 1973). Antibody columns will also be important to purify antigens or remove unwanted contaminants, and both lectin and antibody columns were used in the purification of the rat Thy-1 glycoproteins (Letarte-Muirhead *et al.*, 1975).

In all cases, the strategy would be to carry out all purification steps in the presence of detergent, and then remove detergent at the end if need be. Techniques for removing detergents have been described (Helenius and Simons,

1975). Also, one may wish to change detergents in the course of a purification, and this should be easily accomplished, particularly at any stage involving affinity chromatography at which the changeover could be made with antigen on the column.

In general, there is a wide range of techniques available for the purification of cell-surface antigens, and the main problem in most cases is likely to be the amount of material available.

D. Comparison of Indirect Antibody-Binding Assays with Other Techniques for the Analysis of Cell-Surface Antigens

The radioimmunoassays described above provided a quantitative approach particularly suited to the analysis of complex antisera and purification of the antigens recognized. Some of the problems involved with the more conventional assays are outlined below.

1. Cytotoxicity Assays

Cytotoxicity is the most commonly used technique for analysis of antibodies to cell-surface antigens. The binding of antibody to cells is detected by the fact that it can lead to cytolysis when complement is added. The dead cells can then be counted because they take up or release dyes or other marker compounds (see Klein, 1975, Chap. 4). Undesirable features of this assay are as follows: (1) Quantitation of the number of antigenic sites can never be achieved, nor can the concentration by weight of antibody ever be measured. (2) Absence of lysis does not necessarily mean absence of antigen. This can be due to varying resistance of cells to lysis (Lerner *et al.*, 1971), or to the fact that suboptimal amounts of antigen are present. Complement-mediated lysis is a cooperative phenomenon that does not occur until a certain amount of antibody is bound in the correct orientation for complement fixation. This all means that the specifity of a serum should not be determined by direct cell killing, but by absorption analysis. (3) The class of antibody can influence cytolysis; IgM is more effective than IgG, and some subclasses of IgG do not fix complement at all (Speigelberg, 1974). Thus, the assay could reflect the specificities found in one class of antibody in a serum, while those of another were altogether ignored.

Despite these drawbacks, the cytotoxicity assay has been of fundamental importance, and may be the only assay possible if antisera are very weak [e.g., anti-(HLA) histocompatibility antigen sera]. Cytotoxicity can be relied on, however, only in situations in which specificity is assured by other means, e.g., with alloantisera where the specificities can be genetically defined.

2. *Binding Assays Using Antibody Labeled with Markers Other Than Radioisotopes*

Binding assays can be done as in Fig. 2, but fluorochrome-labeled antibody (Johnson and Holborrow, 1973) or peroxidase-labeled antibody (Antoine and Avrameus, 1974) can be used in the second step. In both cases, this binding can potentially be quantitated, but not automatically and easily, as is the case for the binding of ^{125}I-labeled antibody, which is measured in the gamma counter. Thus, these techniques cannot rival the radioactive binding assay in its function as a radioimmunoassay measuring antigens by inhibition.

The binding of fluorochrome-labeled antibody can be measured by a laser analyzer (Bonner *et al.*, 1972) as in the fluorescence-activated cell sorter, and this is particularly suited to rapidly measuring the distribution of antibody bound within a cell population. In this regard, it is superior to radioactive binding assays in which autoradiography, which is time-consuming, must be used. Also, the cell sorter is uniquely useful in allowing the controlled isolation of cells that have bound different amounts of antibody.

3. *Radioactive Labeling of Membrane Molecules Followed by Immunoprecipitation*

These methods involve radioactive labeling of membrane molecules by biosynthetic methods or by labeling at the cell surface with a reagent that does not penetrate the cell, followed by solubilization in detergent and immunoprecipitation. The specifically precipitated molecules are then characterized by electrophoresis on polyacrylamide gels in sodium dodecyl sulfate (Schwartz and Nathenson, 1971). Incorporation of isotope by surface labeling is the most commonly used method, and usually involves iodination of tyrosine residues with ^{125}I using the enzyme lactoperoxidase (Marchalonis *et al.*, 1971). Other reagents can also be used (Carraway, 1975), and labeling of carbohydrate residues with [^{3}H]sodium borohydrate after oxidation with galactose oxidase may prove particularly useful (Gahmberg, 1976). With biosynthetic labeling, radioactive amino acids or sugars can be used.

Problems with these techniques are as follows: (1) The methods do not allow measurement of amounts of antibody, and are poorly suited to estimating the number of antigenic sites. In particular, the surface labeling method is entirely nonquantitative, since highly selective labeling of molecules can occur. This is clearly shown by the fact that for a mixture of proteins in solution, labeling with the lactoperoxidase method departs markedly from proportionality with the percentage composition (Gow and Wardlaw, 1975). Also, a small number of dead cells can label very heavily internally, compared with labeling of viable cells at the cell surface (Juliano and Behar-Bannelier, 1975). Thus, there is no foundation for calculating the number of antigenic molecules per cell on the basis of percentage of counts incorporated into a particular polypeptide, as has been done by some workers (Marchalonis *et al.*, 1972; Sherr *et al.*, 1972). (2) There is no criterion for solubilization, and low yields of antigen could go undetected. (3) Problems can occur in immunoprecipitation; the problems can include the nonspecific precipitation of material, and could also involve dissociation of antigen-antibody complexes in the course of washing precipitates if low affinity serum were used (see Section IVB). (4) Distribution of antigen within a population of cells cannot be measured. (5) The identification of a band on a gel gives very little information, and purification is still required. However, immunoprecipitation is a poor technique for following antigen in purification studies, since it is neither quantitative nor suitable when large numbers of assays are required.

These drawbacks allow formidable scope for artifacts if the techniques are uncritically used in trying to identify unknown antigens. Immunoprecipitation can be a very useful technique, however, if one has well-characterized antisera, in that it allows the determination of the molecular relationship among antigens on a very small amount of material (Nathenson and Cullen, 1974). Also, surface labeling studies are essential to determine the orientation of molecules in cell membranes, as shown for the polypeptides of the human erythrocyte (Steck, 1974). Finally, if one simply concentrates on the membrane molecules that are prominently labeled, interesting results may be found. For example, a large molecule on fibroblasts (Hynes, 1973) has been identified in this way, as have some large glycoproteins of mouse lymphocyte cell surfaces (Trowbridge *et al.*, 1975a).

4. An Integrated Approach

To summarize, it can be argued that the radioactive binding assays provide the best tool for the analysis of antisera, and for the assay of cell-surface antigens in their purification. This is likely to be particularly so for complex sera, such as xenoantisera against whole cells or membranes. A useful adjunct would be quantitative fluorescence analysis, as available on the fluorescence-activated cell sorter, for the determination of the distribution of antibody-binding among the cell population studied. Once antigens have been clearly identified and purified, surface labeling and immunoprecipitation studies can be used to obtain information about the orientation of antigen in the membrane. Also, immunoprecipitated antigen obtained after biosynthetic labeling with radioactive amino acids may be used for determination of protein sequence on a microscale (Schechter *et al.*, 1975).

V. DIFFERENTIATION ANTIGENS IN THE RAT

The rat is a convenient laboratory animal for biochemical studies on lymphocyte differentiation antigens, mainly because relatively large numbers of cells can be obtained from a reasonable number of animals (e.g., 10^{11} thymocytes from 70 rats, compared with about 700 mice needed for the same number). Also, many inbred strains of rats are available, and many workers use this animal for studies on immunological functions and tissue transplantation. For genetic studies, the mouse is the favorite animal, and obviously it would also be desirable to extrapolate biochemical studies to this species. This may be possible by first characterizing molecules in the rat and then analyzing the mouse equivalent using cross-reacting antibodies. This approach has been successful in terms of characterizing the molecule that carries the Thy-1 antigenic determinants in rat and mouse, and in this section, results of studies on rat Thy-1 will be summarized. Also, the results of analysis of complex xenoantisera recognizing rat lymphocytes will be discussed.

A. Thy-1 Antigen

1. Comparison with Mouse and Tissue Distribution

The Thy-1 (Θ) antigen was one of the first cell-surface differentiation antigens to be defined on lymphocytes, and was found in mice as the Thy-1.1 (Θ-AKR) and Thy-1.2 (Θ-C3H) alloantigenic determinants (Reif and Allen, 1964). These determinants are coded for by the *Thy-1* locus on chromosome 9 (Klein, 1975).

More recently, it was shown that the Thy-1.1 antigenic specificity can be recognized on rat thymocytes and brain with mouse alloantiserum, but no rat strain with Thy-1.2 determinant has yet been reported (Douglas, 1972; Acton *et al.*, 1974). The mouse and rat Thy-1.1 determinants are very similar, since rat thymocytes and brain give almost complete inhibition of the binding of mouse anti-(Thy-1.1) alloantiserum to AKR mouse thymocytes (Williams *et al.*, 1977). In our studies on rat Thy-1.1, the specificity of the binding assays used was established by absorption with mouse strains congenic for the *Thy-1* locus (Acton *et al.*, 1974).

Other determinants can be recognized on mouse and rat Thy-1 antigens by rabbit antiserum to brain or pure Thy-1, and analysis of these clearly shows that the Thy-1 molecules are not identical between the species. There are Thy-1 xenoantigenic determinants specific to rat and mouse in comparison with each other, and other xenoantigenic determinants that cross-react between the species (Clagett *et al.*, 1973; Thiele and Stark, 1974; Morris and Williams, 1975).

If the tissue distribution of Thy-1.1 or Thy-1 xenoantigenic determinants is examined in the rat, similar results are obtained; these results are summarized in Table V and compared with the previously described distribution of Thy-1 antigen in the mouse. In both species, Thy-1 antigenic determinants are found in large amounts in adult brain and thymus, and in undetermined amounts on fibroblasts. Also, in both, the amount of antigen in brain is low at birth, and rises to adult levels after 3 weeks. Other nonlymphoid tissues have very little antigen. Surprisingly, the distribution of Thy-1 in lymphoid tissue other than

Table V. Expression of Thy-1 Antigen on Tissues of Mice and Rats[a]

Tissue	Absorptive capacity (%)[b]		Cells labeled (%)	
	Mice	Rats	Mice	Rats
Thymus	100	90	95	92
Lymph node	14	0.7	55	5
Spleen	7	3.5	30	15
Bone marrow	<1.5	10	1	40
Adult brain	80	70		
Neonatal brain	1.3	4		
Fibroblasts and epidermal cells	+	+		
Erythrocytes, liver, kidney, heart, lung	<1.0			

[a] References: Reif and Allen (1964); Douglas (1972); Scheid *et al.* (1972); Acton *et al.* (1974); Stern (1973); Morris and Williams (1975); Williams (1976).
[b] Compared on the basis of cell number of wet weight of tissue.

the thymus differs between mouse and rat. Most peripheral T cells in the mouse have the antigen, while virtually all bone marrow cells lack it; in the rat, most lymphocytes in lymph nodes or thoracic duct lymph lack antigen, while many bone marrow cells have large amounts. Thus, the Thy-1 antigen is not a general T-cell marker in the rat, but could be useful as a cell marker in rat bone marrow, where it may define subpopulations of immature cells (Williams, 1976).

The absolute amount of antigen is high in thymus and brain of both mice and rats. The number of molecules exposed at the rat thymocyte cell surface was first calculated in terms of the amount of anti-(Thy-1) antibody binding at saturation (Acton *et al.*, 1974; Morris and Williams, 1975), and more recently was precisely measured by a radioimmunoassay calibrated with pure Thy-1 (Williams *et al.*, 1977). All estimates gave a value of about 600,000 molecules per cell. This indicates that the molecule is a major membrane constituent, since the predominant polypeptides of erythrocyte membranes are found in amounts per cell of this order (Steck, 1974).

2. *Solubilization of the Thy-1 Antigen from Rat Thymocytes and Brain and Hydrodynamic Properties in Deoxycholate**

To solubilize Thy-1 from rat thymocytes, many detergents were tested, and the solubilization was compared with that of Ag-B histocompatibility antigen. Nonionic detergents did not affect the antigenic activity of Thy 1.1 or Ag-B

*General references for this section are: Letarte-Muirhead *et al.* (1974, 1975); Morris *et al.* (1975); Barclay *et al.* (1975).

determinants, but they also gave poor solubilization of the Thy-1 antigen. This was somewhat surprising, since a number of detergents that were ineffective for Thy-1 gave complete release of Ag-B antigen into a supernatant after centrifugation at high speed. In contrast, deoxycholate was effective in solubilizing both Thy-1 and Ag-B antigens from thymocyte membrane. With brain, a similar pattern was observed, with deoxycholate giving good solubilization in comparison with nonionic detergents.

Although nonionic detergents did not solubilize Thy-1, they were useful in the purification of the antigen from brain and thymus. In studies on brain, Lubrol-PX was used to remove much protein and lipid from crude membrane prior to solubilization in deoxycholate, and with thymocytes, Tween-40 was used to prepare crude membrane. In the latter detergent, thymocytes released Thy-1 into a particle that remained in the supernatant at 75,000*g* min, but pelleted at 6,000,000*g* min. Further studies on this show that it contains the major glycoproteins of rat thymocyte membrane (Standring and Williams, unpublished observations).

The hydrodynamic properties of Thy-1 from brain and thymocytes in deoxycholate were indistinguishable. From both tissues, the antigen–detergent complex had a sedimentation coefficient of 2.2–2.4*S*, a partial specific volume of 0.7 ml/g, and a Stoke's radius of 3.0 nm. From these values, it was calculated that the antigen in deoxycholate was somewhat asymmetrical and had a molecular weight of 28,000, including bound deoxycholate. All the Thy-1 antigenic determinants were associated with this molecular form, and if antibody affinity chromatography was carried out against one determinant, all three were coincidentally depleted, showing that all the determinants were on the one molecule.

3. *Purification of Thy-1 from Rat Brain and Thymus**

Purification of Thy-1 from both tissues was carried out in the presence of deoxycholate, using a combination of gel-filtration and affinity chromatography. From thymocytes, the antigen was found in two forms, one that bound to a lentil lectin affinity column (Thy-1L+) and another that did not (Thy-1L−). In all cases, the pure antigen was glycoprotein. When the apparent molecular weight was carefully determined by polyacrylamide gel electrophoresis in sodium dodecyl sulfate, brain Thy-1 gave a value of 24,000, compared with 25,000 for Thy-1L+, and 27,000 for Thy-1L−. The latter form was also heterogeneous to larger apparent molecular weights, which suggested that its failure to bind to lentil lectin was not due to degradation.

For thymocytes, it was clearly shown that Thy-1 was a major cell-surface glycoprotein, and this is illustrated in Fig. 4, which shows gels from an antibody affinity chromatography experiment stained for carbohydrate. The pattern

*General references for this section are: Letarte-Muirhead *et al.* (1975); Barclay *et al.* (1975).

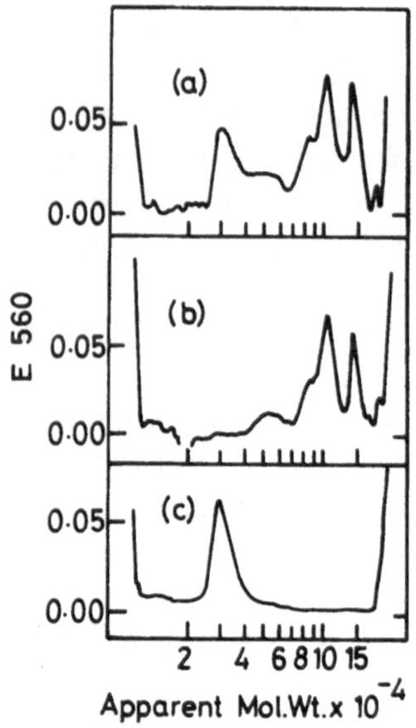

Figure 4. Purification of rat thymocyte Thy-1 with an antibody affinity column. Preparations were subjected to polyacrylamide gel electrophoresis in sodium dodecyl sulfate, and gels were stained for carbohydrate. (a) Extract of thymocyte membrane applied to the antibody column; (b) extract after passage through an anti-(brain-Thy-1) antibody column; (c) material eluted from the antibody column with pH 11.5 buffer. After Letarte-Muirhead *et al.* (1975).

for deoxycholate extract of crude thymocyte membrane is shown in Fig. 4a, while Fig. 4b shows this extract after passage through an anti-(Thy-1) antibody column. In Fig. 4c, the material that was eluted from the antibody affinity column with pH 11.5 buffer in deoxycholate is shown. Thus, the whole of the band staining for carbohydrate at apparent molecular weight 30,000 (Thy-1 is apparently larger on low-percentage acrylamide gels) was Thy-1, and includes Thy-1L+ and Thy-1L−.

4. *Chemical Composition and Antigenicity of Rat Thy-1**

To determine the chemical composition of the Thy-1 glycoproteins, deoxycholate was removed by precipitation with ethanol, in which deoxycholate is soluble. The glycoprotein could then be solubilized in water as a complex of molecular weight 250,000–350,000 which reduced to 29,000 in deoxycholate. Amino acid and carbohydrate composition was determined by standard techniques, and from this it was calculated that about 30% by weight of the molecules was carbohydrate. The compositions are shown in Table VI, in which it can be seen that amino acid compositions are very similar for brain Thy-1 and thymocyte Thy-1L+ and Thy-1L−. In contrast, the carbohydrate compositions were very different between brain and thymocyte Thy-1, with smaller differences being seen between thymocyte Thy-1L+ and Thy-1L−. Thus, between brain and thymus, the glycoprotein may have the same polypeptide chain associated with very different carbohydrate structures.

*The general reference for this section is: Barclay *et al.* (1976).

Table VI. Amino Acid and Carbohydrate Composition of Thy-1 Glycoproteins

	Molecules of each amino acid per 100 molecules of amino acids		
Amino acid	Thy-1 (brain)	Thy-1L+	Thy-1L−
Asx	12.7	12.6	13.0
Glx	9.1	9.1	9.1
His	4.1	3.8	4.0
Lys	6.9	7.2	7.0
Arg	7.5	7.5	7.2
Thr	7.6	8.6	8.3
Ser	7.4	7.1	7.9
Pro	3.6	3.8	3.0
Ala	3.3	2.9	3.2
Cys	3.1	3.2	3.2
Gly	6.0	4.9	5.0
Tyr	2.0	2.0	2.0
Val	7.3	7.4	7.4
Ile	3.9	4.1	4.0
Leu	10.4	11.2	11.1
Phe	4.0	3.7	3.8
Met	1.1	0.9	0.8
Carbohydrate	Molecules of carbohydrate per 100 molecules of amino acids		
Fucose	1.8	1.0	0.9
Mannose	11.9	10.6	9.4
Galactose	1.8	5.5	6.9
Glucose	0.6	1.3	1.1
Glucosamine	8.3	9.4	11.7
Galactosamine	1.0	0.0	0.0
Sialic acid	0.2	1.8	2.2
Percentage by weight of carbohydrate	29	32	35

The composition of Thy-1 suggested that the antigenic determinants may be in the protein part of the molecule, since this appears common to all forms, as is the antigenicity. Two other sets of experiments support this view. First, both the Thy 1.1 and Thy-1 xenoantigenic activities are destroyed by heating for 10 min at temperatures around 70–80°C. This treatment would be expected to destroy protein rather than carbohydrate antigenic determinants. Second, the proteolytic enzyme pronase destroys most of the antigenic activity, in concordance with the destruction of the Thy-1 polypeptide chain as visualized by electrophoresis on polyacrylamide gels in sodium dodecyl sulfate. These points do not completely prove that the antigenic determinants are protein in nature, but they do strongly support this view. From this, one can suggest that the tissue distribution described above is for the polypeptide, not the carbohydrate part of the molecule.

5. *Comparison of Rat and Mouse Thy-1*

There has been considerable disagreement about the molecular nature of mouse Thy-1, and this has been discussed in some detail by Barclay *et al.* (1976). For the present, it is sufficient to say that it is unlikely that gangliosides carry the Thy-1 antigenic determinants, as suggested by Miller and Esselman (1975), and studies have been reported that strongly suggest that mouse Thy-1 is similar to the rat molecule. Using antiserum against rat brain Thy-1 that cross-reacts with mouse Thy-1, Trowbridge *et al.* (1975b) have precipitated a 25,000-molecular-weight band from thymocytes that were labeled with radioactive sugars or surface-labeled by ^{125}I with the lactoperoxidase method. This molecule was present in cell lines that were Thy-1 antigen-positive, but absent from mutants that lacked Thy-1 (Trowbridge and Hyman, 1975). Furthermore, membrane from mouse thymocytes gives a pattern on polyacrylamide gels similar to rat after staining for carbohydrate, and the prominent band that is Thy-1 in the rat is clearly evident in the mouse (Letarte-Muirhead *et al.*, 1975).

6. *Significance of Thy-1 and Future Studies*

Purification of the Thy-1 glycoproteins has not revealed their function, but it has provided relevant information. Quantitative considerations suggest that the glycoproteins are major membrane components in both thymocytes and brain, and it seems likely that they are of functional significance in these tissues. It is also striking that such a dominant molecule should disappear completely in the development of thymocytes to peripheral T lymphocytes in the rat.

The chemical composition has raised the question whether it is the protein or carbohydrate part of the molecule that is functionally important. If the protein part determines a specific function, and the carbohydrate exists only to orient the molecule in the membrane, then a common function for the molecules in brain and thymus is likely. If, however, the protein exists to anchor the molecule in the membrane and to allow a display of carbohydrate ligands for cell–cell interaction, then the specificity of functions between the two tissues may be quite different. Such a role is feasible, since there is currently much attention being given to the possibility that cell–cell interactions are mediated by the recognition of carbohydrate ligands displayed at cell surfaces (Hughes, 1975).

It is difficult to devise experiments to test these possibilities, but there are a number of points of interest that are immediately amenable to study and on which rapid progress should be made. These points include the functional significance of the subpopulation of rat bone marrow cells that have Thy-1 antigen, the histological distribution of Thy-1 antigen in the brain, and the molecular characteristics and orientation of the Thy-1 molecule in the thymocyte membrane.

B. Antigens Recognized by Complex Xenoantisera

In studies on the Thy-1 antigen of rat, a well-defined antiserum was used, and this simplified matters considerably. In the first sections, however, the importance of analyzing more complex sera has been stressed, and claims that radioactive binding assays would allow this have been made. In Oxford, five different complex antisera have been analyzed to some degree or other, and results of these studies give some indication of the success of this approach. Antisera to rat brain, thymocytes, thymocyte membrane, peripheral T lymphocytes, and a rat leukemia have been examined, and in most cases, analysis has been on one bleed of antiserum from one rabbit.

To define lymphocyte-specific antigens, absorption with other tissues was carried out; however, one might argue that this will be difficult to interpret, since it is not known whether tissue homogenates should have similar amounts of membrane to lymphoid cell suspensions. To assess this, the amount of protein from various tissues needed to inhibit a standard binding assay for Ag-B histocompatibility antigen (Williams, 1973) was measured. The values were 8.7 and 4.5 μg for thymus and spleen cell suspensions, and 4.1 and 12.0 μg for liver and kidney homogenate. Also, brain homogenate has a high absorptive capacity for Thy-1 antigen, and thus tissue homogenates should absorb as well as lymphoid cells if they have the appropriate antigen. Another potential source of confusion is the contamination of other tissues with lymphocytes. This did not emerge as a great problem for any tissue except lung, which did give strong absorption of antibody to the two lymphocyte-specific antigens defined below. This absorption was reduced if lung from specific pathogen-free animals was used, and even more so if such animals that had been irradiated were used. The absorptive capacity of lung for these antigens was thus likely to be due to contaminating lymphocytes.

The characteristics of the five sera analyzed will now be discussed in turn.

(a) Rabbit Anti-(Rat Brain) Serum (Morris and Williams, 1975; Morris *et al.*, 1975). Since Thy-1 antigen was known to be present on mouse and rat brain and thymus, analysis of anti-(rat brain) serum in terms of antibodies that would bind to lymphocytes was carried out. Other authors had previously analyzed anti-(rodent brain) sera, and had suggested that there may be a complex set of

molecules uniquely common to brain and lymphoid cells, but not on other tissues (Thiele *et al.*, 1972; Clagett *et al.*, 1973; Thiele and Stark, 1974).

Using the quantitative radioimmune assays and biochemical analysis, it was clearly established that after liver absorption, the only antibody remaining was against the Thy-1 molecule. Three antigenic specificities were recognized as described in Section VA, and these results are in agreement with the cocapping and blocking studies of Thiele and Stark (1974). Thus, the apparent complexity of the brain-thymus antigenic system can be explained in terms of multiple antigenic determinants of one small glycoprotein. There is still a possibility that there may be other antigens uniquely common to brain and lymphoid tissue undetected with the sera that were analyzed, but this remains to be established.

(b) Rabbit Anti-(Rat Thymocyte) Serum (Thompson and Morris, 1976). This antiserum was raised against rat thymocytes by extensive immunization involving complete Freund's adjuvant. Binding of the serum to thymocytes was completely absorbed by brain homogenate, and partially absorbed by liver, kidney, heart, and lung homogenate. After extensive liver absorption, the antibody remaining recognized an antigen of tissue distribution identical to Thy-1. The antibody was also absorbed by pure Thy-1 glycoprotein, and the only detectable lymphocyte specific antibody in this serum was against Thy-1.

(c) Rabbit Anti-(Rat Thymocyte Membrane) Serum (Morris and Williams, 1977). This antiserum was raised against crude thymocyte membrane prepared by the Tween-40 detergent method (Letarte-Muirhead *et al.*, 1975), and involved immunization in complete Freund's adjuvant. The serum analyzed contained about 700 μg/ml of antibody against cell-surface components of thymocytes, and 70% of this was specific for lymphoid cells. Surprisingly, brain homogenate gave no absorption, and anti-(Thy-1) antibody could not be detected in the serum, even though the membrane immunogen contained large amounts of Thy-1 glycoprotein. The main antigens recognized were unique to lymphoid cells compared with brain, erythrocytes, heart, liver, lung, or kidney, and thymocytes or peripheral T lymphocytes had much more antigen than bone marrow or B lymphocytes. This difference was greater than 20-fold by absorption analysis, but it remains to be established whether the antigens are effective T-lymphocyte markers. This serum may be recognizing the same antigens as detected by the anti-(rat T lymphocyte) serum of Goldschneider and McGregor (1973).

For this antiserum, the number of antibodies that would bind to thymocytes at saturation was determined using $F(ab')_2$ antibody that had been extensively absorbed with liver and bone marrow cells, and the value obtained was 120,000 molecules/cell. By quantitative absorption, as described in Section IVA3, the amount of antibody bound per cell was 80,000 molecules. These values suggest that a limited number of cell-surface molecules are involved, since at least 1.5×10^6 molecules of antibody can bind at a thymocyte cell surface (Morris and Williams, 1975).

The antigens recognized by this antiserum can be released into a high-speed supernatant by deoxycholate; also, they bind to lentil lectin affinity columns, and can be eluted with α-methyl D-glucopyranoside. After gel-filtration on a Sepharose 6B column, the antigenicity is found as a homogeneous peak in the same place as the large thymocyte glycoproteins shown in Fig. 4 (i.e., those of apparent molecular weight 110,000-150,000). Possibly the antigen involved is one of these glycoproteins.

(d) Rabbit Anti-(Rat Peripheral T Lymphocyte) Serum (Fabre and Williams, 1977). This antiserum was raised against rat thoracic duct lymphocytes that had been depleted of cells with large amounts of surface immunoglobulin using the rosetting method of Parish and Hayward (1974). The immunization schedule did not involve complete Freunds adjuvant, and was of limited duration as typically recommended for immunosuppressive antilymphocyte serum (Lance *et al.*, 1973). The antiserum was immunosuppressive, as assessed by kidney graft survival.

The antiserum contained about 250 μg/ml of antibody that would bind to thymocytes or thoracic duct lymphocytes, and about 70% of this was lymphocyte-specific in comparison with brain, erythrocytes, heart, liver, lung, or kidney. After absorption with liver, most of the antibody recognized antigens on thymocytes and peripheral T lymphocytes, but also on bone marrow and B lymphocytes. The antigens were also on macrophages, and can be regarded as being white blood cell-specific rather than lymphocyte-specific. Surprisingly, no antibody against the antigens defined by serum (c) could be recognized, and the distinction between the sera is clearly seen in Fig. 5. Bone marrow cells give very poor absorption of antibody in liver-absorbed serum (c), and good absorption of liver-absorbed serum (d), while thymocytes give good absorption of both.

A minor antibody specificity in serum (d) was for antigens on peripheral rat lymphocytes and absent from thymocytes, and this could be similar to that defined by Goldschneider (1975).

The amount of antibody from liver-absorbed serum (d) binding to the main antigen on thymocytes was measured by the quantitative absorption method, and a value of 70,000 molecules/cell was obtained, a little lower than the value for antigens recognized by serum (c). In solubilization studies, the results were also similar, and deoxycholate released the antigen into a supernatant after high-speed centrifugation; also, antigenic activity bound to, and was specifically eluted from, a lentil lectin affinity column. In gel-filtration on a Sepharose-6B column, the main antigen recognized by serum (d) ran as a homogeneous peak that overlapped with that of the antigen recognized by serum (c), but moved slightly ahead of this peak at both the leading and trailing edges. Thus, this antigen was also associated with the large glycoproteins of the thymocyte membrane shown in Fig. 4.

(e) Rabbit Anti-(Rat Leukemia) Serum (Thompson and Morris, 1976). This serum was raised against a rat leukemia that arose in a PVG/c strain rat the spleen

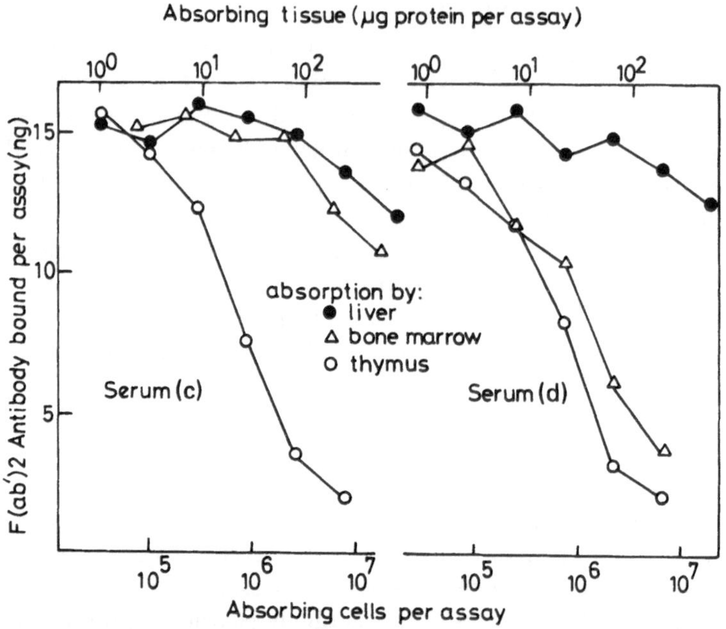

Figure 5. Xenoantigens on rat lymphocytes. Immunoglobulin was prepared from sera (c) and (d) (see text) and degraded with pepsin to F(ab′)2. This was absorbed with liver homogenate in bulk, and then again with increasing amounts of the tissues as shown. Residual antibody after absorption was assayed using thymocyte target cells and saturating ^{125}I-horse F(ab′)2 anti-(rabbit F(ab′)2) antibody.

of which had been exposed to ^{185}W irradiation. This leukemia has a large amount of cell-surface Thy-1 antigen (Acton *et al.*, 1974). The immunization schedule with the leukemia involved the use of complete Freund's adjuvant. Absorption with liver homogenate showed 30% of the antibody to be substantially lymphocyte-specific, and little if any was leukemia-specific. The range of antigens recognized by this serum was more complex than those in (a)–(d) above, and absorption analysis showed the presence of anti-(Thy-1) antibody plus antibody against specificities similar to the major ones in serum (c) and serum (d) above.

(f) General Points with Regard to the Complex Sera. All the antisera described above contained antibody of which a considerable portion was specific for lymphocytes in comparison with the other tissues. This is consistent with the idea that much of the lymphocyte cell surface is differentiated with respect to other membranes.

The results of absorption analysis were surprising in their simplicity and in the differences among antigens recognized by different sera. Thus, sera (b) and (c) were raised against similar immunogens, yet contained quite different major antibody populations. Also, serum (c) might have been expected to contain antibody as in serum (d) and vice versa. Similar results were seen in the studies of Pressman and co-workers on antisera to mouse plasmacytomas that are summarized in Table II. IgM and IgA or IgG plasmacytomas stimulated the production of different antisera, yet all the antigens recognized (except Ig) were shared by all the plasmacytomas. These results can be interpreted in terms of the possibility that antibodies against a limited number of antigens become dominant in a particular serum. Thus, all the anti-(lymphocyte) sera analyzed probably contain a wide range of antibodies to different antigens, with one or two specificities dominating. In absorption analysis, this is simplified in that one works with dilute serum, and also one observes only inhibition of most of the antibody. Thus, a second antibody at the level of 10% or less compared with a dominant specificity would go undetected. If this is correct, one might expect considerable variation among individual animals and with different immunization schedules. This possibility may be exploited to identify different antigens. Also, one could biochemically fractionate membrane molecules into glycoprotein and nonglycoprotein fractions of various sizes obtained by gel-filtration and immunize with these different fractions. In this way, a variety of different antigens may become the dominant immunogen in different animals.

Regardless of all this, it does appear that antigens can be identified and possibly purified using xenoantisera. The antigens recognized by sera (c) and (d) look particularly interesting, and the preliminary biochemical studies suggest that it will be possible to purify them. If this is achieved, then subsequent analysis of other sera will be greatly simplified.

Within the next decade, the major lymphocyte-specific components of the membrane should be identified and purified. Discovery of their biological functions may take a little longer.

VI. SUMMARY

Many alloantigens and xenoantigens of lymphocytes are not found generally on other tissues, and this suggests that much of the lymphocyte cell surface is differentiated in comparison with other cell membranes. These differentiation antigens are probably molecules that mediate lymphocyte-specific functions, and are also of interest in that they provide markers for different lymphoid cell types and may be important as target antigens for immunosuppressive anti-(lymphocyte) sera. The purification of differentiation antigens will be important in allowing their molecular properties to be discovered, and will also lead to the production of strong, specific antisera that can be used in functional studies.

Radioimmunoassays have been developed for the analysis of anti-(lymphocyte) sera, and these assays provide advantages in purification studies over other techniques. The features of these assays are discussed, and studies of differentiation antigens of rat lymphocytes are described. These include the purification and characterization of the rat Thy-1 antigen, and preliminary studies on two other rat lymphocyte differentiation antigens.

ACKNOWLEDGMENTS

The work described herein has been carried out in most enjoyable collaboration with the following workers, in chronological order: Drs. Jens C. Jensenius, Ron T. Acton, Michelle Letarte-Muirhead, Roger J. Morris, A. Neil Barclay, and John W. Fabre. The expert technical assistance of Marilyn Simpkins and Jane Addis has been of great value throughout, and the support and encouragement of Professor R.R. Porter are gratefully acknowledged.

VII. REFERENCES

Acton, R.T., Morris, R.J., and Williams, A.F., 1974, *Eur. J. Immunol.* **4**:598.
Allan, D., Auger, J., and Crumpton, M.J., 1972, *Nature (London) New Biol.* **236**:23.
Antoine, J.C., and Avrameus, S., 1974, *Eur. J. Immunol.* **4**:468.
Bachvaroff, R., Galdiero, F., and Grabar, P., 1969, *J. Immunol.* **103**:953.
Barclay, A.N., Letarte-Muirhead, M., and Williams, A.F., 1975, *Biochem. J.* **151**:699.
Barclay, A.N., Letarte-Muirhead, M., Williams, A.F., and Faulkes, R.A., 1976, *Nature (London)* **263**:563.
Bennett, D., Boyse, E.A., and Old, L.J., 1972, in: *Cell Interactions, Lepetit Collog. 3rd* (L.G. Silvestri, ed.), North Holland Publishing Co., Amsterdam, p. 247.
Bonner, W.A., Hulett, H.R., Sweet, R.G., and Herzenberg, L.A., 1972, *Rev. Sci. Instrum.* **43**:404.
Boyse, E.A., and Old, L.J., 1969, *Annu. Rev. Genet.* **3**:269.
Boyse, E.A., Old, L.J., and Stockert, E., 1968a, *Proc. Nat. Acad. Sci. U.S.A.* **60**:886.
Boyse, E.A., Miyazawa, M., Aoki, T., and Old, L.J., 1968b, *Proc. R. Soc. London Ser. B.* **170**:175.
Boyse, E.A., Old, L.J., and Scheid, M., 1971, *Amer. J. Pathol.* **65**:439.
Bretscher, M.S., 1973, *Science* **181**:622.
Bron, C., and Sauser, D., 1973, *J. Immunol.* **110**:384.
Buck, D.W., and Bodmer, W.F., 1975, in: *Human Gene Mapping* Vol. 6, Kaiser, Basel, p. 87.
Cantor, H., and Boyse, E.A., 1975, *J. Exp. Med.* **141**:1376.
Cantor, H., and Weissman, I., 1976. *Prog. Allergy* **20**:1.
Carraway, K.L., 1975, *Biochem. Biophys. Acta* **415**:379.
Clagett, J., Peter, H.H., Feldman, J.D., and Weigle, W.O., 1973, *J. Immunol.* **110**:1085.
Clarke, S., 1975, *J. Biol. Chem.* **250**:5459.
Colley, D.G., Malakian, A., and Waksman, B.H., 1970, *J. Immunol.* **104**:585.
Crumpton, M.J., and Parkhouse, R.M.E., 1972, *FEBS Lett.* **22**:210.
Cullen, S.E., David, C.S., Shreffler, D.C., and Nathenson, S.G., 1974, *Proc. Nat. Acad. Sci. U.S.A.* **71**:648.

De Witt, C.W., and McCullough, M., 1975, *Transplantation* **19**:310.
Douglas, T.C., 1972, *J. Exp. Med.* **136**:1054.
Fabre, J.W., and Morris, P.J., 1974, *Tissue Antigens* **4**:238.
Fabre, J.W., and Williams, A.F., 1977, *Transplantation*, in press.
Feldman, M., Beverley, P.C.L., Dunckley, M., and Kontiainen, S., 1975, *Nature (London)* **258**:615.
Flaherty, L., and Bennett, D., 1973, *Transplantation* **16**:505.
Ford, W.L., 1975, *Prog. Allergy* **19**:1.
Gahmberg, C.G., 1976, *J. Biol. Chem.* **251**:510.
Goldschneider, I., 1975, *Cell. Immunol.* **16**:269.
Goldschneider, I., and McGregor, D.D., 1973, *J. Exp. Med.* **138**:1443.
Golub, E.S., 1971, *Cell. Immunol.* **2**:353.
Gow, J., and Wardlaw, A.C., 1975, *Biochem. Biophys. Res. Commun.* **67**:43.
Hammerling, G.J., Mauve, G., Goldberg, E., and McDevitt, H.O., 1975, *Immunogenetics* **1**:428.
Helenius, A., and Simons, K., 1975, *Biochem. Biophys. Acta* **415**:29.
Herzenberg, L.A., and Herzenberg, L.A., 1973, in: *Handbook of Experimental Immunology* (D.M. Weir, ed.), 2nd Ed., Blackwell's, Oxford, Chap. 13.
Howard, J.C., and Scott, D.W., 1974, *Immunology* **27**:903.
Hughes, R.C., 1975, *Essays Biochem.* **11**:1.
Hunter, W.M., 1973, in: *Handbook of Experimental Immunology* (D.M. Weir, ed.), 2nd Ed., Blackwell's, Oxford, Chap. 17.
Hynes, R.O., 1973, *Proc. Nat. Acad. Sci. U.S.A.* **70**:3170.
Ivanyi, P., 1970, *Curr. Top. Microbiol. Immunol.* **53**:1.
Jensenius, J.C., and Williams, A.F., 1974a, *Eur. J. Immunol.* **4**:91.
Jensenius, J.C., and Williams, A.F., 1974b, *Eur. J. Immunol.* **4**:98.
Johnson, G.D., and Holborrow, E.J., 1973, in: *Handbook of Experimental Immunology* (D.M. Weir, ed.), 2nd Ed., Blackwell's, Oxford, Chap. 18.
Juliano, R.L., and Behar-Bannelier, M., 1975, *Biochem. Biophys. Acta* **375**:249.
Kabat, E.A., and Mayer, M.M., 1968, *Experimental Immunochemistry*, 2nd Ed., C.C. Thomas Publishers, Springfield, Illinois, p. 22.
Klein, J., 1975, *Biology of the Mouse H-2 Complex*, Springer-Verlag, New York.
Komuro, K., Hakura, K., Boyse, E.A., and John, M., 1975, *Immunogenetics* **1**:452.
Lamelin, J.P., Lisowska-Bernstein, B., Matter, A., Ryser, J.E., and Vassali, P., 1972, *J. Exp. Med.* **136**:984.
Lance, E.M., Medawar, P.B., and Taub, R.N., 1973, *Adv. Immunol.* **17**:1.
Lerner, R.A., Oldstone, M.B.A., and Cooper, N.R., 1971, *Proc. Nat. Acad. Sci. U.S.A.* **68**:2584.
Letarte-Muirhead, M., Acton, R.T., and Williams, A.F., 1974, *Biochem. J.* **143**:51.
Letarte-Muirhead, M., Barclay, A.N., and Williams, A.F., 1975, *Biochem. J.* **151**:685.
Lis, H., and Sharon, N., 1973, *Annu. Rev. Biochem.* **42**:541.
Marchalonis, J.J., Cone, R.E., and Santer, V., 1971, *Biochem. J.* **124**:921.
Marchalonis, J.J., Cone, R.E., and Atwell, J.L., 1972, *J. Exp. Med.* **135**:956.
Meunier, J.C., Olsen, R. W., and Changeux, J.P., 1972, *FEBS Lett.* **24**:63.
Miller, H.C., and Esselman, W.J., 1975, *J. Immunol.* **115**:839.
Morris, R.J., and Williams, A.F., 1975, *Eur. J. Immunol.* **5**:274.
Morris, R.J., and Williams, A.F., 1977, *Eur. J. Immunol.*, submitted.
Morris, R.J., Letarte-Muirhead, M., and Williams, A.F., 1975, *Eur. J. Immunol.* **5**:282.
Muramatsu, T., Nathenson, S.G., Boyse, E.A., and Old, L.J., 1973, *J. Exp. Med.* **137**:1256.
Nathenson, S.G., and Cullen, S.E., 1974, *Biochem. Biophys. Acta* **344**:1.
Neauport-Sautes, C., Lilly, F., Silvestre, D., and Kourilsky, F.M., 1973, *J. Exp. Med.* **137**:511.
Nossal, G.J.V., Warner, N.L., Lewis, H., and Sprent, J., 1972, *J. Exp. Med.* **135**:405.

Obata, Y., Ikeda, H., Stockert, E., and Boyse, E.A., 1975, *J. Exp. Med.* **141**:188.
Owen, J.J.T., 1973, in: *Defence and Recognition, MTP International Review of Science, Biochemistry Series One*, Vol. 10, Butterworth, London, p. 35.
Parish, C.R., and Hayward, J.A., 1974, *Proc. R. Soc. London Ser. B.* **187**:47.
Raff, M.C., 1971, *Transplant. Rev.* **6**:52.
Reif, A.E., and Allen, J.M.V., 1964, *J. Exp. Med.* **120**:413.
Rogers, A.W., 1973, *Techniques of Autoradiography*, 2nd Ed., Elsevier, Amsterdam, Chap. 9.
Schechter, I., McKean, D.J., Guyer, R., and Terry W., 1975, *Science* **188**:160.
Scheid, M., Boyse, E.A., Carswell, E.A., and Old, L.J., 1972, *J. Exp. Med.* **135**:938.
Schwartz, B.D., and Nathenson, S.G., 1971, *J. Immunol.* **107**:1363.
Sherr, C.J., Baur, S., Grunke, I., Zeligs, J., Zeligs, B., and Uhr, J.W., 1972, *J. Exp. Med.* **135**:1392.
Shigeno, N., Arpels, C., Hammerling, U., Boyse, E.A., and Old, L.J., 1968, *Lancet* **2**:320.
Shreffler, D.C., and David, C.S., 1975, *Adv. Immunol.* **20**:125.
Singer, S.J., and Nicholson, G.L., 1972, *Science* **175**:720.
Snell, G., 1958, *J. Nat. Cancer Inst.* **21**:843.
Sparks, F.C., Ting, C.C., Hammond, W.G., and Herberman, R.B., 1969, *J. Immunol.* **102**: 842.
Speigelberg, H.L., 1974, *Adv. Immunol.* **19**:259.
Steck, T.L., 1974, *J. Cell. Biol.* **62**:1.
Stern, P.L., 1973, *Nature (London) New Biol.* **246**:76.
Stout, R.D., Yutoku, M., Grossberg, A., Pressman, D., and Herzenberg, L.A., 1975, *J. Immunol.* **115**:508.
Takahashi, T., Old, L.J., Hsu, C.J., and Boyse, E.A., 1971, *Eur. J. Immunol.* **1**:478.
Thiele, H.G., and Stark, R., 1974, *Immunology* **27**:807.
Thiele, H.G., Stark, R., and Keeser, D., 1972, *Eur. J. Immunol.* **2**:424.
Thompson, A., and Morris, R.J., 1976, *Immunology*, in press.
Trowbridge, I.S., and Hyman, R., 1975, *Cell* **6**:279.
Trowbridge, I.S., Ralph, P., and Bevan, M.J., 1975a, *Proc. Nat. Acad. Sci. U.S.A.* **72**:157.
Trowbridge, I.S., Weissman, I., and Bevan, M.J., 1975b, *Nature (London)* **256**:652.
Tyan, M.L., 1975, *Transplantation* **19**:327.
Yutoku, M., Grossberg, A.L., and Pressman, D., 1974a, *J. Immunol.* **112**:911.
Yutoku, M., Grossberg, A.L., and Pressman, D., 1974b, *J. Immunol.* **112**:1774.
Van Bekkum, D.W., and Dicke, K.A., 1972, *Ciba. Symp. Ontogeny of Acquired Immunity*, North Holland, Amsterdam, p. 222.
Von Boehmer, H., Sprent, J., and Nabholz, M., 1975, *J. Exp. Med.* **141**:332.
Von Fellenberg, R., and Guggisberg, E., 1972, *J. Immunol.* **108**:1647.
Warner, N.L., 1974, *Adv. Immunol.* **19**:67.
Watanabe, T., Yagi, Y., and Pressman, D., 1971, *J. Immunol.* **106**:1213.
Williams, A.F., 1973, *Eur. J. Immunol.* **3**:628.
Williams, A.F., 1975, *Eur. J. Immunol.* **5**:883.
Williams, A.F., 1976, *Eur. J. Immunol.*, **6**:526.
Williams, A.F., Barclay, A.N., Letarte-Muirhead, M., and Morris, R.J., 1977, *Cold Spring Harbor Symp. Quant. Biol.*, in press.
Zeiller, K., and Dolan, L., 1972, *Eur. J. Immunol.* **2**:439.
Zeiller, K., and Pascher, G., 1973, *Eur. J. Immunol.* **3**:614.

Quantitation of Antibody Genes by Molecular Hybridization

T. H. Rabbitts and C. Milstein

Medical Research Council Laboratory of Molecular Biology
Hills Road, Cambridge, CB2 2QH, England

I. INTRODUCTION

Antibodies were recognized at the turn of the century by their neutralizing effect on injurious microbes or substances foreign to an animal. The ability of the animal to respond to such an invasion in a flexible and specific manner quickly led to imaginative theoretical models to account for this activity. But it was not until the work of Landsteiner that the enormous diversity and exquisite specificity of the antibody system was fully appreciated. For a number of years, the understanding of both diversity and specificity remained a problem suitable only for theoretical speculation, but the birth of protein sequence analysis allowed a fresh look at the antibody problem. It became evident that antibodies were molecules with a defined four-chain basic structure, and in addition, the structural nature of antibody diversity started to unfold with the early comparative amino acid sequence studies of myeloma protein chains. It became clear, therefore, that diversity of antibodies was of genetic origin, and a new wave of theoretical speculation could be put to the test.

The combination of protein sequence and genetic studies, made possible by the discovery of genetic markers, led to a scheme for the arrangement of the antibody genes that is now widely accepted (Fig. 1). Nonetheless, this scheme (see Section IA) hides fundamental gaps in our knowledge, such as the number of germ line genes responsible for antibody specificity. This problem is still controversial but essential to our understanding of the origin of antibody diversity.

The detection and subsequent purification of immunoglobulin mRNA

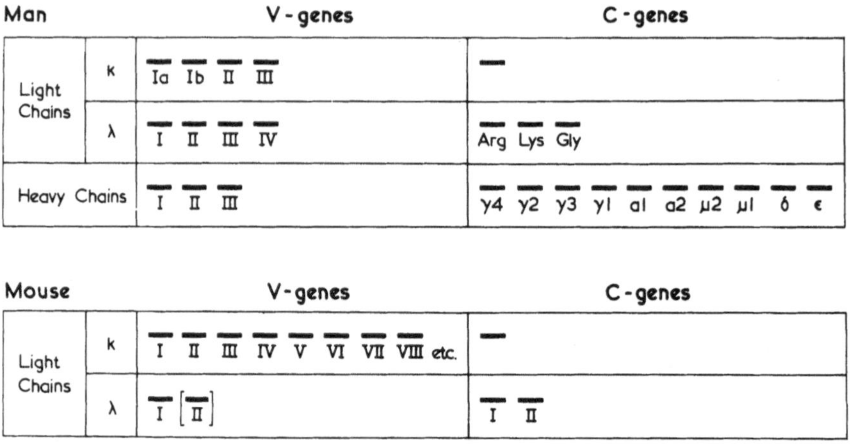

Figure 1. Possible arrangement for a minimum number of genes for human Ig and mouse light chains. The scheme is taken from C. Milstein and Munro (1973). The three unlinked sets of genes coding for the different chains are thought to occur on different chromosomes. A single polypeptide chain results from the expression of a V- and a C-gene from the same set. The number of V-genes depicted is lower than the present estimates of the minimum derived by protein sequences. The second λ V-gene is uncertain.

opened the way to a direct analysis of the genetic diversity of antibody genes by molecular hybridization techniques. The aim of this chapter is to summarize our present views on the results obtained so far and to assess their significance. These studies are quite recent, and therefore the conclusions we can draw at this stage are restricted. In addition, much of the molecular hybridization technique is relatively new, and being so holds problems that are still not well defined. Nevertheless, we believe that a number of observations have reached a stage of reliability that allows us to draw some conclusions on the genetic basis of antibody diversity.

A. Ig Genes

Antibody molecules consist of light and heavy chains. Each of these polypeptides is divided into a variable (V) and a constant (C) section. The V (amino terminal) section consists of about 110–120 residues and carries the antibody combining site. The C section is responsible for the effector properties, such as complement activation and transport across membranes (Porter, 1973). It is now widely accepted that each section is coded for by different genes—the V and the C genes. The genetic information for a single polypeptide is thus encoded (at least conceptually) by two different genes. This two-gene–one-polypeptide hypothesis was first proposed as an *ad hoc* solution to a theoretical paradox (Dreyer and Bennett, 1965). It gained general support by the description of three well-defined basic sequences on human V_κ chains (C. Milstein, 1969) that contrasted with the Mendelian behavior of their corresponding C_κ genes (as defined by their InV markers; Ritter *et al.*, 1966). These markers are due to the presence of either valine or leucine at residue 191 (C. Milstein, 1966; Baglioni *et al.*, 1966) and either valine or alanine at 153 (C. P. Milstein *et al.*, 1974). Clear-cut evidence of the absence of a large number of C_κ and C_λ genes in the mouse has been obtained by molecular hybridization methods, and is fully discussed below.

In summary, a scheme is shown in Fig. 1 for the genetic arrangement of the antibody genes based on the presence of three sets of autosomal genes, for κ, λ, and H chains, respectively. Each set consists of two subsets, each coding for a variety of V and C sections. The multiple C genes of the heavy chains (C_H genes) define the class and subclass of the antibodies.

B. V Genes and Antibody Diversity

For over 20 years, the genetic origin of antibody diversity has been the subject of much controversy. It is not our intention to state, once again, the history of this controversy, and the evolution of the different models proposed to explain the diversity. Two features have led to the realization that the number of V regions required to achieve full diversity may be smaller than previously imagined. The association of two chains, each able to contribute independently to the total number of specificities, had a dramatic effect on the total number of genes required. Thus, 10^2 or 10^3 genes for each chain (H and L) are capable of generating, respectively, 10^4 or 10^6 specificites. Functional randomness of chain combinations has received recent confirmation by the demonstration of the same λ-chain association with different V_H regions (Cesari and Weigart, 1973) and in studies of hybrid cells (Köhler and Milstein, 1976). The repertoire of antibody molecules required to explain antibody specificity is still a matter of controversy. The same antibody molecule may recognize more than one antigen, so that the fine specificity of the antibody has been suggested to be the result of the heterogeneity of the response (Inman, 1974; Richards *et al.*, 1975).

Quite independently of such considerations, a great deal of protein sequence data has accumulated that provides factual evidence on the structural diversity of the chains. A comparison of different V-region sequences showed that these sequences can be arranged into subgroups (C. Milstein, 1969; Gally, 1973); such subgroups may or may not be easy to define. Particularly striking is the observation that the number of postulated subgroups varies considerably among the different V-gene sets within a species, as well as among species within a given set. For example, the V_κ set in the mouse appears to contain so many subgroups that after an analysis of 61 proteins, a minimum of 25 subgroups has been proposed

(Hood *et al.*, 1973). In contrast, the mouse λ chains are remarkably similar and often identical. They appear to belong to only one or two subgroups (Schulenburg *et al.*, 1971; Cesari and Weigart, 1973). It is widely assumed that each well-defined subgroup must be coded for by at least one gene, so that a minimum number of genes can be defined for each V set as in Fig. 1. But the *actual* number of genes coding for each subgroup is a matter of great controversy. As will be seen in Section II, molecular hybridization studies have already contributed interesting new data on this problem.

Proteins within a given subgroup concentrate their differences in well-defined regions called *hypervariable regions* (C. Milstein, 1969; Wu and Kabat, 1970). Hypervariable regions lie near each other in the three-dimensional folding to constitute the antigen binding site (Amzel *et al.*, 1974). For this reason, the origin of the differences among hypervariable regions in chains belonging to the same subgroup is central to the origin of antibody diversity.

C. Immunoglobulin mRNAs

The isolation of the mRNA coding for immunoglobulin chains became possible with the development of cell-free synthesis assays (Stavnezer and Huang, 1971). Progress was fast, and partially purified light-chain mRNA from a variety of sources has been reported (Honjo *et al.*, 1974; Faust *et al.*, 1974; T. M. Harrison *et al.*, 1974; Tonegawa, 1976; Schechter, 1974; Stavnezer *et al.*, 1974). Purity of the preparations is of primary importance for the technique of molecular hybridization. Methods for estimating purity include biological assays, presence of single components in gel electrophoresis, kinetics of hybridization of DNA complementary to the mRNA, and chemical analysis. Only the last two establish chemical purity. The first is based on a comparison of total RNA concentration measured by physical methods and the concentration of the major component by its rate of hybridization (Leder *et al.*, 1973). The second is based on the recovery of specific oligonucleotides from fingerprint analysis (Rabbitts *et al.*, 1975). Structural analysis of the light-chain mRNA has shown that the molecule is a single polynucleotide chain about 1250 bases long. Like many other eukaryotic mRNAs, it includes a poly(A) stretch at the 3′ end that has been shown to be about 200 residues long (Brownlee *et al.*, 1973). A proposed structure is shown in Fig. 2.

Preparations of heavy-chain mRNA have also been reported (Stevens and Williamson, 1973; Cowan and Milstein, 1973; Bernardini and Tonegawa, 1975). Extensive purification, sufficient for preliminary structural studies, has been achieved on a mutant line in which the CHl domain is deleted (Cowan *et al.*, 1976).

The structural analysis has provided final evidence that light- (C. Milstein *et al.*, 1974) and heavy-chain (Cowan *et al.*, 1976) mRNA contain both V- and

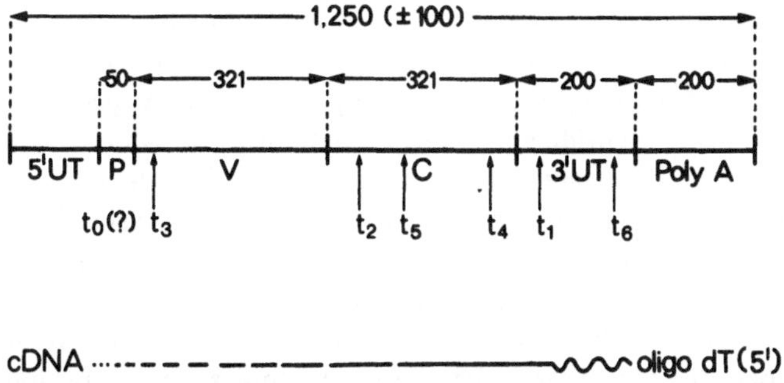

Figure 2. MOPC 21 κ-chain mRNA. The indicated positions of marker oligonucleotides (t_0–t_6) within the different segments of the mRNA are deduced from the results of C. Milstein *et al.* (1974). cDNA made by priming with oligo(dT) is synthesized toward the 5′ end of the mRNA as a heterogeneous population of molecules of variable length.

C-gene products in an integrated molecule. Furthermore, cell hybrids derived by fusion of two immunoglobulin-producing cells have shown that the V and C regions are not scrambled intracellularly (Cotton and Milstein, 1973; Köhler and Milstein, 1975). It appears, therefore, that the most likely level of integration of V and C genes is at the DNA level. Differentiation of immunocytes may therefore involve changes in the primary sequence of the DNA. Experiments to demonstrate such changes by molecular hybridization techniques are under way. In a preliminary report, Tonegawa and Hozumi (1976) describe an experiment that suggests this is the case. This experiment shows that mRNA representing the V and C genes hybridizes to separate fragments of DNA prepared from mouse embryos. When the DNA was prepared from myeloma tissue, however, the V and C regions hybridized with a single DNA size fraction. Determination of the detailed structure and organization of the antibody genes, considered almost intractable until recently, is coming within the limits of present technological developments, thanks particularly to the recent developments in genetic engineering procedures.

D. The DNA Excess Hybridization Technique

The principles of hybridization in vast DNA excess have been well documented (e.g., Bishop, 1972). Briefly, the experimental procedure consists of incubating a vast excess of denatured bulk fragmented DNA with radioactive mRNA or radioactive complementary DNA (cDNA) (see Fig. 2). Samples are removed at different times and used to measure the fraction of the radioactive species that becomes hybridized. The method used for this determination is very important, and will be discussed separately. The data are represented as a "*Cot* curve," which is a semilogarithmic plot of the fraction of radioactive species that is found in the hybrid form at different times at a given DNA concentration (*Co* is the initial DNA concentration in moles of nucleotide per liter and *t* is time in seconds). The $Cot_{1/2}$ value is the half-point of the second-order kinetic transition. The $Cot_{1/2}$ value for the hybridization of a particular RNA species is dependent on the conditions of hybridization, i.e., temperature and salt concentration during the incubation. These are physical factors that affect the rate of hybrid formation. The important point, however, is that the $Cot_{1/2}$ value is proportional to the relative concentration of the sequences complementary to the mRNA or cDNA probe in the bulk DNA (reiteration frequency).

Eukaryotic DNA consists of sequences ranging in reiteration frequency (i.e., in the number of copies) from 10^6 to single copies. Since the hybridization reaction is essentially a kinetic reaction and thus dependent on the collision frequency of similar sequences, the rate of hybridization is dependent on the concentration of a particular sequence in the reaction: for example, the hybridization of a 100-fold repetitive sequence will be two orders of magnitude faster than a nonrepetitive (single-copy) sequence. This is illustrated in Fig. 3, which shows the theoretical *Cot* curves for RNA species coded by repetitive and nonrepetitive genes, as well as a mixture of RNA sequences coded by repetitive and nonrepetitive genes.

The actual reiteration frequency, or gene numbers, can be calculated from these curves, but they are better derived experimentally by comparison with known standards. The kinetic standards most commonly used are the complementary RNA made from *E. coli* DNA, the "unique" fraction of a eukaryotic DNA, and globin mRNA or cDNA. As will be discussed later, none of the standards can be regarded as completely satisfactory.

Two methods are generally used to measure the percentage hybridization.

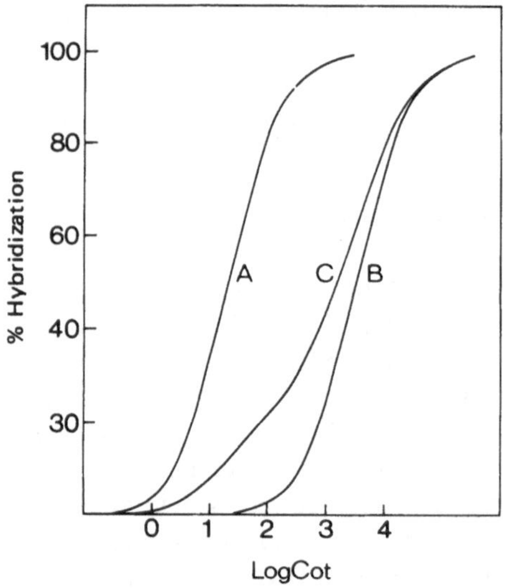

Figure 3. Second-order kinetic curves exemplifying theoretical hybridization in vast DNA excess. (A) $Cot_{1/2}$ of 20 corresponds to about 250 gene copies per haploid genome if probe is mRNA; (B) $Cot_{1/2}$ of 3200, repetition frequency of about one gene; (C) mixed population of an RNA molecule made of 25% sequences complementary to genes repeated about 250 times and 75% sequences complementary to single genes.

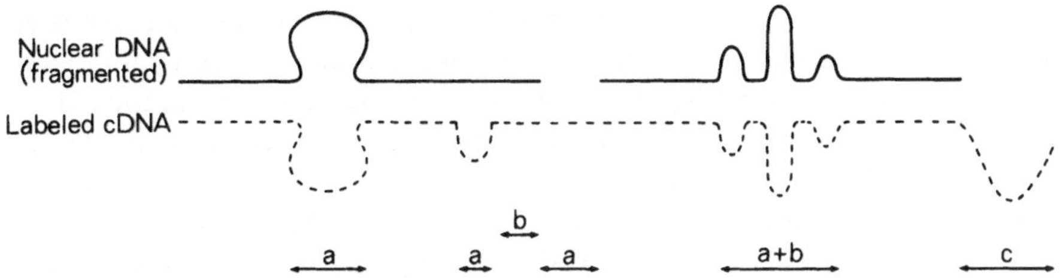

Figure 4. Behavior of partially mismatched hybrids on analysis by hydroxyapatite and nuclease digestion. All the cDNA in this figure will be retained by HAP columns and computed as 100% in the hybrid form. But S_1 nuclease will digest single-strand segments like (a) or (c). Double-strand segments like (b) may be too short to remain as duplexes and be digested by S_1 nuclease. The hybridization percentage will therefore be 100 − (a + b + c).

The first method is to measure the radioactivity released by nuclease digestion of the unhybridized (single-stranded) fraction. The second method is by fractionation of the mixture into double- and single-strand material on hydroxyapatite. Nuclease digestion of RNA is usually carried out with pancreatic ribonuclease, and digestion of cDNA with the single strand-specific S_1 nuclease (Sutton, 1971). Nuclease procedures digest away mismatched and unhybridized tails, and therefore only the actual hybrid region remains intact after the digestion. Hydroxyapatite (HAP) procedures (generally used with cDNA), on the other hand, consist of a two-step elution of material: (1) a low-salt elution of the single-strand component, and (2) a high-salt or high-temperature elution of double-strand material. The noteworthy difference between hydroxyapatite and nuclease (Fig. 4) is that in the former procedure, the double-strand (hybrid) fraction includes single-strand molecular segments such as single-strand tails or mismatched regions. This distinction is important in the interpretation of hybridization with V-region cDNA probes, as will be discussed.

II. HYBRIDIZATION PROPERTIES OF IMMUNOGLOBULIN GENES

A. DNA Excess Hybridization Using mRNA as Probe

All experiments so far have utilized Ig mRNA prepared from a variety of mouse myelomas, and studies have been made of κ and λ L-chain mRNA as well as γ H-chain mRNA. Ig mRNAs have been difficult to obtain in pure form, and the mRNA preparations used have frequently contained only 50–60% Ig mRNA. A number of reports have been published in which mRNA purity was judged only by *in vitro* translation studies that indicated essentially homogeneous Ig mRNA preparations. Chemical analysis (Brownlee *et al.*, 1973), however, has shown that impurities, revealed by ^{32}P-mRNA fingerprints, are not translated in the most commonly used reticulocyte cell-free system. Initial hybridization experiments with such mRNA preparations yielded biphasic hybridization kinetics for the κ-chain mRNA (Delovitch and Baglioni, 1973; Rabbitts *et al.*, 1974a; Storb, 1974; Tonegawa *et al.*, 1974a). Experiments involving H-chain mRNA have also been reported (Premkumar *et al.*, 1974; but see Stevens and Williamson, 1975; Bernardini and Tonegawa, 1974), but the purity of these preparations is even more questionable.

A typical result demonstrating biphasic hybridization kinetics is shown in Fig. 5. Here, the κ-chain mRNA of the myeloma MOPC 21 is hybridized with either liver or myeloma DNA. The curves are identical with both tissues, and the two transitions represent sequences repeated around 250 times and around 1–5 times in the genome. The hybridization curve of 18 S RNA is also shown to illustrate the kinetics of a homogeneous product of a repetitive gene. The interpretations of these biphasic kinetic curves were various. Caution was clearly indicated, however, by a number of observations:

1. Fingerprints of the mRNA showed the presence of contaminating species (Brownlee *et al.*, 1973).
2. Non-Ig mRNAs (e.g., mouse fibroblast) also show biphasic hybridization kinetics (Rabbitts *et al.*, 1974a).
3. Molecular weight estimation of several L-chain mRNAs (Brownlee *et al.*,

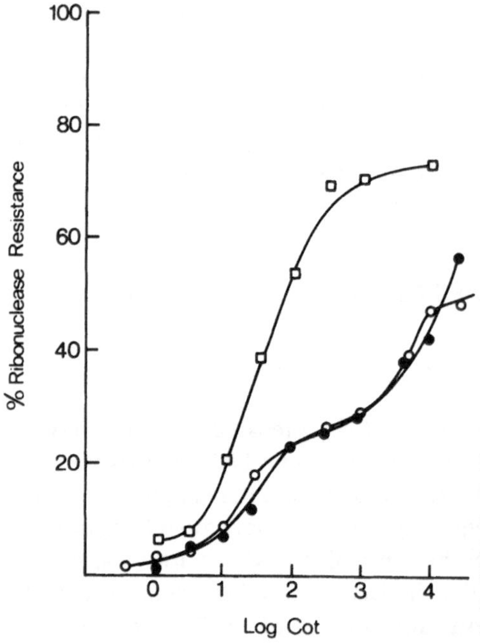

Figure 5. A typical biphasic hybridization curve of a light-chain ^{32}P-mRNA to mouse nuclear DNA. (○) MOPC 21 mRNA + myeloma DNA; (●) MOPC 21 mRNA + liver DNA; (□) 18 S rRNA + myeloma DNA. From Rabbitts *et al.* (1974a).

1973; Mach *et al.*, 1973; Honjo *et al.*, 1974; Stavnezer *et al.*, 1974; Tonegawa *et al.*, 1974b) and globin mRNA (e.g., Gould and Hamlyn, 1973) showed that eukaryotic mRNAs may often possess considerable amounts of apparently noncoding sequences.

Clearly, there was no immediate justification for making any firm conclusions from these kinetic experiments. Consideration had to be given to the hybridization properties of the contaminating RNA species, the V-region sequence, the C-region sequence, and the noncoding sequence. It was necessary first to establish whether the two components were due to separate populations of RNA molecules hybridizing independently with repetitive and nonrepetitive genes, or to single mRNA molecules containing stretches hybridizing with repetitive and nonrepetitive genes, respectively.

In order to investigate the nature of the repetitive component in our mRNA preparations, and in particular to determine the hybridization properties of the V-region sequence, we have reported the following experiment (Fig. 6; Rabbitts *et al.*, 1975). Fragmented myeloma nuclear DNA was denatured and allowed to reanneal, thus yielding a fraction of repetitive DNA. The value of log *Cot* 2 was used because it is the point at which the repetitive component of our preparation of L-chain mRNA is totally hybridized (see Fig. 5). The repetitive DNA fraction was hybridized with ^{32}P-labeled L-chain mRNA, a preparation possessing the hybridization characteristics shown in Fig. 5. Since the repetitive fraction of the nuclear DNA was used, only the repetitive component of the mRNA fraction was thus capable of forming hybrids. These hybrids were retained by a hydroxyapatite column, while the nonhybridized (nonrepetitive) portions were not retained. The fingerprint and the hybridization properties of these two fractions were then examined (Fig. 6). The unfractionated mRNA population showed the characteristic biphasic curve (see Fig. 5), but the two isolated mRNA fractions showed markedly different hybridization properties. The repetitive RNA fraction (i.e., the fraction that hybridized to the repetitive DNA) showed only a rapidly hybridizing transition, while the nonrepetitive RNA fraction showed a single, unique hybridizing transition. The two hybridization components of the initial mRNA preparation can therefore be separated into two distinct populations, one hybridizing with repetitive genes, and the other *only* with nonrepetitive genes. The repetitive component is therefore not a stretch of all molecules, but represents separate molecular species. Since the mRNA was labeled with ^{32}P, it was possible to identify which of the RNA fractions contained the L-chain mRNA by two-dimensional fractionation of the T_1 ribonuclease products (fingerprint). The fraction of RNA hybridizing only with unique genes showed a fingerprint with all the characteristics of the L-chain mRNA (see Fig. 6). It is important to note, as can be done by referring to Fig. 2, that the labeled oligonucleotides in Fig. 6 are derived from all regions of the L-chain mRNA: in particular, the presence of t_3 shows the occurrence of a V-region marker in this

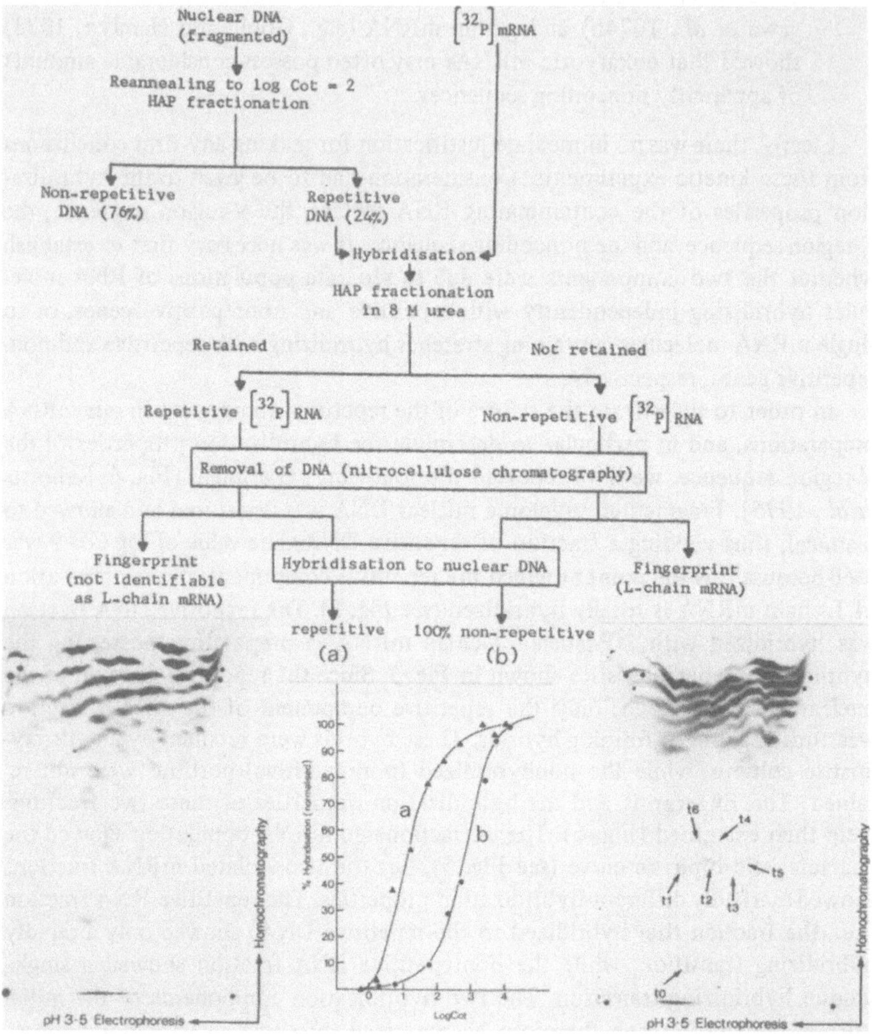

Figure 6. Demonstration that the MOPC 21 κ-chain mRNA does not hybridize with repetitive DNA sequences. (▲) Repetitive RNA fraction; (●) nonrepetitive RNA fraction; Adapted from Rabbitts *et al.* (1975).

RNA fraction. Hence, it was concluded that the entire L-chain mRNA (including the V-region) hybridizes to nonrepetitive genes, and that the repetitive component was due to impurities in the mRNA preparations.

These results explain the different proportions of the repetitive component observed in mRNA hybridization experiments performed by different investigators. We had ourselves observed the proportion of this component to vary with different preparations of the same mRNA. Leder *et al.* (1974) reported having detected very little repetitive component in mRNA prepared from MOPC 41 tumors.

Other investigators have arrived at the conclusion that different κ-chain mRNA species also hybridize only to nonrepetitive genes. Mach *et al.* (1973) reported that the earlier preparations of κ-chain mRNA from MOPC 41 showed biphasic kinetics hybridizing to genes repeated about 250 times and about 2–4 times respectively. Fingerprint evidence had previously shown that polyacrylamide gels in formamide were a powerful further step in the purification procedure (Brownlee *et al.*, 1973). By careful elution of a narrow band from such a denaturing polyacrylamide gel, Mach and co-workers were able to isolate a fraction that hybridized only with nonrepetitive DNA. This fraction was identified as κ-chain mRNA by a cell-free translation assay (Farace *et al.*, 1976). The MOPC 41 tumor used in these experiments is the same as that used by Leder *et al.* (1974); however, the latter workers reported the presence of a component hybridizing with between 30 and 50 genes, as well as that hybridizing with the unique transition. This discrepancy between the two reports is difficult to explain, except as due to the effect of RNA contaminants.

Tonegawa (1976) has also produced recent evidence of homogeneous hybridization curves using both κ-chain and λ-chain mRNA species. Again, early studies of this group had shown biphasic hybridization profiles for the MOPC 70E κ-chain mRNA (Tonegawa *et al.*, 1974a). More highly purified MOPC 321 κ-chain mRNA was again obtained by fractionation using denaturing polyacrylamide gels, and such material was shown to hybridize only to nonrepetitive genes (Tonegawa, 1976). In addition, the λ-chain mRNA of MOPC 104E was found to possess unique hybridization kinetics, and this mRNA showed no hybridization with repetitive genes (Tonegawa, 1976).

It is therefore concluded that no *bona fide* Ig mRNA species has been demonstrated to contain a repetitive component. Furthermore, evidence accumulates to indicate that the V-region and C-region sequences of both κ- and λ-chain mRNA hybridize at similar rates, which correspond to genes repeated at most a few times in the genome. In the future, reports indicating the presence of a repetitive component can be considered significant only if they are shown to be an integral part of the immunoglobulin mRNA molecule.

B. DNA Excess Hybridization Using cDNA as Probe

There have been a variety of experiments with cDNA made by reverse transcriptase copying various L-chain mRNAs using oligo(dT) as primer. These transcripts are shorter than the total length of the mRNA. In general, they do not include more than the 3′ untranslated region and part of the total C region, i.e., about 500 residues. All reports using unfractionated cDNA show simple kinetics which indicate that the C_κ gene is present in only 1-5 copies per haploid genome (Faust *et al.*, 1974; Honjo *et al.*, 1974; Rabbitts, 1974; Stavnezer *et al.*, 1974). The exact quantitation of gene numbers will be discussed in Section IIC.

At this point, it is worth mentioning the sources of the nuclear DNA used in the experiments described. This information is incorporated in Table I. In many instances, the DNA was prepared from both myeloma and liver or spleen, and the hybridization of the cDNA or mRNA was measured with DNA from both sources. No difference in the kinetics of hybridization of the L-chain sequences was detected when either source of DNA was used. This rules out the possibility of specific amplification of immunoglobulin genes in myeloma cells.

The results with cDNA and mRNA are apparently contradictory. The cDNA made from mRNA gives single hybridization kinetics, while the impure mRNA itself gives biphasic kinetics. An early interpretation of this discrepancy was that the repetitive component of the mRNA molecules occurred at the extreme 5′ end, and that only the longest copies of cDNA could detect it (Rabbitts and Milstein, 1975a). The hybridization properties of the longest cDNA copies certainly complicated the picture, and will be discussed separately (see below). It seems clear, however, that the repetitive component of the mRNA is not a fragment of the Ig mRNA itself, but represents a separate molecular species. If the cDNA copies made from mRNA do not include a repetitive component, it follows that the repetitive component is not transcribed into cDNA. This hypothesis has been experimentally substantiated, and the possible origin of the repetitive contaminant has been further discussed (Rabbitts *et al.*, 1975).

In two cases, the cDNA prepared was of sufficient length to include enough of the V region to take part in hybridization reactions. One of these reactions made use of unfractionated cDNA copies of a λ-chain mRNA (see below; Leder *et al.*, 1975); the other was based on a size fractionation of cDNA copies of MOPC 21 κ-chain mRNA (Rabbitts and Milstein, 1975a). Both demonstrate that the V-region sequences of these myelomas hybridize with nonrepetitive genes. In the second case, three size classes of cDNA were prepared, which included: (1) only the C region; (2) the C and V regions; (3) the largest molecule, including the 5′ untranslated region. No difference among these three classes was detectable when they were analyzed by S_1 nuclease (Fig. 7a). Similarly, no difference between classes (1) and (2) was detected on analysis by HAP fractionation (Rabbitts and Milstein, 1975a).

The hybridization kinetics of the MOPC 21 L-chain and globin cDNA to mouse liver nuclear DNA are compared in Fig. 7b. For this experiment, [^{3}H] DNA made from MOPC 21 L-chain mRNA and from mouse globin mRNA were fractionated on alkaline sucrose gradients to produce a population of long cDNA molecules (L-chain cDNA 600–900 bases, globin 600 to full-length cDNA). No

Table I. Summary of Recent Light-Chain V-Gene and C-Gene Numbers Estimated by Hybridization Kinetics

Tumor	mRNA (κ and λ)	Bulk DNA	Hybridization probe	Number of genes detected		Kinetic standard used	References
				V	C		
MOPC 41	κ	Liver Myeloma	cDNA	–	1–5	Mouse DNA	Faust *et al.* (1974)
MOPC 41	κ	Liver Myeloma	cDNA	–	3–4	Unique sequence mouse DNA	Stavnezer *et al.* (1974)
MOPC 41	κ	Spleen Myeloma	cDNA	–	<5	Globin cDNA	Honjo *et al.* (1974)
MOPC 21	κ	Myeloma	cDNA	–	2–3	Mouse DNA	Rabbitts (1974)
MOPC 21	κ	Myeloma	cDNA	1–8	1–8	*E. coli* DNA *P. mirabilis* DNA	Rabbitts and Milstein (1975a) Rabbitts *et al.* (1974b)
	κ	Liver	cDNA	1–5	1–5	Globin cDNA	See Fig. 7.
MOPC 41	κ	Myeloma	^{125}I-mRNA	2–4	2–4	Globin mRNA	Farace *et al.* (1976)
RPC 20	λ	Spleen Myeloma	cDNA	2	2	Globin cDNA	Leder *et al.* (1975)
MOPC 321	κ	Liver	^{125}I-mRNA	3	3	Globin mRNA	Tonegawa (1976)
MOPC 104E	λ	Liver	^{125}I-mRNA	3	3	Globin mRNA	Tonegawa (1976)

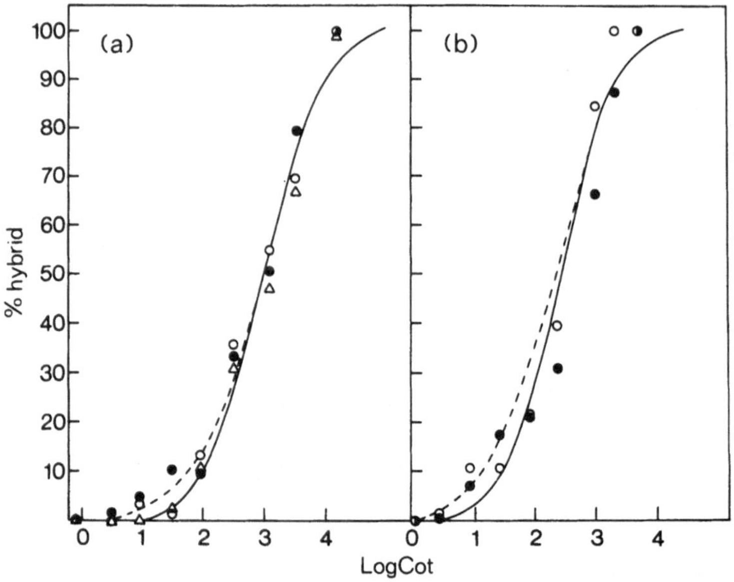

Figure 7. Hybridization of MOPC 21 light-chain cDNA to nuclear DNA. (a) Analyzed by S_1 nuclease. The data from Rabbitts and Milstein (1975a) have been normalized. Three size classes of cDNA were used [number of bases from the oligo(dT)] : (△) 400–600 bases (C); (●) 580–800 bases (B); (○) 750–1080 bases (A). The figure shows that the inclusion of differing portions of the V region does not significantly change the hybridization properties of the cDNA. (b) Analysed by HAP. The cDNAs for the light chain (●) and globin (○) were 600–900 bases long. The experiment is similar to the one described by Rabbitts and Milstein (1975a), except that the nuclear DNA was of liver origin, globin cDNA is included for comparison, and the data have been normalized. The curves shown are theoretically second-order curves. The solid line represents a single gene with a low repetition frequency N (calculated to be from single-copy to a maximum of 8). The dashed line is the theoretical hybridization curve for a mixture: (1) 75% of a gene of repetition frequency N and 25% of a gene of repetition frequency 10 N; (b) 50% mixture of genes as before. The 25% and 50% figures are chosen as representing, in each case, the contribution of V sequences, assuming the cDNA to be about 60% pure.

difference can be detected between them, which further endorses our conclusion that the C_κ and V genes of MOPC 21 are repeated at most a few times in the genome, and in any case not detectably more than the globin gene. It should be noted, however, that the sensitivity of the method does not allow precise statements concerning the contribution of particular sequences to these kinetic curves (see the Fig. 7 caption). This point is dealt with in Section IID4 (see Fig. 9).

1. A Repetitive Component Detected with cDNA of MOPC 21

When the MOPC 21 cDNA was fractionated by size, a very long fraction could be prepared (Rabbitts and Milstein, 1975a). This fraction included copies that corresponded in length to almost the whole κ-mRNA. The yield of this cDNA size class was, however, below 1% of the total cDNA. When the hybridization properties of this size class were tested, the class was found to include a repetitive component (repetition frequency around 200 copies). This component could be detected *only* by hydroxyapatite, not by S_1 nuclease digestion. The smaller fractions of the same cDNA did not contain such a component (Rabbitts and Milstein, 1975a). For these reasons, we conclude that this is a repetitive component *that is not detected in experiments using mRNA as a probe*, but only by the longest cDNA copies, which include segments at the 5′ end of the mRNA. As pointed out (Rabbitts and Milstein, 1975a), however, this component may or may not represent elements of the L-chain mRNA, and conclusions cannot be made until a firm assignment has been achieved.

C. Number of V and C Genes Recognized by Specific mRNAs or the Corresponding cDNA

In the previous sections, we have described experiments showing that the entire mRNAs (i.e., both V- and C-region sequences) of light chains hybridize with unique DNA or to genes repeated at most a few times in the genome. Can we be more precise about the numbers involved? Table I summarizes the data available for the purified mRNA or cDNA hybridization, together with the kinetic standards used to estimate gene number. It is unfortunate that the quoted gene numbers vary considerably from author to author, but it should be noted that the main reason for this variation is that gene number is estimated relative to a standard. Ideally, the standard should be an RNA or DNA of precisely known reiteration frequency and similar to the reiteration of the immunoglobulin genes. No such standard exists. The standards usually employed are mouse unique DNA, mouse globin mRNA, and bacterial DNA. The drawbacks associated with these standards are somewhat similar, but will be dealt with separately.

(a) Mouse Unique DNA. The final kinetic transition of mouse DNA renaturation consists of about 70% of the total DNA (Britten and Kohne, 1968). This is known as the *unique* or *single-copy* DNA fraction. However, this fraction consists of an extremely large number of sequences with heterogeneous reiteration frequencies. They probably range from single-copy sequences to increasingly repetitive sequences. Therefore, the $Cot_{1/2}$ value for this transition may not represent the area of renaturation of hybridization of genes repeated only once per haploid genome.

(b) Mouse Globin mRNA or cDNA. This has been used as a kinetic standard on the basis that the globin genes are present as single copies in the genome. The hybridization data on mouse globin cDNA, however, do not allow such a clear statement. P. R. Harrison *et al.* (1972) found evidence for 0.7–1.4 copies of the mouse globin genes using an mRNA fraction consisting of both α- and β-globin, but further studies by this group (P. R. Harrison *et al.*, 1974) did not allow a greater accuracy than 1–5 genes for the mouse globin genes. Other studies have produced similar estimates of globin gene number (Ross *et al.*, 1974). Clearly,

the use of this kind of kinetic experiment is not accurate enough to measure absolute values of gene numbers.

(c) Bacterial DNA. This is the best-documented single-copy DNA, but it is not an internal standard. Furthermore, the genome size of bacteria is much smaller than the eukaryotic genome. Adjustments of DNA concentrations are required, and uncertainties arise.

That the number of V genes and the number of C genes for each set of experiments is of the same order of magnitude also deserves some comment. It is quite possible that in all cases, the number of V and C genes (see Table I) is the same, e.g., 1. But it is also possible that the numbers are not identical, and that the values given for each set of experiments represent the average number of V and C genes that are detected. This introduces further inaccuracies. Nevertheless, we consider 10 V genes for all the individual cases listed in Table I as a maximum upper limit. A value of 1-5 V genes is more likely.

D. Hybridization Kinetics and Gene Pool Size

Normally, the hybridization experiments have been carried out under what may be termed highly stringent conditions, in which mismatching and infidelity of hybrid formation are minimized. Under these conditions, it is possible that only closely related V-gene sequences were able to cross-hybridize and thus recognize each other, while less similar genes would remain undetected. Unfortunately, we do not know what degree of cross-reaction is likely to occur, and therefore it is important to attempt to estimate the extent of cross-hybridization of V genes under a given set of hybridization conditions. The effect of mismatching on cross-hybridization of cDNA with globin mRNA of different species has been studied (Leder *et al.*, 1973; Gummerson and Williamson, 1974). To gain more pertinent information on this problem, we have measured, under various experimental conditions, the hybridization of mouse cDNA (made from the MOPC 21 κ-chain mRNA) with DNA prepared from the nuclei of rat, rabbit, and human tissues. Since the species differences among the amino acid sequences of the κ-chain C regions are known, the experiments provide a model for the cross-hybridization properties of different V genes within a single species. Schecter (1975) has studied the cross-hybridization between cDNA of one mouse myeloma κ chain and mRNAs of different L chains. The results are consistent with lack of cross hybridization between mRNAs with very different V regions (MOPC 41 and 321, Table II) but complete cross-hybridization between closely related sequences (MOPC 63 and 321). The data are unfortunately complicated by the unexpected hybridization of the λ chain in mRNA.

Table II outlines the data on the difference in amino acid sequences of the various C and V regions between mouse MOPC 21 L-chain and those of rat, rabbit, and human. The difference between the mouse and rat C_κ sequences (a minimum of 31 base changes per 100 amino acid residues) is bigger than the difference between the V_κ sections of human light chains belonging to the same subgroup (see Table II). The situation in the mouse κ subgroups is less straight-

Table II. Differences between Light Chain Sequences (Minimum Base Changes Coding for 100 Amino Acid Residues in Light Chains)[a]

A. Mouse C_κ region and C_κ regions of

Rat	31
Human	50
Rabbit	69

B. Individual mouse myeloma light-chain V regions

	MOPC 173	MOPC 21	MOPC 41	MOPC 70	MOPC 321	MOPC 63
MOPC 21	61					
MOPC 41	38	55				
MOPC 70	52	58	57			
MOPC 321	52	48	56	26		
MOPC 63	50	46	54	24	8	
T 124	50	50	54	25	4	9

C. Range of variation among human V regions of same and different subgroups

	$V_{\kappa Ia}$	$V_{\kappa II}$	$V_{\kappa III}$
$V_{\kappa Ia}$[b]	16–27		
$V_{\kappa II}$	56–66	28	
$V_{\kappa III}$	44–58	44–49	13–22

[a]Data from: (A) Starace and Querinjean (1975); (B) Schiff and Fougereau (1975); (C) C. Milstein and Pink (1970).
[b]The original κ_I subgroup was subdivided into κ_{Ia} and κ_{Ib} (C.P. Milstein, 1973).

forward, since most V_κ sequences examined thus far appear to be fairly diverse, and do not easily fall into a small number of well-defined subgroups (Hood *et al.*, 1973). It is possible that the sequence difference between V regions in the same subgroup is even smaller in mouse than in human, but that the total number of V_κ subgroups in mouse is much larger than in human (Cohn *et al.*, 1974).

On the other hand, the difference between the C_κ sequences of mouse and human (50 minimum base changes) and between mouse and rabbit (69 minimum base changes) is similar to or greater than the differences among V regions belonging to different human and mouse subgroups (see Table II). In summary, a measure of the hybridization properties of the C region of MOPC 21 to mouse, rat, rabbit, and human nuclear DNA should mimic the hybridization properties of a mouse V region to other mouse V region genes of sequences closely and more distantly related.

Such hybridization studies were restricted to the C region by using a cDNA fraction of suitable size (Table III). The hybridization reaction was allowed to proceed for a certain time, and the extent of hybridization was then measured by HAP fractionation or S_1 digestion. The stringency of hybridization was varied by using different temperatures and salt concentrations. The stringency of hybrids so derived was determined by comparing S_1 nuclease digestion with HAP fractionation.

Table III. Hybridization of Mouse C_κ-DNA with DNA of Different Species[a]

Hybridization conditions			Percentage hybridization (high *Cot*)[b] measured by:	
Temp. (C)	Salt	Source of of DNA	Hydroxyapatite column	S_1 nuclease digestion
70°	0.24 M PB[c]	Mouse	65	56
		Rat	61	20
		Human	13	4
		Rabbit	21	4
65°	0.48 M PB	Mouse	69	
		Human	28	
		Rabbit	32	
60°	0.48 M PB	Mouse	62	
		Human	36	
55°	0.48 M PB	Mouse	77	
		Human	45	
		Rabbit	56	

[a] The cDNA was a fraction prepared by alkaline sucrose gradient and shown by acrylamide gels to be 100–600 bases long (average 500).
[b] *Cot* = 10,000.
[c] Sodium phosphate buffer, pH 6.8.

1. Effect of Mismatching on Hybridization Levels

Under standard annealing conditions, mouse and rat DNA hybridized MOPC 21 cDNA to a similar extent when the hybridization was assayed by hydroxyapatite. For example (see Table III), at 70°C and 0.24 M sodium phosphate buffer (pH 6.8), the mouse:mouse hybrid contained 65% of the available cDNA, while the mouse:rat hybrid contained 61%. However, a considerable fraction of the hybrids formed with the rat DNA must include stretches of unpaired bases due to sequence differences. Stretches of this type are revealed by S_1 nuclease analysis (see Fig. 2), and by this procedure, the percentage hybridization of the mouse:rat hybrid drops to 20%, compared with 56% for the mouse:mouse hybrid.

According to protein sequence data, the mouse and rat C regions should differ by at least 10% of the bases (31 bases in 100 amino acids). This value is an absolute minimum that does not take into consideration base changes that do not lead to amino acid changes. Such "silent" changes are likely to be quite frequent, and could raise the difference between mouse and rat to a maximum of 35%. The sequence of the 3′ untranslated stretch in the Ig mRNA is a further important unknown. Recent work indicates that in the case of globin, the final base-change differences are likely to be intermediate between the minimum and the maximum of the value indicated by the amino acid sequence differences (Proudfoot and Brownlee, 1976). Extrapolation of these considerations implies a difference between the mouse and rat C regions of around 15-20%.

Investigation of the melting characteristics of the mouse:mouse and the mouse:rat hybrids indicated a slightly lower value of dissimilarity. The melting temperature (T_m) of a hybrid is known to be related to the amount of mismatched bases. Mismatching causes instability, and thus lowers the temperature at which a hybrid melts. The greater the mismatching, the greater the lowering of T_m. Previously, we have shown that the T_m of the mouse:rat hybrid is about 75°C, compared with 88°C for the reannealed rat DNA (Rabbitts and Milstein, 1975b). There is considerable variation in the literature concerning the relationship between mismatching and T_m; for example, 1% mismatching depresses the T_m of a hybrid by 1.6°C according to Ullman and McCarthy (1973), or by 1°C according to Bonner *et al.* (1973). The measured drop in T_m between mouse:rat hybrids would therefore represent between 8% and 13% mismatching according to these two relationships. Since the minimum predicted difference (based on amino acid sequence differences) is about 15%, we are probably justified in assuming that the mouse:rat hybrids contain about 8-15% mismatching. In terms of protein sequences, therefore, this could include proteins differing by up to 30 residues in 100.

How different can DNA sequences be before we fail to detect them under the hybridization conditions used? Again, useful information is gained by consideration of the high *Cot* hybridization values given in Table III. Unlike the case with rat DNA, our standard hybridization conditions (70°C, 0.24 M PB) support very poor cross-hybridization of mouse cDNA with either human or rabbit DNA (when assayed by HAP). Virtually no hybridization is observed when the hybrids are digested with S_1 nuclease, as expected from the very limited homology of the mouse, rabbit, and human sequences. By lowering the stringency of hybridization (i.e., by lowering the temperature and raising the salt concentration), we can see that the amount of cross-hybridization gradually increases. For example, Table III shows that human DNA hybridizes 13% mouse cDNA at 70°C, 28% at 65°C, 36% at 60°C, and 45% at 55°C. Relative to the homologous mouse:mouse hybridization (i.e., normalizing the homologous reaction to 100%), these values represent 20% at 70°C, 40% at 65°C, and 58% at 60 and 55°C. These values indicate that it is necessary to lower the stringency of hybridization well below our standard conditions before wide cross-hybridization is observed. They also suggest that by lowering the stringency, genes from different subgroups might be detected using a common probe. The potentiality of this conclusion is discussed at the end of this chapter.

These experiments on the characterization of the hybridization potential of our system are vital to the interpretation of data on cDNA of a variety of different mouse L-chain mRNA species. Farace *et al.* (1976) describe an experiment with the κ-mRNA of MOPC 41 using lower stringency hybridization conditions, and conclude that the number of V genes observed did not increase. The actual potential of their conditions was not examined by model experiments, and since they are quite different from our own, are rather difficult to assess quantitatively.

2. *Effect of Mismatching on Hybridization Rates*

In addition to the lowering of T_m, mismatching affects the rate of hybridization and, consequently, the *Cot* curves. Model studies have indicated that mismatching lowers the rate of hybridization, but the extent of this effect is somewhat complicated by the choice of hybridization conditions (McCarthy and Farquhar, 1972; Bonner *et al.*, 1973). Therefore, a measure of gene reiteration by means of partially mismatching probes may underestimate the pool size by a factor that will depend on the degree of mismatching. For example, a probe such as mouse cDNA should hybridize to rat DNA with a $Cot_{1/2}$ value about 2.5 times higher than to mouse DNA. It should be noted that this difference is near the sensitivity of the procedure, and corresponds to an increase in gene numbers from, say, 1 to 2.5.

To study the effect of mismatching on hybridization rates under our experimental conditions, we have examined the relative rates of hybridization of the light-chain cDNA in the homologous reaction (i.e., mouse DNA vs. mouse cDNA) and in the heterologous reaction (i.e., rat DNA vs. mouse cDNA). This

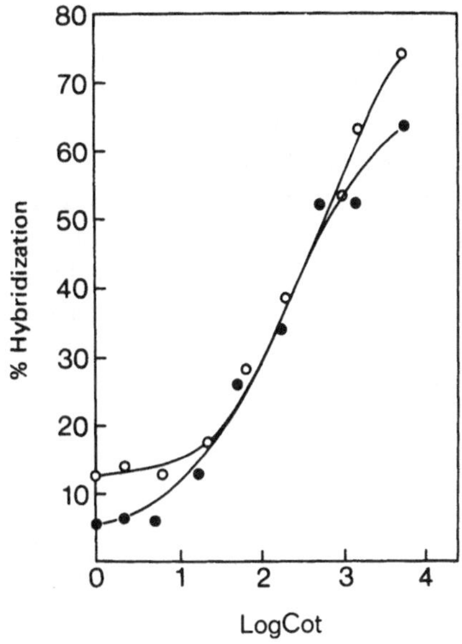

Figure 8. Effect of mismatching on the rate of cDNA hybridization. Mouse C_{κ}-^{3}H-cDNA was made from MOPC 21 L-chain mRNA with reverse transcriptase and oligo(dT) as primer. The size fraction of 100–500 bases was selected. Hybridization was at 70°C in 0.24 M phosphate buffer using liver nuclear DNA of rat and Balb/C mouse. (●) Rat; (○) mouse.

experiment was carried out at our standard hybridization conditions (70°C and 0.24 M PB). Figure 8 shows that the rates of the homologous and heterologous reactions are very similar. Minor differences are, however, reflected in the difference in the final percentage hybridization between mouse:mouse and mouse:rat hybrids (see Table III). This result has obvious implications in terms of possible cross-hybridization of V genes, particularly as regards putative members of a V-region subgroup. We should expect not too dissimilar rates of hybridization of a given cDNA sequence (in our case, the MOPC 21 sequence) with the homologous V gene and with heterologous V genes that differ from the MOPC 21 sequence by around 8–15% of the bases.

Our own evidence with cDNA indicated that the number of detected sequences for both V and C genes was less than 8 (Fig. 7 and Rabbitts and Milstein, 1975a). Thus, the Balb/C mouse genome does not seem to contain a large number of germ-line sequences identical to or differing by 8–15% bases from the MOPC 21 myeloma V-region gene sequence.

3. Competitive Hybridization and Sequence Homology

A different approach to the problem of V-gene cross-hybridization relied on hybridization competition. The experiments involved the use of various unlabeled κ-mRNA species to compete against the hybridization of radioactive MOPC 70E mRNA with mouse liver DNA (Tonegawa *et al.*, 1974a,b). The homologous cold mRNA (i.e., MOPC 70E) was found to reduce to about 55%

the hybridization of radioactive 70E mRNA in the part of the kinetic curve in which only the L-chain unique hybridizing component was involved. Using this value as 100% competition, it was found that MOPC 321 mRNA reduced by 60% the 70E hybridization, while MPC 11 mRNA reduced it by 47%. As we have discussed, the C_κ gene hybridized with unique kinetics, so that one expects just over 50% competition as the contribution of the C_κ gene (and the 3′ noncoding sequence; see Fig. 2). This amount is approximately the amount of competition exhibited by MPC 11 mRNA. Thus, it seems reasonable to conclude that the V region of MPC 11 mRNA does not compete (i.e. cross-hybridize) with the70E sequence. This is consistent with preliminary sequence data of the proteins (Smith, 1973; McKean *et al.*, 1973), which show that they differ at 31 positions out of the first 49 residues. Experiments on cross-species hybridization indicate that such extensive dissimilarity makes it very unlikely that cross-hybridization could occur between the sequences under the experimental conditions used. The competition of MPC 11 is thus likely to be the effect of C_κ sequences only.

On the other hand, the 70E and 321 sequences show the same degree of homology as found among V_κ regions within a human subgroup (see Table II). The competition hybridization data (Tonegawa *et al.*, 1974b) show that 321 mRNA is 60% as effective as the homologous 70E mRNA competition of the hybridization to mouse liver DNA. This result cannot be taken to indicate hybridization to the same gene, since similar competition should then be attainable with *both* 70E and 321 mRNA. On the contrary, it is possible that the experiments with 70E and 321 mRNA concern two partially cross-hybridizing genes; the partial inhibition of 70E by 321 could therefore reflect the partial sequence homology of the two genes. Nevertheless, the experiment shows that the number of cross-hybridizing genes is not measurably higher than the number of C genes.

4. V_λ Genes

The uncertainty that surrounds the possible ability to detect cross-reacting V_κ is a major problem in the interpretation of the hybridization data. The case of the mouse V_λ sequences, however, presents on face value a much more straightforward situation. Nineteen mouse λ chains have been sequenced; from these, 12 have identical V-region sequences, while the others have maximally 4 amino acid replacements (Cesari and Weigert, 1973) and 8 replacements in a rather special case (Schulenburg *et al.*, 1971, and Fig. 1). Furthermore, the changes are clustered in the hypervariable regions in a manner similar to the V_κ sequences. Thus far, there are 8 different sequences known for V_λ chains. Since all 8 have been detected among 19 randomly chosen λ chains, however, it is likely that other variants will be found as more proteins are investigated. A strict germ-line theory of their origin would require a minimum of 8 V_λ genes and probably considerably more. Our estimates of cross-hybridization of heterologous sequences (see Section IID1) indicate that (1) all the V_λ sequences thus far seen should cross-hybridize efficiently, and (2) the rate of hybridization of the different V_λ genes with a radioactive V_λ probe should be similar to the homologous sequence. Thus, hybridization kinetics of V_λ sequences should give a direct answer to the question of whether there are more or less V_λ-genes than V_λ protein sequences. Two such studies have been made (Leder *et al.*, 1975; Tonegawa, 1976). The former study involved the use of cDNA made against RPC 20 mRNA (from a tumor producing a λ chain with a single amino acid change from the major group of λ chains); this cDNA had an average length of 830 nucleotides, and thus most of the molecules would contain some V-region sequence. The hybridization of this cDNA to mouse tumor and spleen DNA (hybrid formation was assayed by S_1 nuclease) gave values consistent with 2 copies per haploid genome when compared with the hybridization of globin cDNA. Thus, it was concluded that the C_λ and V_λ sequences were represented 1 or 2 times per genome (Leder *et al.*, 1975).

This result seems to be incompatible with the expectation of at least 8 germ-line V_λ genes required by a strict germ-line theory. The conclusion depends, however, on the amount of V_λ sequences present in the cDNA population used in the experiments. If the λ-mRNA is 90% pure, 830 bases will contain around 30% V-region complementary sequence (this calculation assumes a λ-mRNA structure similar to the MOPC 21 κ chain; see Fig. 2). Since the maximum amplitude of the *Cot* curve (effective protection at the high *Cot* end point) given for this cDNA is about 70%, the actual effect of the V region is only about 20%. At such a level, it is rather difficult to confidently exclude the possibility that such a small proportion is not hybridizing with, for example, 10 genes (see below).

Support for the very limited number of V_λ genes comes from experiments with iodinated mRNA (Tonegawa, 1976). In this case, MOPC 104E λ-mRNA hybridized with mouse liver DNA with a single kinetic transition more or less indistinguishable from that of mouse globin mRNA (Fig. 9), giving a nominal reiteration frequency of 2 or 3. Although no independent measure of the purity of the mRNA has been made, the procedure for its preparation and the simple kinetics argue for a reliable preparation, although the author's estimate of 90% purity may be an overestimate. Figure 9 (see also Fig. 7) illustrates some of the difficulties discussed for the accurate interpretation of otherwise excellent experimental data (i.e., that the difference between the three theoretical curves is not substantially different from the actual experimental points). All these numerological arguments should not, however, overshadow the significance of the coincidence between the two sets of data (globin and L-chain mRNAs).

A more detailed analysis of the λ-mRNA hybridization was also carried out by competition hybridization (Tonegawa, 1976). In these experiments, λ-chain

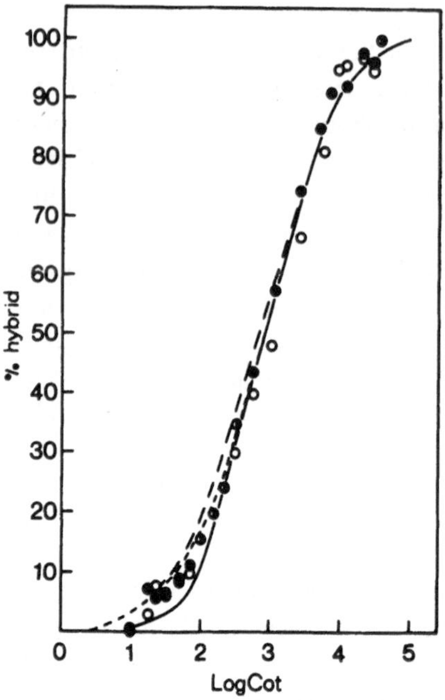

Figure 9. Kinetics of hybridization of λ-chain mRNA and globin mRNA to mouse liver DNA. (○) Mouse globin ^{125}I-mRNA; (●) M104 λ-chain ^{125}I-mRNA. The experimental points taken from Tonegawa (1976) have been normalized to 100%. The solid line is a theoretical second-order kinetic curve derived for an RNA with a repetition frequency N (around 1–4 genes). The two dashed lines are theoretical curves due to mixtures of RNAs with repetition frequency 10 N and N in the proportions of 25–75%. (short dashes) and 45–55% (long dashes). The V gene of a 100% pure light chain constitutes around 30–45% of the non-poly(A) stretch (see Fig. 2).

[^{125}I] mRNA from MOPC 104E was in competition with unlabeled 104E and unlabeled H 2020 λ-mRNA. The data showed virtually no difference in the ability of the two RNA species to compete out the radioactive mRNA, indicating complete cross-hybridization of the two mRNA types. Such cross-hybridization confirms the gene numbers obtained by the kinetic experiment (i.e., 2 or 3). Once again, the detectable V_λ genes appear to be lower in number than the described λ chains.

III. CONCLUSIONS

The hybridization data discussed in this article may be summarized as follows:

1. cDNA copies of mouse C_κ regions of a number of different mRNA species have been shown to hybridize with 1–5 genes per haploid genome.
2. The detected reiteration frequency of the V_κ gene of MOPC 21, MOPC 321, and MOPC 41 is similar to the respective C_κ portion. Those V genes therefore appear to be repeated at most a few times in the haploid genome.
3. The presence of a highly reiterated component detected in earlier studies has been associated with impurities of the mRNA preparations.

4. Hybridization of mouse λ-mRNA and cDNA thereof indicated a limited number of V_λ and C_λ genes.
5. Control hybridization experiments indicate our ability to detect cross-hybridization (in standard hybridization conditions) of sequences that differ by at least 30–45 bases per 100 amino acid residues.

The results discussed in this chapter throw light on the number of genes coding for V-region subgroups, and so far, there is no reason to believe that the total number of genes is significantly greater than the total number of subgroups derived by protein sequence studies. It follows that in cases in which a low number of subgroups have been defined by protein chemistry data, the total number of genes should be low. Since cross-hybridization within a subgroup is to be expected, reliable data on the mouse and human heavy chains, as well as the human κ chain, may provide further clues on this problem.

The data as a whole have relevance to the problem of the origin of antibody diversity, because they strongly suggest that the number of V-region sequences that we can detect by hybridization is lower than the number of amino acid sequences predicted or found by studies of myeloma proteins. Although this conclusion is not totally free of uncertainties and difficulties (as discussed above), it implies that somatic processes contribute to immunoglobulin (and hence antibody) diversity. The present state of the hybridization experiments indicates that the extent of this contribution is likely to be significant.

Somatic mutation bridges the gap between the number of genes and the number of chains required for optimum diversity. The magnitude of this gap is unknown, but is likely to depend on the evolutionary equilibrium among a number of variables (C. Milstein and Munro, 1973). The origin of the antibody diversity will eventually be defined by quantitative evaluation of these variables in each species. The total number of germ-line genes is the most obvious parameter, and molecular hybridization is the method of choice to define it. A measure of the total gene pool is not an easy task, but there are indications that estimates of this type are not impossible. It would emerge from the accumulation of hybridization data on all the subgroups and in different species. More interesting, methods might be developed for such measurements by making use of cross-hybridization techniques. Our ability to detect cross-hybridization among sequences as diverse as the C regions of human, rabbit, and mouse is encouraging in this respect.

IV. REFERENCES

Amzel, L., Poljak, R., Saul, F., Varga, J., and Richards, F., 1974, *Proc. Nat. Acad. Sci. U.S.A.* **71**:1427.
Baglioni, C., Alexio-Zonta, L., Cioli, D., and Carbonara, A., 1966, *Science* **152**:1519.
Bernardini, A., and Tonegawa, S., 1974, *FEBS Lett.* **41**:73.

Bishop, J.O., 1972, *Biochem. J.* **126**:171.

Bonner, T.I., Brenner, D.J., Neufeld, B.R., and Britten, R.J., 1973, *J. Mol. Biol.* **81**:123.

Britten, R.J., and Kohne, D.E., 1968, *Science* **161**:529.

Brownlee, G.G., Cartwright, E.M., Cowan, N.J., Jarvis, J.M., and Milstein, C., 1973, *Nature (London) New Biol.* **244**:236.

Cesari, I.M., and Weigert, M., 1973, *Proc. Nat. Acad. Sci. U.S.A.* **70**:2112.

Cohn, M., Blomberg, B., Geckeler, W., Raschke, W., Riblet, R, and Weigert, M., 1974, in: *The Immune System* (E.E. Sercaz, A.R. Williamson, and C.F. Fox, eds.), Academic Press, New York and London, p. 89.

Cotton, R.G.H., and Milstein, C., 1973, *Nature (London)* **244**:42.

Cowan, N.J., and Milstein, C., 1973, *Eur. J. Biochem.* **36**:1.

Cowan, N.J., Secher, D.S., and Milstein, C., 1976, *Eur. J. Biochem.* **61**:355.

Delovitch, T., and Baglioni, C., 1973, *Cold Spring Harbor Symp. Quant. Biol.* **38**:739.

Dreyer, W.J., and Bennett, J.C., 1965, *Proc. Nat. Acad. Sci. U.S.A.* **54**:864.

Farace, M.G., Aellen, M.F., Briand, P.A., Faust, C.H., Vassalli, P., and Mach, B., 1976, *Proc. Nat. Acad. Sci. U.S.A.* **73**:727.

Faust, C.H., Diggelman, H., and Mach, B., 1974, *Proc. Nat. Acad. Sci. U.S.A.* **71**:2491.

Gally, J.A., 1973, in: *The Antigens* (M. Sela, ed.), Vol. 1, Academic Press, New York and London, p. 283.

Gould, H.J., and Hamlyn, P.H., 1973, *FEBS Lett.* **30**:301.

Gummerson, K.S., and Williamson, R., 1974, *Nature (London)* **247**:265.

Harrison, P.R., Hell, A., Birnie, G.D., and Paul, J., 1972, *Nature (London)* **239**:219.

Harrison, P.R., Birnie, G.D., Hell, A., Humphries, S., Young, B.D., and Paul, J., 1974, *J. Mol. Biol.* **84**:539.

Harrison, T.M., Brownlee, G.G., and Milstein, C., 1974, *Eur. J. Biochem.* **47**:621.

Honjo, T., Packman, S., Swan, D., Nau, M., and Leder, P., 1974, *Proc. Nat. Acad. Sci. U.S.A.* **71**:3659.

Hood, L., McKean, D., Farnsworth, V., and Potter, M., 1973, *Biochemistry* **12**:741.

Inman, J., 1974, in: *The Immune System* (E.E. Sercaz, A.A. Williamson, and C.F. Fox, eds.), Academic Press, New York and London, p. 37.

Köhler, G., and Milstein, C., 1975, *Nature (London)* **256**:495.

Leder, P., Ross, J., Gielen, J., Packman, S., Ikawa, Y., Aviv, H., and Swan, D., 1973, *Cold Spring Harbor Symp. Quant. Biol.* **38**:753.

Leder, P., Honjo, T., Packman, S., Swan, D., Nau, M., and Norman, B., 1974, *Proc. Nat. Acad. Sci. U.S.A.* **71**:5109.

Leder, P., Honjo, T., Swan, D., Packman, S., Nau, M., and Norman, B., 1975, in: *Molecular Approaches to Immunology* (E.E. Smith and D.S. Ribbons, eds.), Academic Press, New York and London. p. 173.

Mach, B., Faust, C.H., and Vassalli, P., 1973, *Proc. Nat. Acad. Sci. U.S.A.* **70**:451.

McCarthy, B.J., and Farquhar, M.N., 1972, in: *Evolution of Genetic Systems Brookhaven Symp. Biol.*, No. 23, p. 1, Gordon & Breach, New York.

McKean, D., Potter, M., and Hood, L., 1973, *Biochemistry* **12**:760.

Milstein, C., 1966, *Biochem. J.* **101**:338.

Milstein, C., 1969, *FEBS Lett.* **2**:301.

Milstein, C., and Munro, A. J., 1973, in: *Defence and Recognition* (R.R. Porter, ed.), International Review of Science, Butterworth, London, p. 199.

Milstein, C., and Pink, J.R.L., 1970, in: *Progress in Biophysics and Molecular Biology*, J.A.V. Butler and D. Noble, eds.), Vol. 21, Pergamon Press, Oxford and New York, p. 209.

Milstein, C., Brownlee, G.G., Cartwright, E.M., Jarvis, J.M., and Proudfoot, N.J., 1974, *Nature (London)* **252**:354.
Milstein, C., Adetugbo, K., Cowan, N.J. Kohler, G., Secher, D.S., and Wilde, C.D., 1976, *Cold Spring Harbor Symp. Quant. Biol.*, in press.
Milstein, Celia P., 1973, *FEBS Lett.* **30**:40.
Milstein, Celia P., Steinberg, A.G., McLaughlin, C., and Solomon, A., 1974, *Nature (London)* **248**:160.
Porter, R.R., 1973, in: *Defence and Recognition* (R. R. Porter, ed.), Vol. 10, International Review of Science, Butterworth, London, p. 158.
Premkumar, E., Shoyab, M., and Williamson, A.R., 1974, *Proc. Nat. Acad. Sci. U.S.A.* **71**:99.
Proudfoot, N.J., and Brownlee, G.C., 1976, *Nature* **263**:211.
Rabbitts, T.H., 1974, *FEBS Lett.* **42**:323.
Rabbitts, T.H., and Milstein, C., 1975a, *Eur. J. Biochem.* **52**:125.
Rabbitts, T.H., and Milstein, C., 1975b, *Trans. Biochem. Soc.* **3**:870.
Rabbitts, T.H., Bishop, J.O., Milstein, C., and Brownlee, G.G., 1974a, *FEBS Lett.* **40**:157.
Rabbitts, T.H., Milstein, C., and Brownlee, G.G., 1974b, *Symp. 9th Meeting Fed. Eur. Biochem. Soc.*, p. 141.
Rabbitts, T.H., Jarvis, J.M., and Milstein, C., 1975, *Cell* **6**:5.
Richards, F., Konigsberg, W., Rosenstein, R., and Varga, J., 1975, *Science* **187**:130.
Ritter, H., Ropartz, C., Rousseau, P.Y., Rivat, L., and Walker, H., 1966, *Blut* **13**:373.
Ross, J., Gielen, J., Packman, S., Ikawa, Y., and Leder, P., 1974, *J. Mol. Biol.* **87**:697.
Schechter, I., 1974, *Biochemistry* **13**:1875.
Schechter, I., 1975, *Proc. Nat. Acad. Sci. U.S.A.* **72**:2511.
Schiff, C., and Fougereau, M., 1975, *Eur. J. Biochem.* **59**:525.
Schulenburg, E., Simms, E., Lynch, R., Bradshaw, R., and Eisen, H., 1971, *Proc. Nat. Acad. Sci. U.S.A.* **70**:2112.
Smith, G.P., 1973, *Science* **181**:941.
Starace, V., and Querinjean, P., 1975, *J. Immunol.* **115**:59.
Stavnezer, J., and Huang, R.-C.C., 1971, *Nature (London) New Biol.* **230**:172.
Stavnezer, J., Huang, R.-C.C., Stavnezer, E., and Bishop, J.M., 1974, *J. Mol. Biol.* **88**:43.
Stevens, R.H., and Williamson, A.R., 1973, *J. Mol. Biol.* **78**:517.
Stevens, R.H., and Williamson, A.R., 1975, *Proc. Nat. Acad. Sci. U.S.A.* **72**:467.
Storb, U., 1974, *Biochem. Biophys. Res. Commun.* **57**:31.
Sutton, W.D., 1971, *Biochim. Biophys. Acta* **240**:522.
Tonegawa, S., 1976, *Proc. Nat. Acad. Sci. U.S.A.* **73**:203.
Tonegawa, S., and Hozumi, N., 1976, in press.
Tonegawa, S., Bernardini, A., Weimann, B.J., and Steinberg, C., 1974a, *FEBS Lett.* **40**:92.
Tonegawa, S., Steinberg, C., Dube, S., and Bernardini, A., 1974b, *Proc. Nat. Acad. Sci. U.S.A.* **71**:4027.
Ullman, J.S., and McCarthy, B.J., 1973, *Biochim. Biophys. Acta* **294**:416.
Wu, T., and Kabat, E., 1970, *J. Exp. Med.* **132**:211.

Complement Receptors

Celso Bianco

The Rockefeller University
New York, New York 10021

and

Victor Nussenzweig

Department of Pathology, New York University School of Medicine
New York, New York 10016

I. INTRODUCTION AND HISTORICAL BACKGROUND*

In the beginning of this century, it was noted by many investigators that in the presence of immune serum, protozoa, bacteria, and other particles adhered to leukocytes and platelets, both *in vivo* and *in vitro* (reviewed by D.S. Nelson, 1963). This attachment of parasites promoted their clearance from the blood and was part of the mechanism of defense against infection. Progress in the understanding of these observations was very slow and controversial, however, probably because several different phenomena were involved, in which antibody and complement participated in varying degrees.

In 1953, R.A. Nelson observed the adherence of microorganisms sensitized with antibody and complement to human erythrocytes, and coined the

*Abbreviations in this chapter: (AMCC) antibody-mediated cell cytotoxicity; (C1–4) complement components 1–4; (factors P, B, and D) complement components of the alternative pathway; (CRI and II) complement receptors I and II; (CRL) complement-receptor lymphocytes; (E) sheep erythrocytes; (EA) sheep erythrocytes coated with rabbit antibodies of undetermined class; (EAC) sheep erythrocytes coated with antibody and complement; (EIgG, EIgM) sheep erythrocytes coated with IgG or IgM; (CRA) complement-mediated complex-release activity; (CoF) cobra venom factor; (LPS) lipopolysaccharide.

term *immune-adherence* to describe the phenomenon. In a series of classic studies, R.A. Nelson, M. Siqueira, D.S. Nelson, K. Nishioka, and others clarified the mechanism of this reaction (D.S. Nelson, 1963). They established the criteria for distinguishing immune adherence from other adherence and hemagglutination reactions, developed convenient methods for detecting immune adherence, and showed that particle-bound C3 was probably the ligand involved in the reaction. In these studies, primate erythrocytes and nonprimate platelets were used as indicator particles. Although a few observations suggested that immune-adherence receptors were present on other leukocytes, and could play a role in resistance to infection and in the promotion of phagocytosis, immune adherence nonetheless remained for many years mostly a convenient tool for measuring complement-fixation and detecting small amounts of antibody and antigen.

It was only in 1968 that it was independently established in three different laboratories that C3 receptors were also present on the plasma membrane of leukocytes.

Lay and Nussenzweig (1968) used a different method to detect immune adherence: rosette or cluster formation between sensitized particles and leukocytes. This powerful and simple technique permitted the identification of complement receptors, and also of receptors for the Fc portion of IgG at the level of single cells. In contrast, the most commonly used methods were based on hemagglutination, which detected the presence or absence of immune-adherence receptors only at the level of cell populations. Through the systematic use of the rosette method, with EA or EAC as particles, Lay and Nussenzweig found receptor sites for C3 on the plasma membrane of mouse macrophages, PMNs, monocytes, and in a subpopulation of lymphocytes from the spleen and lymph nodes. Their findings also suggested that the role of C3 receptors in phagocytosis was to promote adherence of the particle to the phagocytes, rather than to trigger the ingestion process (Lay and Nussenzweig, 1969). Further studies by Bianco *et al.* (1970) and Eden *et al.* (1971, 1973b), using the same approach and techniques, showed that B lymphocytes bear complement receptors, and provided direct evidence that C3b was the ligand involved. The key observations were that rosette formation between lymphocytes and EAC depended on the amount of C3 used to prepare EAC, and that cluster formation was inhibited and reversed by antibodies to C3, and by C3b itself.

Also in 1968, Gigli and Nelson studied the role of complement in the engulfment of sensitized erythrocytes by neutrophils and monocytes. They showed that the presence of C4 and C3 on E was required both for immune adherence and immune phagocytosis by guinea pig leukocytes. C1 and C2 could be removed from the erythrocytes without changing their reactivity. The binding of the late complement components (C5-8) did not enhance ingestion of sensitized erythrocytes, nor influence immune adherence. Most important, they treated the red cells with the enzyme C3b-inactivator, which cleaves C3b into two fragments (C3c and C3d), one of which (C3d) remains on the red cell. After treatment, neither immune adherence nor immune phagocytosis took place. This finding was interpreted as indicating that only a portion of C3 (C3c) provided the opsonic signal. As discussed in Section IVB, it is probable that the ingestion of EAC observed by Gigli and Nelson was actually mediated by the IgG antibodies bound to the erythrocytes, rather than by C3b itself.

Results similar to those of Gigli and Nelson were also reported by Huber *et al.* (1968), using as target cells monolayers of human monocytes. They made the important observation that IgG and C3 had synergistic effects on phagocytosis.

Interest in complement receptors has grown considerably in recent years. Perhaps the most important reason was the demonstration that they were a marker for B lymphocytes (Bianco *et al.*, 1970; Bianco and Nussenzweig, 1971). This finding and other observations (Pepys, 1972) suggested that complement receptors played a role in the immune response, and participated in the regulation of interaction among lymphocytes, macrophages, and complement-containing immune aggregates. An additional level of complexity for the understanding of the physiological function of complement receptors was added with the finding that C4b (Bokisch and Sobel, 1974; Ross and Polley, 1975) and two regions of C3 (C3c and C3d) could be independently recognized by leukocytes (Okada and Nishioka, 1973; Eden *et al.*, 1973c; Ross *et al.*, 1973).

Another reason for the increasing interest in this area was that the rosette techniques constituted the basis for the development of new methods for the isolation and depletion of cell populations (Bianco *et al.*, 1970), as well as for identification of cells in tissue sections (Dukor *et al.*, 1970).

In this review, we will deal with some aspects of C3-complement receptor interaction. We have not attempted to cover the literature, but only to discuss work performed in recent years, particularly in areas related to our own research. For more background, we recommend other reviews (Shevach *et al.*, 1973; Nussenzweig, 1974; Bianco, 1976).

II. THE LIGAND

C3 consists of two polypeptide chains (α and β) of mol. wt. 120,000 and 70,000, linked by disulfide bonds (Bokisch *et al.*, 1975). It is quantitatively and functionally the most important of the components of the complement system. Its concentration in serum is between 1 and 2 g/liter, which is close to the amount of all other complement components from the classical and alternative pathways combined. Complement receptors of leukocytes bind split products of C3 (C3b, C3c, and C3d) and C4 (C4b), which are incorporated into immune complexes after interaction with the complement system. Most studies on the generation of these C3 peptides and their association with immune complexes have been performed with particulate antigens. They have been the subject of many reviews (e.g., Müller-Eberhard, 1975), and for this reason will be dealt with here only very briefly. In contrast, the mechanisms of generation of *soluble* complexes containing C3, although probably also of direct relevance to several areas of basic immunology and immunopathology, have been largely ignored. This subject will be discussed in somewhat greater detail. A more comprehensive review has been published elsewhere (Takahashi *et al.*, 1976).

A. Interaction of Complexes Prepared with Soluble Antigens with the Complement System

Miller and one of us (Miller and Nussenzweig, 1975) recently observed that the complement system has a remarkable effect on Ag–Ab aggregates. When immune-precipitates are treated with fresh serum, high-molecular-weight soluble complexes containing Ag, Ab, C3, C4, and other complement components are released into the medium. Using a simple assay (CRA), it was possible to gain insight into the events leading to the incorporation of C3 onto the complexes. The experimental system consisted of incubating fresh serum at 37°C with washed precipitates. Either the Ag or Ab was radioiodinated, and CRA was measured kinetically. As shown in Fig. 1, in a few minutes, most of the radioactivity was released from the precipitate and appeared in the supernatant. In control tubes, in which complement activity had been destroyed, most counts remained in the pellet.

Solubilization of immune aggregates occurred in all Ag–Ab systems tested, with polysaccharides or proteins as antigens, and with 7 S or 19 S antibodies from rabbits or mice. However, the *rate* of solubilization varied considerably in the different Ag–Ab systems. One of the parameters that affected the rate of solubilization was the affinity of the Ab for the Ag in the precipitate. Solubilization proceeded faster with Ab of low affinity (Czop and Nussenzweig, 1976).

CRA is mediated by the complement system. It occurs at 37°C, but not at 25°C. C3b has a central role in CRA as an effector molecule, and also probably as part of the enzyme (C3-convertase) that catalyzes C3 conversion and generation of C3b. In Fig. 2, we present our concept of the process of solubilization (Takahashi *et al.*, 1976). It is based on the results of recent experiments performed in our laboratory and on current ideas on the mechanism of activation of the alternative pathway.

Solubilization can occur in two ways: exclusively through the alternative pathway, or through the combined activity of the classical and alternative pathways. Under conditions in which only the alternative pathway operates—e.g., in the absence of Ca^{2+}, or if C2- or C4-deficient sera are used—the process is slower and much less efficient.

The essential feature of CRA is the generation of a properdin- and factor

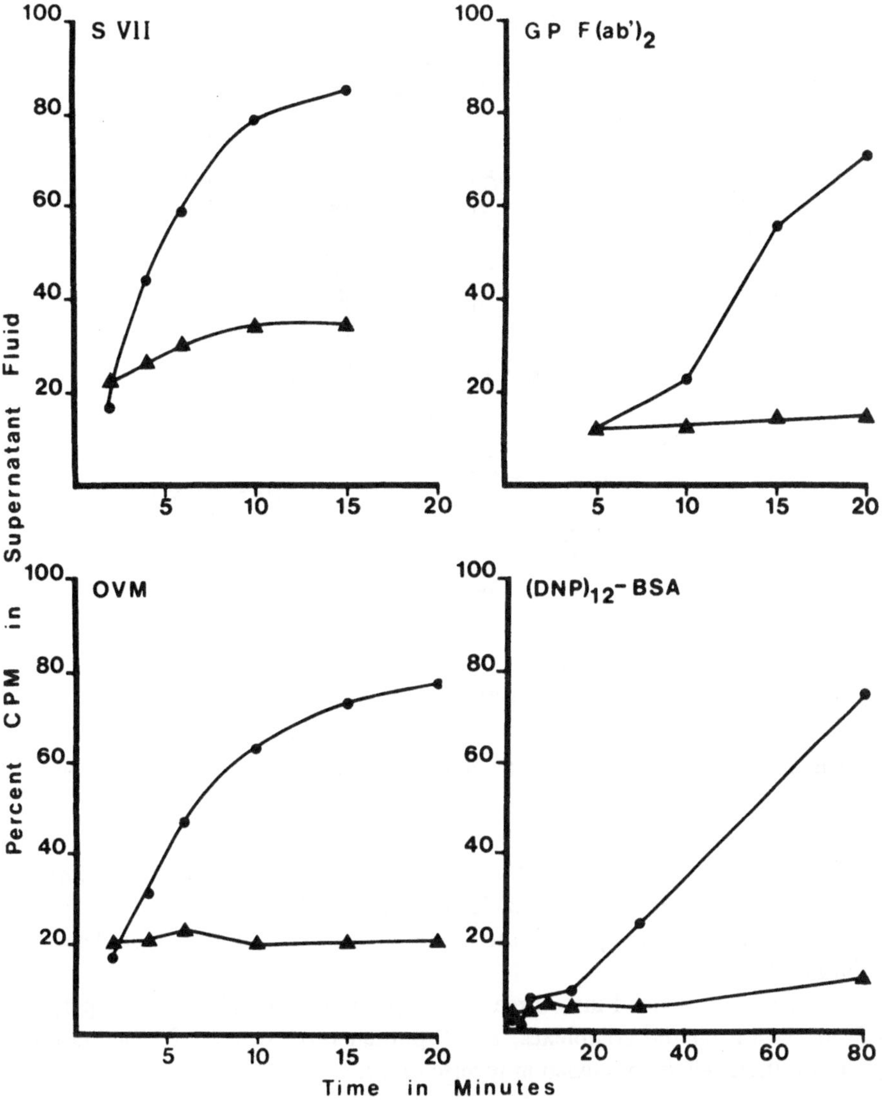

Figure 1. Immune precipitates prepared at equivalence. Antibodies to BSA, guinea-pig $F(ab')_2$ fragments, pneumococcal polysaccharide type VII, and dinitrophenylated (DNP)-BSA were obtained from rabbit antisera. Antibodies to ovomucoid were derived from mice. Either the antigen or the antibodies were radiolabeled. The immune precipitates were incubated with 300 μl of a 1:2 dilution of fresh rabbit or mouse serum as a source of complement. Samples (50 μl) were withdrawn at certain time intervals, diluted with 250 μl cold saline, and centrifuged at 1200g at 4°C for 10 min. Both pellets and supernatant fluids were counted in a gamma counter. Results are expressed as the percentage of total counts per minute found in the supernatant fluids. Controls consisted of the same complexes incubated in serum heated at 56°C for 30 min. Notice that the kinetics of solubilization vary in different systems. Also, the absolute amount of complexes that can be solubilized by a given volume of serum is quite variable (Czop and Nussenzweig, 1976).

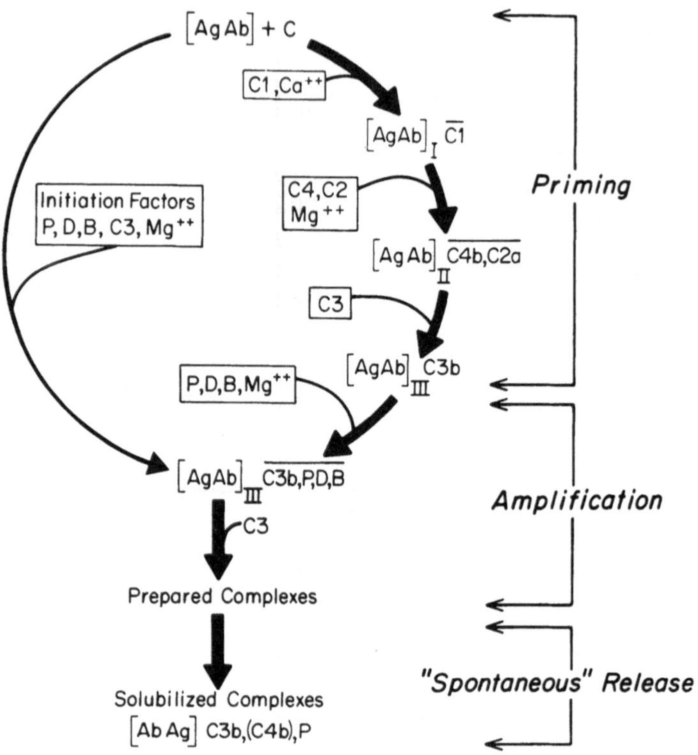

Figure 2. Proposed mechanism of solubilization of immune complexes by complement.

B-dependent C3-convertase *on* the complexes. When this immune complex-associated enzyme reacts with C3, large amounts of C3 (probably C3b) are incorporated into the complexes, the lattice is disrupted, and the complexes are solubilized.

CRA can be divided into three stages: priming, assembly of a B-dependent C3-convertase on the complexes, and "spontaneous" release. To facilitate exposition, these will be discussed in reverse order.

1. "Spontaneous" Release

During solubilization, several intermediates can be generated by treatment of immune complexes with fresh serum at 37°C for limited periods of time. One of the end products ("prepared complexes"), containing large amounts of C3, could be isolated from serum and quantitatively solubilized in salt solutions at 37 or 25°C. Therefore, some further rearrangements of the lattice, subsequent to the binding of complement to the complexes, must take place. This "spontaneous" release occurs in the absence of Ca^{2+}, Mg^{2+}, or complement components in the fluid phase.

Binding of C3 (C3b) to the immune precipitate is very rapid. After 5 min of incubation at 37°C, the immune precipitate may contain 1 or 2 molecules of C3 per molecule of antibody. A large proportion of C3 is very closely associated with the IgG. The bonds between C3 peptides and IgG could not be disrupted after incubation of the Ag-Ab-C3 precipitates in 1% SDS containing 8 M urea at 56°C for 1 hr. High-molecular-weight aggregates of C3 and Ab were detected by electrophoresis in 5% acrylamide gels. After complete reduction, and in the presence of 8 M urea, the aggregates were resolved into their components. We found that the α chain of C3 had been degraded into peptides smaller than 70,000, while the β chain appeared to be largely intact. It is likely that the cleavage of the α chain was caused by C3b-inactivator and other serum proteases (Takahashi *et al.*, 1976).

Interestingly, although the solubilized complexes contain very large amounts of C3, they have a very low affinity for cells with complement receptors (Miller *et al.*, 1973). The reason is not clear. One explanation is that the C3-complement receptor interaction is very weak, and can be observed only after multiple cooperative binding. The number of C3 molecules on each separate soluble immune aggregate may not be great enough to bind to the cells in a stable manner. Alternatively, the C3 molecule moieties on the complexes may have been modified or may be sterically hindered by the Ag, Ab, or other components of the complement system. In any case, this is an important point that is relevant to the fate of these complexes *in vivo*, and should be further investigated.

2. Assembly of the C3-Convertase

The stage preceding the formation of the "prepared" complexes, which can be "spontaneously" solubilized, consists in the assembly of a C3-convertase *on* the complexes, followed by its interaction with C3. This C3-convertase is factor B-dependent, since its enzymatic activity can be quantitatively inhibited by treating the intermediate with an antiserum to factor B. This finding is in agreement with the observation that the solubilization of immune complexes is strictly dependent on factors P, B, and D, C3, and Mg^{2+}, and does not occur in serum lacking any one of these factors. On the other hand, the deletion of components of the classical pathway (C1, C4, C2, or Ca^{2+}) only slows down the reaction. The reason solubilization cannot take place, or is extremely inefficient, through the classical pathway alone may be the presence of limiting amounts of C2 normally found in serum. Perhaps the number of $C\overline{1,4,2}$ sites generated on the complexes is very small as compared with the number of $\overline{C3b,B}$ sites. Alternatively, the special arrangements of these different convertases on the complexes may not be the same.

3. *Priming*

CRA results from the interaction of complex-bound $\overline{C3b,B}$ with C3. As mentioned, the assembly of this enzyme is influenced by the classical pathway. Comparing the kinetics of CRA in the presence and in the absence of the classical pathway components, it became clear that when C1, C4, C2, or Ca^{2+} was not present, a much longer lag phase was observed. In many experiments, after this initial delay, the rate of the reaction in the presence or absence of the classical complement components was identical. For this reason, we suggest in Fig. 2 that the main role of the classical pathway is to initiate the reaction in an efficient way. It is possible that through the interaction of $C\overline{1,4,2}$, with C3, some C3b molecules are deposited onto the aggregate. These C3b molecules could serve as nuclei for assembly of the $\overline{B}$-dependent C3-convertase. The ensuing reaction with more C3 would lead to more deposition of C3b in neighboring sites, and the expansion of this process would lead to solubilization.

In short, solubilization of Ag–Ab aggregates is a *combined* function of the properdin and classical pathways. C3b plays a key role in the reaction, both in the assembly of the C3-convertase and in causing the rearrangement of the lattice. After further reaction with serum, the α chain of the immune complex-bound C3b is split. The products that remain associated with the aggregate have not yet been characterized. It is not known whether some fragments of C3 are released into the medium, or whether all portions of the split molecule remain associated with each other and with the Ag–Ab.

B. Interaction of Particulate Immune Complexes with the Complement System

When erythrocytes bearing $C\overline{1,4,2}$ on their membranes interact with C3, several events can be distinguished. C3 is broken down into two peptides, C3a (mol. wt. 9000) and C3b (mol. wt. 180,000). The C3b molecules either bind to the surface of the red cell or remain in the fluid phase and are hemolytically inactive. The mechanism of binding of nascent C3b to the membrane of the cell (or to the immune complexes) is not known. It is generally assumed that the bonds between C3b and the substrate are hydrophobic, and that molecules of different nature can serve as acceptors. Among the C3b molecules that bind to the surface of the cell, only a few participate in the generation of C5-convertase, the function of which is to cleave C5 and thus continue the process leading to the lysis of the cell. Most of the nascent C3b molecules are fixed onto the cell membrane around the C3 and C5-convertase site (reviewed in Müller-Eberhard, 1975).

Cells bearing C3b are positive in immune adherence. Tamura and Nelson (1967) and Ruddy and Austen (1969) described an enzyme in serum, C3b-inactivator, that blocks the immune-adherence property of C3b-bearing erythrocytes. This enzyme was later found to be identical to the conglutinogen-activating factor (KAF) described by Lachmann and his collaborators (Lachmann and Müller-Eberhard, 1968).

The mode of action of C3b-inactivator is not entirely clear. When it interacts with cell-bound C3b, a large fragment (mol. wt. 140,000) is released that has the characteristics of C3c or of β1A found in aged serum. The small portion of C3 remaining on the cell surface antigenically resembles the C3d fragment of aged serum, or serum treated with CoF. However, there is no direct evidence that they are identical. Gitlin *et al.* (1975) recently reported that the reaction *in the fluid phase* between C3b and C3b-inactivator takes place in two steps. The first cleavage of C3b is completed in a few minutes, generating a peptide of molecular weight 155,000. This fragment, designated $C3b^i$, is further degraded by other serum enzymes, and the final product resembles C3c (mol. wt. 140,000). Several questions remain unanswered. For example, during which step of enzymatic activity is C3d generated? Also, it is not clear what the relationship is between these events and those that take place following the interaction of *cell-bound* C3b with C3b-inactivator, i.e., which of the small peptides remains associated with the cell surface.

III. COMPLEMENT RECEPTORS

A. Definitions

For the purpose of this review, complement receptors will be operationally defined as plasma membrane structures that are able to interact specifically with a fragment of C3 or C4 in a reversible manner. This definition excludes the many binding sites present on cell walls and cell membranes to which C3 and other complement components bind sequentially after activation. This nonspecific interaction with a short-lived C3 site may be very strong and resist treatment with 8 M urea, 6 M guanidine, 1% 2-mercaptoethanol, high concentrations of salt, and some detergents (Stossel *et al.*, 1975). Erythrocytes from certain species (e.g., sheep) have no complement receptors, but bind C3 during complement fixation. They are excellent indicators in rosette assays, carrying fragments of C3 firmly attached to their membrane and exposing various regions of the molecule.

The existence of two types of plasma membrane receptors for C3, CRI and CRII, is well documented.

CRI (also called *b* receptors) correspond to the "immune-adherence" receptors of erythrocytes from humans and primates and of platelets of other mammals.

They bind C4b, and C3b generated by the classical or by the alternative pathway of C fixation. Further cleavage of red cell-bound C3b by the C3b-inactivator abolishes binding to CRI of the red cell now bearing only C3d.

The initial studies on immune adherence always focused on C3. Cooper (1969) demonstrated, however, that EAC4b are also immune-adherence positive. The minimum number of molecules of C3b or of C4b attached to indicator particles necessary for immune adherence to occur is about the same (Bokisch and Sobel, 1974). C4b is also cleaved by a serum enzyme that may be identical to C3b-inactivator to a form that is inactive in immune adherence (Cooper, 1975). C3b, C3c, and C4b added in the fluid phase can inhibit the binding of EIgMC3b to the CRI receptor. C3d is not inhibitory. These findings suggest that the ligand that interacts with CRI is C3c or C4b, and that these two complement peptides may be structurally related (Ross and Polley, 1975).

CRII (also called *d* receptor) is specific for the C3d fragment of C3. Both EIgMC3b and EIgMC3d bind to this receptor. Therefore, the C3d portion of C3 that combines with CRII is at least partially exposed in C3b. Binding to the CRII can be inhibited by fluid-phase C3b and C3d.

B. Detection

Many methods for the detection of complement receptors have been developed in recent years. However, most of the background work that established their properties utilized the rosette assay, in which erythrocytes coated with several complement components and fragments are mixed with the cell population being tested. The typical rosettes are scored under the microscope. The test is very simple, and the diversity of reagents available allows the preparation of various red cell intermediates. Methods for preparation of reagents to detect complement receptors are described elsewhere (Bloom and David, 1976).

Table I describes the various forms of immune complexes and their abilities to bind to CRI or CRII receptors. EAC can be prepared either with purified complement components or with whole serum as a source of complement. In the latter case, conversion of C3b to C3d is decreased by shortening the incubation periods with serum and by the use of Suramin, a drug that inhibits the action of the C3b-inactivator (Lachmann *et al.*, 1972). On the other hand, complexes prepared with purified complement components, in the absence of C3b-inactivator, will contain only C4b or C3b.

The reaction between complement receptors and C3 components frequently occurs across species. One notable exception is that EAC prepared with human complement does not provide a reliable reagent to detect complement receptors of mouse leukocytes (Bianco *et al.*, 1970).

Other methods for the detection of complement receptors have been devel-

Table I. Binding Characteristics of Various Immune Complexes

Red cell intermediates	Source of complement	Binding to receptor type: CRI	CRII
EIgG		–	–
EIgM		–	–
EIgMC3b	Mouse, C5-deficient, short incubation, Suramin	+	+
EIgMC3d	As above, long incubation	–	+
EIgMC14	Purified, human	+	–
EIgMC1423b	As above	+	+
EIgMC1423d	As above, followed by C3b inactivator	–	+

oped: (1) Radiolabeled soluble immune complexes containing C3 (Eden *et al.*, 1973a) are incubated with the cells, and the amount of cell-associated radioactivity is determined. (2) Soluble fragments of C3 are incubated with the cell population under study. Their binding to complement receptors is detected either by radiolabeling C3 (Theophilopoulos *et al.*, 1974a) or by the addition of fluoresceinated antiserum to C3 (Ross and Polley, 1975). (3) Indicator particles other than erythrocytes can also be used. Zymosan particles (Mendes *et al.*, 1974; C. Huber and H. Wigzell, 1975), and fluoresceinated *Salmonella typhi* incubated with human serum as a source of complement (J.A. Gelfand *et al.*, 1976), have also been successfully used for the identification of cells bearing complement receptors. The sensitivity of these methods varies widely. The availability of fluoresceinated reagents has allowed the use of automated systems for the quantitation of complement receptor–bearing cells.

Anatomical areas containing cells with complement receptors can also be identified *in situ*. Frozen sections of lymphoid tissues will bind complement-coated erythrocytes, permitting the histological identification of B areas in lymphoid organs of mice (Dukor *et al.*, 1970) and in human patients (Shevach *et al.*, 1973).

C. Distribution

Table II shows the distribution of complement receptors among cells of mammals. To our knowledge, no studies have yet been performed with cells from

Table II. Distribution of Complement Receptors Among Cells

Cell type	Origin	Animal species	Complement receptors	Type of complement receptor: CRI	Type of complement receptor: CRII	References[a]
B lymphocytes	Peripheral blood and lymphoid organs	Human	Present	+	+	1–3
		Mouse	Present	+	+	1,4
		Guinea pig	Present	ND[b]		1
		Rabbit	Present	ND		1,5
		Rat	Present	ND		1
Plasma cells	Spleen	Mouse	Absent[c]			1,6
T lymphocytes	All lymphoid organs	Mouse	Absent			1,7
Polymorphs	Peripheral blood	Human	Present	+	–	2,3
		Mouse	Present	+	+	4,8
Immature neutrophils	Blood and bone marrow	Mouse	Present	–	+	4
Eosinophils	Peripheral blood	Human	Present	+	+	9
	In vitro colonies	Mouse	Absent			10

Mononuclear phagocytes						
promonocytes	*In vitro* colonies	Mouse	Present	ND		10
monocytes	Peripheral blood	Human	Present	+	+	11,12
macrophages	Lung	Human	Present	+	+	13
macrophages	Liver	Mouse	Present	ND		14
macrophages	Peritoneal cavity	Mouse	Present	+	–[d]	15
activated macrophages	Peritoneal cavity	Mouse	Present	+	–	15
macrophages	Peritoneal cavity	Guinea pig	Present	+	+	16
Megakaryocytes	Bone marrow	Guinea pig	Present	+	–	17
Platelets	Peripheral blood	Nonprimate mammals	Present	+	–	18
		Human and primates	Absent			18
Erythrocytes	Peripheral blood	Nonprimate mammals	Absent			18
		Human and primates	Present	+	–	18
Mast cells		Mouse	Absent			19

[a] (1) Bianco *et al.* (1970); (2) Eden *et al.* (1973c); (3) Ross *et al.* (1973); (4) Ross *et al.* (1976); (5) Calkins *et al.* (1975); (6) Ramasamy and Williams (1975); (7) Bianco and Nussenzweig (1971); (8) Lay and Nussenzweig (1968); (9) Gupta *et al.* (1976b); (10) Rabellino and Metcalf (1975); (11) Ross and Polley (1975); (12) Ehlenberger and Nussenzweig (1975); (13) Reynolds *et al.* (1975); (14) Munthe-Kaas *et al.* (1975); (15) Griffin *et al.* (1975); (16) Wellek *et al.* (1975); (17) Fedorko (personal communication); (18) reviewed in D.S. Nelson (1963); (19) Tigelaar *et al.* (1971).

[b] Not determined to our knowledge.

[c] Only a few plaque-forming cells have complement receptors. They may represent immature antibody-secreting cells.

[d] The presence of CRII receptors is referred to by Ross *et al.* (1976).

other vertebrates or from invertebrates. In mammals, the receptors have been detected on the plasma membrane of most formed elements of the blood, but not on T cells (see below). Species differences have been reported for both the distribution and the type of receptors. For instance, humans and primates have CRI on erythrocytes, and not on platelets. Other mammals have the receptor on platelets, and not on erythrocytes. Also, the type of receptor present, CRI or CRII, may vary according to the species. Polymorphs in humans have CRI-type receptors, while in mice, immature neutrophils carry CRII and polymorphs carry both CRI and CRII. Complement receptors have also been detected in some fibroblast cell lines, such as WI-38 (Ueki *et al.*, 1974), and in human renal glomerulus (M.C. Gelfand *et al.*, 1975).

Certain features seem to be conserved in many species. B lymphocytes of mouse and man carry CRI and CRII receptors. In several species, phagocytic cells such as monocytes, macrophages, and polymorphs have at least the CRI receptor. Cells bearing exclusively CRII receptors have been found in few instances: chronic lymphocytic leukemia, lymphoid cell lines (Ross and Polley, 1975), and immature neutrophils of the mouse (Ross *et al.*, 1976).

Contradictory information about the presence of CRII on monocytes and macrophages has been reported. Human peripheral blood monocytes, human lung macrophages, starch-elicited guinea pig macrophages, and mouse peritoneal macrophages bear CRI and CRII as detected with red cell intermediates prepared with purified complement components. When whole serum was used as a source of complement, however, only CRI were detected on macrophages from human lung (Reynolds *et al.*, 1975) or from the peritoneal cavity of the mouse (Griffin *et al.*, 1975). The reason for this discrepancy is not clear. It may be that the red cell intermediate prepared with whole serum bears a modified form of C3. Whatever the interpretation, in the model closest to the *in vivo* situation, i.e., when whole serum is the source of complement, there exists on the immune complex a form of C3 that is not recognized by monocytes and macrophages. During the *in vitro* construction of the complexes with purified complement components, some event with major significance for the fate of the complex *in vivo* does not occur.

The findings of Schreiber and Frank (1972) may be relevant to this question. They injected guinea pigs with EIgM, prepared with homologous red cells. Although C3 determinants could be detected on the circulating sensitized erythrocytes, they were cleared very slowly, with a half-life identical to that of normal erythrocytes. In other words, the form of C3 that was on the erythrocytes was not recognized by phagocytic cells. Also, soluble immune complexes, prepared in the presence of fresh serum, contain large amounts of C3, and may have low affinity for cells with complement receptors (see Section IIA).

Lymphocytes with complement receptors (CRL) have been well characterized in the mouse, and appear to be B lymphocytes for the following reasons:

Precursors of CRL are found in the bone marrow, and their appearance in lymphoid organs is not thymus-dependent (Dukor *et al.*, 1971). They are found in large numbers in nude mice. Their density is somewhat lower than that of lymphocytes that do not bear complement receptors, and they bind readily to nylon wool (Bianco *et al.*, 1970). This property has been employed to remove mouse B lymphocytes from mixtures of cells (Julius *et al.*, 1973). Most or all CRL are Ig^{+}. In human peripheral blood, most CRL have IgD and/or IgM, but not IgG or IgA, on the membrane (see below). Mouse CRL are Thy-1-negative (Bianco and Nussenzweig, 1971) and bear receptors for immune complexes (Fc receptors) (Eden *et al.*, 1973a). They can be either short- or long-lived (Bianco *et al.*, 1970), and recirculate from blood to lymph (Nussenzweig, 1974). In lymphoid organs, CRL localize in certain areas, such as the follicles of the white pulp of the spleen, the cortex of the lymph nodes, and the follicles of the Peyer patches. CRL are rarely found in the thymus, and they appear to be scarce in the T-dependent areas of the lymphoid organs (Dukor *et al.*, 1970).

The presence of complement receptors on some mouse T lymphocytes has been reported by Arnaiz-Villena and Hay (1975). In this case, the characterization of T cells was based on their reaction with a nonconventional reagent, i.e., a rabbit antiserum to mouse brain. The antiserum killed some cells with complement receptors. However, this can also be interpreted as a lack of specificity of this antiserum. Similarly, a small percentage of lymphocytes from human peripheral blood appear to have membrane receptors for sheep erythrocytes, a T-cell marker, and also complement receptors (Shevach *et al.*, 1974). In a few patients with leukemia, the circulating lymphocytes showed this unusual pattern of reactivity (Lin and Hsu, 1976; Shevach *et al.*, 1974). It is not possible to decide at the moment, in view of the absence of absolute criteria for identification, whether these cells represent an unusual subpopulation of B lymphocytes or T lymphocytes.

Although most studies indicate that CRL are B lymphocytes (Jondal *et al.*, 1973; Hallberg, 1975; Yata *et al.*, 1973), not all B lymphocytes have complement receptors. For example, plasma cells may not bear complement receptors. The loss of C3 receptors during B-cell maturation is also suggested by the observation that in rat lymph, IgA-containing large lymphocytes lack complement receptors (Mason, 1976b). Gut-homing Ig^{+} lymphoblasts in mouse mesenteric lymph nodes also lack complement receptors (McWilliams *et al.*, 1975). In addition, it is a common observation that in the mouse spleen and lymph nodes, there are more Ig-bearing cells than CRL.

Among lymphocytes from human peripheral blood, the finding of a very large number of Ig^{+} CR^{-} cells has been reported. However, Lobo *et al.* (1975) and Winchester *et al.* (1975) recently showed that the percentage of human PBL bearing surface Ig is actually lower, the higher number being due to the presence of cells with passively absorbed Ig. Among the lymphocytes with *tightly* bound

Ig, the large majority were found to have IgD and/or IgM on their membrane, and also to bear complement receptors (Ehlenberger *et al.*, 1976). Among lymphocytes of the thoracic duct of the rat, more than 80% of the Ig^+ cells bear IgM on the membrane, and virtually all are CR^+. In contrast, the few IgG^+ cells could be either CR^+ or CR^- (Mason, 1976a). The concurrent presence of IgM/IgD and complement receptors on the lymphocyte membrane may imply a functional relationship in B-cell triggering.

CR^+ Ig^- cells have also been detected in humans. According to Ross (1976), this population of cells is nonphagocytic, and can be found in relatively large numbers in the tonsils.

D. Ontogenesis and Relationship to the Major Histocompatibility Complex

Complement receptors may be present only during certain stages in the life history of a cell. For example, while most B lymphocytes carry the receptor, only a small part of the plasma cells show receptor activity. IgM-bearing cells with no complement receptors have been found in human fetal liver (Gupta *et al.*, 1976a). Suggestive evidence of loss of complement receptors during cell maturation was observed after stimulation of mouse B cells *in vitro* with endotoxin (Gormus *et al.*, 1974). After 72 hr in culture, when IgM secretion was at its peak, only 39% of blasts had complement receptors, while at 24 hr, 86% were positive.

Mouse bone marrow precursors incubated with ubiquitin, a small polypeptide extracted from many cells, develop complement receptor activity in a few hours (Scheid *et al.*, 1975). Furthermore, stimulation of the adenylate cyclase system and an increase in cAMP levels had similar effect. Also, established myeloid leukemic cell lines, known to respond to certain inducers, differentiate into mature granulocytes and macrophages bearing complement receptors (Lotem and Sachs, 1974).

The appearance of cells bearing membrane Ig in the spleens of newborn mice precedes that of CRLs (M.C. Gelfand *et al.*, 1974a). It is not known whether Ig^+ CR^- turn into Ig^+ CR^+ cells or whether a new cell type appears in the spleen. Furthermore, M.C. Gelfand *et al.* (1974b) found that the percentage of CRLs in the spleens of mice at 2 weeks of age is influenced by *H-2*. They suggested that a gene in *H-2* controls the development of complement receptors on the membrane. Since at 2 weeks of age, serum levels of C3 are also influenced by *H-2* (Ferreira and Nussenzweig, 1975), these two phenomena might be causally related. For this reason, Ferreira and one of us repeated some of the experiments of M.C. Gelfand *et al.* (1974b). We (Ferreira and Nussenzweig, 1976) found that although the percentage of CRLs in the spleens of mice was influenced by their *H-2* type, their absolute number was not. The reason is that the cellularity of the spleens of mice during ontogeny is markedly influenced by *H-2*. For example, at

15 days of age, the spleens of DBA/2J mice may contain 5 times as many cells as the spleens of AKR/J mice. Therefore, while the percentage of CRLs in AKR/J mice is much higher than in DBA/2J, in absolute numbers, the spleens of DBA/2J mice contain more CRL. The nature of cells that are under genetic control by *H-2* is not clear. From our observations, they are not CRLs, nor are they Thy-1-positive. They could be either "null" cells or hemopoietic cells, or Ig^+ CR^- lymphocytes, as suggested by the data of Gelfand *et al.* (1974b).

E. Nature

The biochemical nature of the receptors for C3 is unknown. Also, there is no evidence that the receptors are identical in all cell types, except that a single antiserum could block CRI on both human lymphocytes and erythrocytes (Ross *et al.*, 1973).

The evidence that CRI and CRII are present in independent sites of the plasma membrane of lymphocytes is quite convincing. In studies performed with human lymphocytes, each of the two receptors could be blocked by separate antisera. Also, the binding of erythrocytes coated with C3b to CRI could not be blocked by C3d added to the fluid phase; similarly, binding of C3d-coated erythrocytes to the CRII receptors could be blocked by fluid-phase C3d, but not by C3c. Furthermore, in cocapping experiments, CRI and CRII localized at different poles of the cells (Ross and Polley, 1975).

The binding to complement receptors is temperature-dependent. At 4°C, very few complement-coated erythrocytes bind to PMNs, macrophages, or lymphocytes (Lay and Nussenzweig, 1968). The number of erythrocytes bound increases with increase in temperature, and at 37°C, maximum binding is reached. At 0°C, the percentage of lymph-node lymphocytes binding soluble immune complexes is one-third of that observed at 37°C (Eden *et al.*, 1973a). These differences in binding with temperature changes may be related to the fluidity of the membrane. This hypothesis is supported by the observation that aggregation of the receptors on the lymphocyte plasma membrane may be necessary for the binding to occur (Dierich and Reisfeld, 1975).

In most systems studied, no requirement for Ca^{2+} or Mg^{2+} for binding to CR could be demonstrated. In the mouse, however, binding of EAC to macrophages attached to a glass surface requires Mg^{2+} (Lay and Nussenzweig, 1968).

The evidence that proteins of the cell membrane are essential for the expression of complement receptor activity is provided by studies using proteases. Trypsin destroys receptor activity on macrophages and lymphocytes (Lay and Nussenzweig, 1968). Papain is also effective (Hoffman, personal communication). Chymotrypsin, however, does not destroy complement receptors of mouse peritoneal macrophages (Nogueira and Cohn, 1976).

The trypsin sensitivity of the receptor for complement is especially useful in distinguishing binding via C3 from binding via the Fc portion of IgG in cells carrying both receptors (Lay and Nussenzweig, 1968).

The receptors for complement are independent of several other well-identified plasma membrane structures. Binding to lymphocyte complement receptors is not blocked by anti-Ig (Bianco and Nussenzweig, 1971) or by soluble immune complexes bound to Fc receptors (Eden *et al.*, 1973a; Theophilopoulos *et al.*, 1974b). On mouse peritoneal macrophages, blocking of Fc receptor by an antiserum to macrophages did not interfere with binding to C3 receptors (Bianco *et al.*, 1975). Antisera to products of the *I* region of the *H-2* complex also did not affect binding to C3 receptors (Dickler and Sachs, 1974).

Recently, some reports have indicated that antisera to *H-2* (Arnaiz-Villena *et al.*, 1975; Schlesinger and Chaouat, 1975) and to *HLA* (Arnaiz-Villena and Festenstein, 1976) were able to interfere with the interaction of EAC with complement receptors of lymphocytes. In the case of *HLA*, the conclusions were based on experiments in which mononuclear cells isolated from the blood were pretreated with specific antisera to the 4a and 4b histocompatibility antigens. This treatment specifically blocked rosette formation between the lymphoid cells and EAC prepared with mouse serum as a source of complement. In collaboration with Ferreira and Fotino (Ferreira *et al.*, 1977), we repeated these experiments using other antisera against the 4a and 4b histocompatibility antigens. We found that our antisera did not inhibit rosette formation with lymphocytes in suspension, or with human monocytes bound to cover slips. These negative results were obtained both with the native antisera, which strongly agglutinated the leukocytes, and with high concentrations of Fab fragments of the IgG fraction of these antisera. The reasons for these contradictory results remain to be explained. It could be that the products of the *HLA* 4a, 4b system are large molecules with several immunogenic–antigenic sites, one of which is associated with complement receptors. Another possibility is that the inhibition observed by Arnaiz-Villena and Festenstein (1976) was a nonspecific consequence of the specific binding of the antibodies to the 4a and 4b antigens on the cell membrane.

Epstein-Barr virus (EBV) is a lymphotropic herpes virus the main target of which is the human B lymphocyte. Only B lymphocytes appear to have specific EBV receptors (Jondal and Klein, 1973; Greaves *et al.*, 1975). Recently, Klein has suggested that complement receptors of lymphocytes are either identical to or closely associated with EBV receptors (Klein, 1976).

Attempts to isolate C3 receptors have not yet been successful. Most detergents destroy receptor activity. Large lymphocyte membrane fragments obtained after nitrogen cavitation and treatment with 2 M KBr have been shown to retain C3-binding activity (Dierich and Reisfeld, 1975). Complement receptor activity measured as inhibition of platelet release reaction has also been isolated from rabbit platelets by affinity chromatography of NP-40 lysates on zymosan-

C3 or sheep erythrocytes coated with C3. Several active peaks were detected. However, these preparations did not inhibit binding of EAC to platelets (Henson and Neshyba, 1976).

The difficulties encountered in fractionation of plasma membrane receptors for complement have prompted Stossel (1975) to postulate that these receptors do not exist. However, the characteristics of the binding of C3 to complement receptors, described in different sections of this review, fulfill all criteria required to define a plasma membrane receptor, that is: (1) Complement receptors bind specifically certain fragments of C3, and are present only in well-defined cell populations. (2) The binding of C3 fragments to complement receptors is reversible and amenable to saturation kinetics studies. (3) The binding can be prevented by antibodies to the ligand. (4) Binding of the ligand is prevented by antibodies to the plasma membrane receptors. Furthermore, antibodies to other membrane structures do not interfere with binding. (5) Complement receptors are sensitive to certain proteases and not to others. They are resynthesized by the cells (see Section IIIF). (6) CRI and CRII are freely mobile on the plane of the membrane, and can be induced to cap independently on lymphocytes.

The biochemical nature of the receptors, whether they are single or multicomponent structures, and include only protein or other constituents, is not known.

F. Resynthesis

Studies performed by Rabinovitch and DeStefano (1973) with mouse macrophages maintained in culture for prolonged periods of time indicated that complement receptors were unstable. When thioglycollate-induced macrophages were cultivated in serum-free medium, the receptor disappeared after 24 hr. Complement receptor activity lasted for a week in cultures containing 10% fetal calf serum. These findings cast doubts on the ability of macrophages to synthesize the receptor.

That a large number of lymphocyte lines carry complement receptors (Shevach *et al.*, 1972) indicates that the receptors are synthesized by these cells, and not acquired passively from other cells or from the medium. In these cell lines, the receptor is expressed throughout the cell cycle (Paperhausen *et al.*, 1975).

In relation to macrophages, we have approached the problem directly (Gold and Bianco, manuscript in preparation). Normal and thioglycollate-induced mouse peritoneal macrophages were trypsinized and then cultivated in serum-free medium. Figure 3 shows the results obtained with thioglycollate-induced macrophages. Newly synthesized receptors for complement could be detected as early as 6 hr after trypsinization. This recovery could be blocked by cycloheximide.

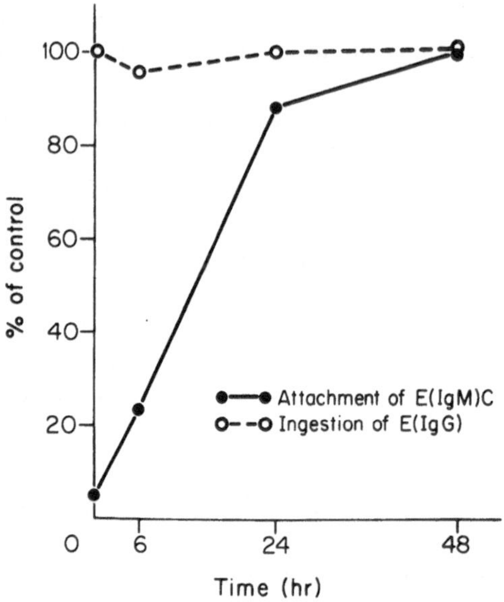

Figure 3. Kinetics of the reappearance of plasma membrane receptors for complement on mouse peritoneal macrophages after trypsin treatment. Macrophages were obtained 4 days after intraperitoneal injection of Brewer thioglycollate medium, adhered to glass cover slips, treated with 1 mg trypsin/ml for 20 min at 37°C, washed with medium containing 1 mg ovomucoid/ml and incubated at 37°C in Dulbecco modified Eagle's MEM containing 0.05% lactoalbumin hydrolysate. The index is defined as the number of erythrocytes bound or ingested by 100 macrophages. From Gold and Bianco (manuscript in preparation).

The viability of the cells treated with the protein synthesis inhibitor was higher than 95%, as evidenced by phagocytosis of opsonized erythrocytes. Similar results were found with unstimulated macrophages.

It is possible that the results of Rabinovitch were caused by the large amounts of neutral proteases secreted by stimulated macrophages (Gordon *et al.*, 1975).

IV. BIOLOGICAL FUNCTION

The extensive distribution of complement receptors among cells is an indication of their importance in the recognition and handling of immune complexes. The initial descriptions of complement receptors on erythrocytes suggested that they played a passive role as transporters of immune complexes. Now, the functional significance of these receptors is recognized in many other areas.

The consequences of the interaction between cells and immune complexes depends on several factors: (1) The specificity of the plasma membrane receptors available for interaction. (2) The nature of the immune complexes, i.e., the form of C4 or C3 bound to the complexes, and the presence of other ligands (e.g., IgG) able to interact with other plasma membrane receptors. As discussed in Section IIA, during the interaction of complement with soluble immune complexes, several enzymes are assembled on the complexes, and different intermediates are formed. They consist of macromolecular aggregates containing complement components. The precise composition of these complexes, and the spatial relationships among the various constituents, are not known. However, C3 and C4 are part of the aggregates, and may interact with complement receptors. On the other hand, the presence of complement components may hinder the interaction between Fc receptors and the Fc portion of the Ig that is part of the aggregate (Eden *et al.*, 1973a; Theophilopoulos *et al.*, 1974b). (3) The presence in the fluid phase of materials able to compete for binding of the complexes, such as C3b or IgG, and of enzymes, such as C3b and C4b-inactivator, that modify C3b and C4b. During the buildup and destruction of these complexes, they will be able to interact only with certain cell types, or with no cells. Since some cells bear complement receptors only during certain stages of differentiation, the ability to interact with the immune complexes will be limited to these periods. Furthermore, if the interaction occurs in an inflammatory area, proteolysis of the plasma membrane receptors and/or the immune complexes may occur. The picture that emerges is therefore that of a very complex interplay of many elements.

In the following sections, we consider only selected situations in which a role for complement receptors has been reasonably well defined.

A. Control of the Traffic of Cells and Immune Complexes

Complement receptors may contribute to the follicular localization of antigen (Bianco *et al.*, 1970), an antibody-dependent mechanism that brings antigenic substances to certain areas of lymphoid organs, presumably for the induction of the immune response (reviewed in Unanue, 1972). The Ag–Ab complexes found accumulated in these areas are associated with the plasma membrane of cells, perhaps via complement receptors. This hypothesis is supported by the findings of Dukor *et al.* (1974) and Papamichail *et al.* (1975), who showed that *in vivo* decomplementation of mice with CoF completely prevented trapping of aggregated human globulin within follicular areas and germinal centers of the spleen (see Section IVE).

B. Phagocytosis

A variety of evidence *in vivo* and *in vitro* has shown that C3, as well as IgG, are opsonins; i.e., they enhance phagocytosis. Important progress in the understanding of the mechanism of opsonization occurred when it was realized that phagocytes possess separate membrane receptors for both IgG (Fc receptors) and C3. These findings introduced the idea that particles bearing IgG and C3 are ingested by the phagocytes *because* they bear membrane receptors for these molecules. Interiorization results from the bridging between the ligands on the particles with the respective membrane receptors (reviewed in Rabinovitch, 1970; Ehlenberger and Nussenzweig, 1976). Since phagocytosis occurs in two steps—attachment of the particle to the phagocyte and ingestion—Mantovani *et al.* (1972) studied the roles of the Fc and C3 receptors in these two phases of the process. The results suggested that particle-bound C3 was primarily involved in attachment, whereas only IgG was capable of promoting ingestion. This finding was confirmed in different systems, involving macrophages, monocytes, and PMNs from man, mouse, and guinea pig.

This functional discrimination occurs at the level of the individual phagocytic cell. When EIgMC- and IgG-coated pneumococci are simultaneously bound to the same mouse peritoneal macrophage, only the IgG-coated particles are ingested (Griffin *et al.*, 1975).

Furthermore, it has been demonstrated that particle-bound C3 and IgG act *synergistically* in promoting phagocytosis (Huber *et al.*, 1968; Ehlenberger and Nussenzweig, 1975). This was shown in experiments in which comparisons were made of the ingestion by human monocytes and PMNs of red cells sensitized with IgG anti-E (EIgG), with IgM anti-E and C3 (EIgMC3), and with IgM, C3, and IgG prepared by incubating EIgMC3 with IgG anti-E. EIgMC3s were bound and formed large rosettes with human PMNs. However, virtually no erythrocytes were ingested. On the other hand, EIgGs were ingested, but large amounts of antibody were required. EIgGs with 6×10^3 or fewer IgG molecules per red cell were not ingested at all. EIgMC3 · IgGs with 10^3 molecules of C3, together with 2×10^3 molecules of IgG, were ingested more efficiently than EIgGs sensitized with 60×10^3 molecules of IgG. Very similar results were obtained with monolayers of human monocytes. EIgMC3s were not ingested. IgG was 10–30 times more effective in inducing phagocytosis when the red cells had been previously sensitized with C3. The experiments described above were carried out by overlaying a monolayer of phagocytes with sensitized particles; under these conditions, a minimum of shear forces existed between red cell and phagocyte. The synergistic effect of C3 was even greater when the cells were kept in suspension. In this situation, most human monocytes ingested EIgMC3 · IgG sensitized with 150 molecules of Ig, but completely ignored EIgG sensitized with 15×10^3 molecules of IgG (Ehlenberger and Nussenzweig, 1977).

Particle-bound C3 enhances phagocytosis by its ability to bring the particle in close contact with the phagocyte. Actually, a variety of agents that augment contact between particle and phagocyte, such as centrifugation, neuraminidase treatment of the red cells, and protamine or dextran in the medium, mimic the effect of C3 (Ehlenberger and Nussenzweig, 1977). A similar effect was obtained by Rabinovitch, by pretreating red cells with glutaraldehyde, which increased their adhesiveness to macrophages (Rabinovitch, 1967). Also, there is a strict parallelism between the nature of the C3 receptor of the phagocyte (CRI and/or CRII), rosette formation with particles coated with C3b and C3d, and phagocytosis. For example, human PMNs have receptors exclusively for the C3c region of C3b (CRI). Monocytes have, in addition, receptors for C3d (CRII). Accordingly, monocytes, but not PMNs, will bind, form rosettes, and efficiently ingest particles sensitized with IgG and C3d.

In summary, C3 and IgG have synergistic effects in phagocytosis, and supplement each other's function. IgG, through its Fc fragment, stimulates particle interiorization, but is less efficient at inducing binding. C3 mediates binding, but does not promote ingestion. The presence of both opsonins on a particle is clearly advantageous for efficient phagocytosis.

One consequence of these findings is that particle-bound C3 may *appear* to trigger ingestion directly, in cases in which ingestion without C3 is negligible. For example, as mentioned, EIgGs coated with 6×10^3 molecules of IgG do not bind, and are not ingested by PMNs but will be avidly phagocytosed if a few molecules of C3 are added to the particle to promote its binding to the phagocyte. Moieties such as these (low doses of IgG) can be considered *potential* triggers of phagocytosis. Their presence on a particle is only apparent *after* C3 deposition, or after particle and phagocytes are brought together by other means.

If our interpretation is correct, it implies that microbes can be ingested in the absence of antibody if two conditions are fulfilled: (1) that they have surface molecules that can "nonspecifically" induce phagocytosis, and (2) that they establish effective contact with the phagocyte. For example, if the alternative pathway of complement activation can be initiated by the bacteria or virus in the absence of antibody, these microorganisms would be optimally opsonized by deposition of C3 on their surfaces.

Recent observations show that red cells bearing IgM and C3b are avidly ingested by *activated* mouse macrophages, while they mostly bind to the normal macrophages (Bianco *et al.*, 1975). The importance of this finding is that it provides a practical marker for identifying activated macrophages, and it suggests that during differentiation of leukocytes, the function of C3 receptors may change, and perhaps mediate ingestion (Fig. 4).

C. Antibody-Mediated Cell Cytotoxicity

AMCC has been the subject of intensive investigation. In this system, specific antibodies mediate the lysis of target cells by unsensitized leukocytes *in vitro*. The effector cells have been shown to carry receptors for C3 and for the Fc

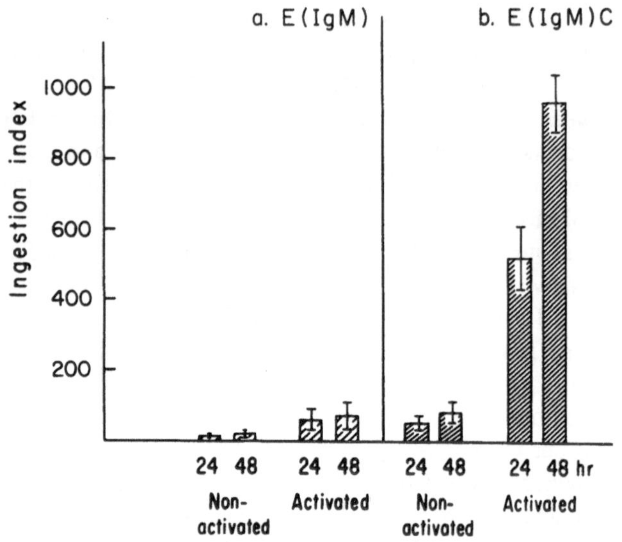

Figure 4. Ability of activated mouse peritoneal macrophages to ingest sheep erythrocytes coated with IgM (a) and mouse complement (b). Activated macrophages were obtained 4 days after intraperitoneal injection of Brewer thioglycollate medium. Cells were cultivated on glass cover slips for 24 or 48 hr before the assay. The ingestion index is the number of erythrocytes ingested by 100 macrophages. Reprinted with permission from Bianco *et al.* (1975).

Table III. Antibody-Mediated Cell Cytotoxicity: Absence of Cytotoxicity Toward C3-Coated Bystander Cells[a]

Target cells[b]		
^{51}Cr-labeled	Unlabeled	Target cell lysis (%)[c]
E (chicken) IgG	E (sheep) IgMC	48.8
E (sheep) IgMC	E (chicken) IgG	0
Controls		
E (sheep) IgMC + IgG	–	40.1
E (chicken) IgG	–	52.3
E (sheep) IgG	–	45.7

[a] Adapted from Lustig and Bianco (1976).
[b] Target cells were chicken erythrocytes coated with BSA and mouse antibodies, and sheep erythrocytes coated with rabbit IgM and mouse complement.
[c] ^{51}Cr release was measured after 18 hr of incubation of the target cells with mouse spleen cells at a ratio of 1:12.5.

fragment of IgG (reviewed by Perlmann and Holm, 1969). C3 by itself, in the absence of IgG, is unable to mediate cytotoxicity (Perlmann *et al.*, 1975; Lustig and Bianco, 1976). Table III summarizes an experiment in which two different target cell populations, one coated with IgG, the other with IgM and complement, were placed in the same mixture together with the effector cells. One or the other set of target cells was labeled with ^{51}Cr. It can be seen that only the IgG-coated targets were lysed. The complement-coated target cells were not lysed as bystanders. Even though C3 cannot mediate cytotoxicity it enhances the lytic effect, probably by bridging together target and effector cells. This potentiation is more evident at low effector cell–target cell ratios. Up to 5-fold more lysis was observed on addition of C3 to target cells (Lustig and Bianco, 1976). The effect of complement may be crucial *in vivo*, because serum and IgG can inhibit AMCC in the absence of target cell–bound C3 (MacLennan *et al.*, 1973). Recently published experiments confirm the previous observations, and show that complement potentiates cytotoxicity in the presence of serum in a system involving human effector cells (Scornik, 1976).

D. Release of Mediators

Interaction of complement receptors with the ligand may directly or indirectly initiate the secretion of mediators by platelets, neutrophils, monocytes, and lymphocytes. It has long been known that rabbit platelets treated with immune complexes containing C3 release vasoactive amines and nucleotides (reviewed by Osler and Siraganian, 1972; Henson, 1972).

Human neutrophils bind to Sepharose coated with C3. This leads to increased production of superoxide anions. If IgG is present simultaneously on the beads, degranulation and release of lysosomal constituents occur. If the beads are treated with $F(ab')_2$ anti-C3, no binding occurs. Degranulation is blocked by treatment with $F(ab')_2$ anti-IgG (Goldstein *et al.*, 1976). In other words, it appears that as in the cases of phagocytosis and AMCC, C3 and IgG cooperate in the triggering of certain PMN functions.

The experiments of Schorlemmer *et al.* (1976) indicate that mouse macrophages cultivated in the presence of purified C3b selectively release some lysosomal enzymes in the medium. The effect occurs apparently without cell damage, and is dose- and time-dependent. Maximum effects occur only after 48–72 hr in culture.

The production and release of enzymes and vasoactive amines after stimulation by C3b and other complement cleavage products could explain the ability of leukocytes and platelets to cause local tissue damage during inflammation.

Guinea pig lymphoid cells, cultivated with EAC or C3b, produce a lymphokine chemotactic for monocytes (Wahl *et al.*, 1974; Sandberg *et al.*, 1975). Also, the binding of EAC to human B lymphocytes induced the release of a chemotactic factor, and of a mitogenic lymphokine, without concomitant blastogenesis (Mackler *et al.*, 1974).

E. Role in Induction of the Immune Response

The suggestion that C3 might play a role in immune responses is based on experiments of Pepys and his colleagues (Pepys, 1972, 1974; Pepys *et al.*, 1976a,b). They showed that the injection of CoF in mice had a suppressive effect on the IgG, IgA, and IgE responses to some thymus-dependent, but not thymus-independent, antigens. The effect of CoF appeared to be a consequence of C3 depletion, rather than antigenic competition (CoF is a potent antigen in mice). Furthermore, the depletion of complement by CoF did not cause gross changes in the histology of lymphoid organs, or in the number and distribution of cells with complement receptors. Subsequently, it was shown that in CoF-treated mice, the pattern of localization of aggregated IgG or a polysaccharide (SIII) in lymphoid organs was profoundly modified (Dukor *et al.*, 1974; Papamichail *et al.*, 1975). In normal mice, part of these antigens are retained for some days in the follicles of the spleen if they are injected intravenously. In CoF-treated animals, uptake in the follicles was suppressed. When C3 levels were restored to normal, the capacity to localize aggregated IgG in the splenic germinal centers was restored. The immunological significance of the phenomenon of follicular localization of antigen is not clear. It has been postulated that the antigen-retaining cells have an important role in the recruitment of B lymphocytes *in vivo*, and that their function is to present the antigen to immunocompetent cells (Nossal *et al.*, 1968). The development of follicles is known to be thymus-dependent, and they may be the site for the generation of B memory cells (Thorbecke *et al.*, 1974). On the basis of these results, we believe that the effects of C3 depletion on the immune response may be the indirect result of a change in the pattern of traffic of B lymphocytes, and of the Ag-Ab-complement complexes formed between the antigen and natural or immune antibodies (Nussenzweig *et al.*, 1973). According to this view, the role of complement receptors would be nonspecific and serve only to concentrate the antigen, in the form of Ag-Ab-complement complexes, onto B lymphocytes and macrophages. Of course, it is imperative that these immune complexes remain on the surface membrane of cells with complement receptors in order to be able to trigger other cells. As previously discussed, the interaction between complement receptors and C3 associated with complexes does not trigger interiorization if IgG is absent (see Section IVB), as is usually the case in initial stages of the immune response.

This "focusing" hypothesis is supported by the findings of Möller and Coutinho (1975), who performed experiments with several polyclonal mitogens such as LPS. They compared the effectiveness of LPS and LPS with bound C3 as a mitogen to spleen cells *in vitro*. They consistently found that LPS that had bound C3 caused a *shift* in the dose–response curve; i.e., much lower concentrations of LPS were necessary for a maximum response.

Dukor and his colleagues proposed a different and intriguing hypothesis on the role of complement receptors in the immune response (Dukor and Hartmann, 1973). Their concept was based on the general idea that the triggering of B cells might require two signals, only one of them given by the antigen. Mainly on the basis of the finding that many polyclonal mitogens, and thymus-independent antigens, are also capable of directly activating the complement system, they proposed that complement receptor–C3 interaction is a *necessary* second signal to activate B cells. Although it appears that in some experimental conditions (Hartmann and Bokisch, 1975), but not all (Sandberg *et al.*, 1975), C3b may indeed be a mitogen, other findings are difficult to explain on the basis of Dukor's hypothesis:

1. A few patients with homozygous deficiency of C3 have "normal" levels of immunoglobulin, and can make antibodies to both thymus-dependent and thymus-independent antigens (reviewed in Rosen, 1975).
2. *In vitro* antibody responses to thymus-independent and thymus-dependent antigens (Coutinho, 1975; Waldmann and Lachmann, 1975) can be obtained in serum-free media. Therefore, no exogenous source of C3 is necessary for *in vitro* antibody responses. However, C3 may be synthesized during the time that the cells are in culture. The addition of native IgG antibodies to C3 to the cultures did inhibit the response to some thymus-dependent antigens (Feldmann and Pepys, 1974), but this effect could not be mediated by the $F(ab')_2$ fragment of the antibody (Waldmann and Lachmann, 1975). It seems that the immune complexes generated between C3 that had been synthesized or released by the cells and the IgG antibodies to C3 inhibited the immune response nonspecifically. In short, antibody responses *in vitro* can occur in the absence of C3.
3. According to Mason (1976a), complement receptors are not required for the generation from B cells of a thymus-dependent 7S antibody response. This was studied in an adoptive transfer system using thoracic duct lymphocytes from primed rats as a source of precursors. Mason found that if he removed CR^+ cells from the immune population, the adoptive transfer of a 7S antibody response was reduced, but not abolished. The precursors of 19S antibody-forming cells were found, however, only in the CR^+ subpopulation of lymphocytes.
4. Although several antigens capable of directly activating B cells can also convert C3 through the alternative pathway, there are several exceptions (Janossy *et al.*, 1973). Recent observations show that C3 activation, T-

independent immunogenicity, and B-cell stimulation are not correlated properties (Diamantstein and Blitstein-Willinger, 1975; Elin *et al.*, 1976). A striking example is CoF, a very potent immunogen in mice. CoF is a very effective activator of C3. Nevertheless, it failed to elicit neutralizing or precipitating antibodies in thymectomized mice, and must therefore be regarded as a T-dependent antigen (Pryjma and Humphrey, 1975).

Therefore, a specific role for complement receptors and C3 in cell cooperation has not yet been established. Because of the importance of C3 and complement receptors in phagocytosis, traffic of cells, and immune complexes, however, it is likely that complement activation influences the immune response.

V. CONCLUDING REMARKS

Multiple physiological and pathological activities are mediated by immune complexes. Some depend on the direct interaction of these complexes with cell membranes. The widespread distribution of complement receptors and Fc receptors among leukocytes strongly suggests that they are important in the recognition of IgG and C3 in the immune complexes.

In some better-defined experimental models, in which the antigen is a particle, complement receptors and Fc receptors have synergistic function. Complement is an important regulating moiety in the interaction between complexes and cell membranes. This seems to be the case with phagocytosis by neutrophils, monocytes, and macrophages; in antibody-mediated killing of target cells by leukocytes; and in the induction of release of lysosomal enzymes by neutrophils when in contact with sensitized particles. In these examples, the cell function appears to be mediated by Fc–Fc receptor interaction, while complement receptors serve mainly or exclusively to approximate the ligand to the cell membrane. Most cells and particles have an overall negative charge, and can be expected to repel each other over short distances. Overcoming such a barrier may represent a considerable obstacle for the recognition by the cell of antibody molecules bound to particulate antigens. C3–complement receptor interaction may serve to overcome this electrostatic repulsion. Actually, in the case of phagocytosis by neutrophils, antibodies are quite inefficient in inducing particle-binding, and opsonization with C3 may be a *necessary* condition for ingestion, although C3 by itself does not trigger phagocytosis.

On the other hand, the complement cascade, and C3 in particular, has a pronounced effect on the degree of aggregation, solubility, and composition of immune complexes made with soluble antigens. The binding of these complexes to Fc receptors and complement receptors of leukocytes and platelets will depend primarily on the availability of the ligand (Fc of IgG, as well as C3 and

C4 moieties) on the immune aggregates. Complement fixation may affect this interaction, and consequently the traffic of immune complexes, in several ways. First, it will cause the incorporation of large amounts of C3 (and C4) and of several enzymes on the complexes. Second, the presence of large complement peptides on the aggregate may sterically prevent the Fc–Fc receptor interaction, and therefore inhibit cell activities that are Fc-mediated. It is therefore possible, though entirely speculative, that in certain complement deficiencies, the catabolism of immune complexes, and in particular the binding to cells with complement receptors and Fc receptors, will be altered, and this may contribute to disease. In addition, the solubilization effect of complement on immune aggregates raises interesting questions regarding the mechanism of lattice formation and precipitation, the nature and sites of interaction between Ab and C3, and the effect of such interaction on the primary Ag–Ab bonds.

ACKNOWLEDGMENTS

This work was supported in part by NIH grants CA19056, AL-08499, and CA16247. Celso Bianco is the recipient of a NCI-DHEW Research Career Development Award.

VI. REFERENCES

Arnaiz-Villena, A., and Festenstein, H., 1976, *Nature (London)* **258**:732.
Arnaiz-Villena, A., and Hay, F.C., 1975, *Immunology* **28**:719.
Arnaiz-Villena, A., Halloran, P., David, C.S., and Festenstein, H., 1975, *J. Immunogenet.* **2**:415.
Bianco, C., 1976, in: *Biological Amplification Systems in Immunity* (N. Day and R. Good, eds.), Plenum Press, New York, in press.
Bianco, C., and Nussenzweig, V., 1971, *Science* **173**:154.
Bianco, C., Patrick, R., and Nussenzweig, V., 1970, *J. Exp. Med.* **132**:702.
Bianco, C., Griffin, F.M., and Silverstein, S.C., 1975, *J. Exp. Med.* **141**:1278.
Bloom, B., and David, J., 1976, *In Vitro Methods of Cell-Mediated Immunity*, 2nd Ed, Academic Press, New York, in press.
Bokisch, V.A., and Sobel, A.T., 1974, *J. Exp. Med.* **140**:1336.
Bokisch, V.A., Dierich, M.P., and Müller-Eberhard, H.J., 1975, *Proc. Nat. Acad. Sci. U.S.A.* **72**:1989.
Calkins, C.E., Carboni, J.M., and Waksman, B.H., 1975, *J. Immunol.* **115**:1339.
Cooper, N.R., 1969, *Science* **165**:396.
Cooper, N.R., 1975, *J. Exp. Med.* **141**:890.
Coutinho, A., 1975, *Transplant. Rev.* **23**:49.
Czop, J., and Nussenzweig, V., 1976, *J. Exp. Med.* **143**:615.
Diamantstein, T., and Blitstein-Willinger, E., 1975, *Immunology* **29**:1087.

Dickler, H.B., and Sachs, D.H., 1974, *J. Exp. Med.* **140**:779.
Dierich, M.P., and Reisfeld, R.A., 1975, *J. Immunol.* **114**:1676.
Dukor, P., and Hartmann, K.H., 1973, *Cell Immunol.* **7**:349.
Dukor, P., Bianco, C., and Nussenzweig, V., 1970, *Proc. Nat. Acad. Sci. U.S.A.* **67**:991.
Dukor, P., Bianco, C., and Nussenzweig, V., 1971, *Eur. J. Immunol.* **1**:491.
Dukor, P., Dietrich, F.M., Gisler, R.H., Schumann, G., Bitter-Suermann, D., 1974, in: *Progress in Immunology, II*, vol. 3 (L. Brent and J. Holborow, eds.), North-Holland Publishing Co., Amsterdam, p. 99.
Eden, A., Bianco, C., and Nussenzweig, V., 1971, *Cell. Immunol.* **2**:658.
Eden, A., Bianco, C., and Nussenzweig, V., 1973a, *Cell. Immunol.* **7**:459.
Eden, A., Bianco, C., Nussenzweig, V., and Mayer, M.M., 1973b, *J. Immunol.* **110**:1452.
Eden, A., Miller, G.W., and Nussenzweig, V., 1973c, *J. Clin. Invest.* **52**:3239.
Ehlenberger, A.G., and Nussenzweig, V., 1975, *Fed. Proc. Fed. Amer. Soc. Exp. Biol.* **34**:854.
Ehlenberger, A.G., and Nussenzweig, V., 1977, *J. Exp. Med.*, in press.
Ehlenberger, A.G., McWilliams, M., Phillips-Quagliata, J.M., Lamm, M.E., and Nussenzweig, V., 1976, *J. Clin. Invest.* **57**:53.
Elin, R.J., Sandberg, A.L., and Rosenstreich, D.L., 1976, *J. Immunol.*, **117**:1238.
Feldmann, M., and Pepys, M.B., 1974, *Nature (London)* **249**:159.
Ferreira, A., and Nussenzweig, V., 1975, *J. Exp. Med.* **141**:513.
Ferreira, A., and Nussenzweig, V., 1976, *J. Immunol.*, **117**:771.
Ferreira, A., Fotino, M., and Nussenzweig, V., 1977, *Eur. J. Immunol.*, in press.
Gelfand, J.A., Fauci, A.S., Green, I., and Frank, M.M., 1976, *J. Immunol.* **116**:595.
Gelfand, M.C., Elfenbein, G.J., Frank, M.M., and Paul, W.E., 1974a, *J. Exp. Med.* **139**:1125.
Gelfand, M.C., Sachs, P.H., Lieberman, R., and Paul, W.E., 1974b, *J. Exp. Med.* **139**:1142.
Gelfand, M.C., Frank, M.M., and Green, I., 1975, *J. Exp. Med.* **142**:1025.
Gigli, I., and Nelson, R.A., 1968, *Exp. Cell Res.* **51**:45.
Gitlin, J.D., Rosen, F.S., and Lachmann, P.J., 1975, *J. Exp. Med.* **141**:1221.
Goldstein, I., Kaplan, H.B., Radin, A., and Frosch, M., 1976, *J. Immunol.*, **117**:1282.
Gordon, S., Unkeless, J.C., and Cohn, Z.A., 1975, in: *Immune Recognition, Proceedings of the Ninth Leukocyte Culture Conference* (A.S. Rosenthal, ed.), Academic Press, New York, p. 589.
Gormus, B.J., Crandall, R.B., and Shands, J.W., Jr., 1974, *J. Immunol.* **112**:770.
Greaves, F.M., Brown, G., and Rickinson, A.B., 1975, *Clin. Immunol. Immunopathol.* **3**:514.
Griffin, F.M., Bianco, C., and Silverstein, S.C., 1975, *J. Exp. Med.* **141**:1269.
Gupta, S., Pahwa, R., Reilly, R., Good, R.A., and Siegal, F.P., 1976a, *Proc. Nat. Acad. Sci. U.S.A.* **73**:919.
Gupta, S., Ross, G.D., Good, R.A., and Siegal, F.P., 1976b, *J. Allergy Clin. Immunol.* **57**:189.
Hallberg, T., 1975, *Acta Pathol. Microbiol. Scand. Sect. C., Suppl.*, No. 250.
Hartmann, K.U., and Bokisch, V.A., 1975, *J. Exp. Med.* **142**:600.
Henson, P.M., 1972, in: *Biological Activities of Complement* (D.G. Ingram, ed.), Karger, Basel, p. 173.
Henson, P.M., and Neshyba, J., 1976, *J. Immunol.*, **116**:1736.
Huber, C., and Wigzell, H., 1975, *Eur. J. Immunol.* **5**:432.
Huber, H., Polley, M.J., Linscott, W.D., Fudenberg, H.H., and Müller-Eberhard, H.J., 1968, *Science* **162**:1281.
Janossy, G., Humphrey, J.H., Pepys, M.B., and Greaves, M.F., 1973, *Nature (London) New Biol.* **246**:108.
Jondal, M., and Klein, G., 1973, *J. Exp. Med.* **138**:1365.

Jondal, M., Wigzell, H., and Aiuti, F., 1973, *Transplant. Rev.* **16**:163.
Julius, M.H., Simpson, E., and Herzenberg, L.A., 1973, *Eur. J. Immunol.* **3**:645.
Klein, G., 1976, *N. Engl. J. Med.* **293**:26.
Lachmann, P.J., and Müller-Eberhard, H.J., 1968, *J. Immunol.* **100**:691.
Lachmann, P.J., Elias, D.E., and Moffet, A., 1972, in: *Biological Activities of Complement* (D.H. Ingram, ed.), S. Karger, Basel, p. 202.
Lay, W.H., and Nussenzweig, V., 1968, *J. Exp. Med.* **128**:991.
Lay, W.H., and Nussenzweig, V., 1969, *J. Immunol.* **102**:1172.
Lin, P.S., and Hsu, C.C.S., 1976, *Clin. Exp. Immunol.* **23**:209.
Lobo, P.I., Westervelt, F.B., and Horwitz, D.A., 1975, *J. Immunol.* **114**:116.
Lotem, J., and Sachs, L., 1974, *Proc. Nat. Acad. Sci. U.S.A.* **71**:3507.
Lustig, H., and Bianco, C., 1976, *J. Immunol.* **116**:253.
Mackler, B.F., Altman, L.C., Rosenstreich, D.L., and Oppenheim, J.J., 1974, *Nature (London)* **249**:834.
MacLennan, I.C.M., Howard, A., Gotch, F.M., and Quie, P.G., 1973, *Immunology* **25**:459.
Mantovani, B., Rabinovitch, M., and Nussenzweig, V., 1972, *J. Exp. Med.* **135**:780.
Mason, D.W., 1976a, *J. Exp. Med.* **143**:1122.
Mason, D.W., 1976b, *J. Exp. Med.* **143**:1111.
McWilliams, M., Phillips-Quagliata, J.M., and Lamm, M.E., 1975, *J. Immunol.* **115**:54.
Mendes, N.F., Mike, S.S., and Peixinho, Z.F., 1974, *J. Immunol.* **113**:531.
Miller, G.W., and Nussenzweig, V., 1975, *Proc. Nat. Acad. Sci. U.S.A.* **72**:418.
Miller, G.W., Saluk, P.H., and Nussenzweig, V., 1973, *J. Exp. Med.* **138**:495.
Möller, G., and Coutinho, A., 1975, *J. Exp. Med.* **141**:647.
Müller-Eberhard, H.J., 1975, *Annu. Rev. Biochem.* **44**:697.
Munthe-Kaas, A.C., Berg, T., Seglen, P.O., and Seljelid, R., 1975, *J. Exp. Med.* **141**:1.
Nelson, D.S., 1963, *Adv. Immunol.* **3**:131.
Nelson, R.A., 1953, *Science* **118**:733.
Nogueira, N., and Cohn, Z.A., 1976, *J. Exp. Med.*, **143**:1402.
Nossal, G.J.V., Abbot, A., Mitchell, J., and Lummers, Z., 1968, *J. Exp. Med.* **127**:277.
Nussenzweig, V., 1974, *Adv. Immunol.* **19**:217.
Nussenzweig, V., Bianco, C., and Eden, A., 1973, in: *3rd International Convocation on Immunology, Specific Receptors of Antibodies, Antigens and Cells* (D. Pressman, ed.), S. Karger, Basel, p. 317.
Okada, H., and Nishioka, K., 1973, *J. Immunol.* **111**:1444.
Osler, A.G., and Siraganian, R.P., 1972, *Prog. Allergy* **16**:450.
Papamichail, M., Gutierrez, C., Embling, P., Johnson, E., Holborow, E.J., and Pepys, M.B., 1975, *Scand. J. Immunol.* **4**:343.
Paperhausen, P., Papageorgiou, P., and Hirschhorn, K., 1975, *J. Immunol.* **114**:519.
Pepys, M.B., 1972, *Nature (London)* **237**:157.
Pepys, M.B., 1974, *J. Exp. Med.* **140**:126.
Pepys, M.B., Wansbrough-Jones, M.H., and Mirjah, D.D., 1976a, *Clin. Exp. Med.* **23**:378.
Pepys, M.B., Wansbrough-Jones, M.H., Mirjah, D.D., and Dash, A.C., 1976b, *J. Immunol.*, **116**:1746.
Perlmann, P., and Holm, G., 1969, *Adv. Immunol.* **11**:117.
Perlmann, P., Perlmann, H., and Müller-Eberhard, H.J., 1975, *J. Exp. Med.* **141**:287.
Pryjma, J., and Humphrey, J.H., 1975, *Immunology* **28**:569.
Rabellino, E., and Metcalf, D., 1975, *J. Immunol.* **115**:688.
Rabinovitch, M., 1967, *Exp. Cell Res.* **46**:19.
Rabinovitch, M., 1970, in: *Mononuclear Phagocytes* (R. van Furth, ed.), Blackwell Scientific Publications, Oxford, p. 299.
Rabinovitch, M., and DeStefano, M.J., 1973, *J. Immunol.* **110**:695.

Ramasamy, R., and Williams, H., 1975, *Immunology* **28**:577.
Reynolds, H.Y., Atkinson, J.P., Newhall, H.H., and Frank, M.M., 1975, *J. Immunol.* **114**:1813.
Rosen, F.S., 1975, in: *Immunogenetics and Immunodeficiency* (B. Benacerraf, ed.), University Park Press, Baltimore, p. 229.
Ross, G.D., 1976, in: *Clinical Evaluation of Immune Function in Man* (G. Siskind and S. Litwin, eds.), Grune and Stratton, New York, in press.
Ross, G.D., and Polley, M.J., 1975, *J. Exp. Med.* **141**:1163.
Ross, G.D., Polley, M.J., Rabellino, E.M., and Grey, H.M., 1973, *J. Exp. Med.* **138**:798.
Ross, G.D., Rabellino, E.M., and Polley, M.J., 1976, *Fed. Proc. Fed. Amer. Soc. Exp. Biol.* **35**:254.
Ruddy, S., and Austen, K.F., 1969, *J. Immunol.* **102**:533.
Sandberg, A.L., Wahl, S.M., and Mergenhagen, S.E., 1975, *J. Immunol.* **115**:139.
Scheid, M.P., Goldstein, G., Hammerling, U., and Boyse, E.A., 1975, in: *Membrane Receptors of Lymphocytes* (M. Seligmann, J.L. Preud'Homme, and F.M. Kourilsky, eds.), North-Holland Publishing Co., Amsterdam, p. 353.
Schlesinger, M., and Chaouat, M., 1975, *Eur. J. Immunol.* **5**:27.
Schreiber, A.D., and Frank, M.M., 1972, *J. Clin. Invest.* **51**:583.
Scornik, J.C., 1976, *Science* **192**:563.
Shevach, E.M., Herberman, R., Frank, M.M., and Green, I., 1972, *J. Clin. Invest.* **51**:1933.
Shevach, E.M., Jaffe, E.S., and Green, I., 1973, *Transplant. Rev.* **16**:3.
Shevach, E.M., Edelson, R., Frank, M., Lutzner, M., and Green, I., 1974, *Proc. Nat. Acad. Sci. U.S.A.* **71**:863
Schorlemmer, H.U., Davies, P., and Allison, A.C., 1976, *Nature (London)* **261**:48.
Stossel, T.P., 1975, *Semin. Hematol.* **12**:83.
Stossel, T.P., Field. R.J., Gitlin. J.D., Alper, C.A., and Rosen, F.S., 1975, *J. Exp. Med.* **141**:1329.
Takahashi, M., Czop, J., Ferreira, A., and Nussenzweig, V., 1976, *Transplant. Rev.* **32**: 121.
Tamura, N., and Nelson, R.A., 1967, *J. Immunol.* **99**:582.
Theophilopoulos, A.N., Bokisch, V.A., and Dixon, F.J., 1974a, *J. Exp. Med.* **139**:696.
Theophilopoulos, A.N., Dixon, F.J., and Bokisch, V.A., 1974b, *J. Exp. Med.* **140**:877.
Thorbecke, G.J., Romano, T.J., and Lerman, S.P., 1974, in: *Progress in Immunology II*, Vol. 3 (L. Brent and J. Holborow, eds.), North-Holland Publishing Co., Amsterdam, p. 25.
Tigelaar, R.E., Vaz, N.M., and Ovary, Z., 1971, *J. Immunol.* **106**:661.
Ueki, A., Itagashi, Y., Hyodoh, F., and Kimoto, T., 1974, *Virchows Arch. B.* **18**:101.
Unanue, E.R., 1972, *Adv. Immunol.* **15**:95.
Wahl, S.M., Iverson, G.M., and Oppenheim, J.J., 1974, *J. Exp. Med.* **140**:1631.
Waldman, H., and Lachmann, P.J., 1975, *Eur. J. Immunol.* **5**:185.
Wellek, B., Helmut, H.H., and Wolfgang, O., 1975, *J. Immunol.* **114**:1643.
Winchester, R.J., Fu, S.M., Hoffman, T., and Kunkel, H.G., 1975, *J. Immunol.* **114**:1210.
Yata, Y., Tsukimoto, I., and Tachibana, T., 1973, *Clin. Exp. Immunol.* **14**:319.

Induction of Tumor-Immune Responses and Their Interaction with the Developing Tumor

Robert William Baldwin and Richard Adrian Robins

Cancer Research Campaign Laboratories
University of Nottinghan
Nottingham, NG7 2RD, England

I. INTRODUCTION

The central thesis of tumor immunology is that host responses to tumor-associated antigens exert a degree of immunological control over a developing tumor. This concept has developed principally from studies on experimental animal tumors induced by chemical carcinogens or oncogenic viruses, and to a lesser extent with naturally occurring tumors, in which it has been established that immunological rejection of tumors can sometimes be induced in suitably presensitized syngeneic recipients (Sjögren, 1965; Baldwin, 1973). Furthermore, immune rejection responses can be demonstrated in the tumor-bearing host, so that while the primary tumor implant is beyond host control, a concomitant challenge with the same tumor may be rejected, provided it is not too large (Gershon *et al.*, 1967; Vaage, 1971). This has led to a further postulate, which proposes that the failure of immunocompetent hosts to reject a nascent tumor results from specific immune defects induced by tumor-associated products influencing primarily the cell-mediated arm of the tumor-immune response (I. Hellström and K.E. Hellström, 1969; K.E. Hellström and I. Hellström, 1974; Baldwin and Robins, 1975).

In this chapter, we will consider the overall responses in the induction of tumor immunity and consider how the effector phase of the tumor-immune response can be influenced by tumor-associated factors. The principal objective will be to describe the types of immune response that are relevant in the host with a developing tumor and to consider evidence suggesting that tumor antigen-containing factors released by a developing tumor diminish the effectiveness of immune rejection responses.

Two general points should be made at this stage. First, although tumor-rejection antigens can be identified on many types of tumors by their capacity to elicit immunity in normal hosts to a subsequent challenge with viable tumor cells, this is not a universal feature of malignant cells. For example, rat hepatomas induced by aminoazo dyes are almost always immunogenic, in that immunological rejection of tumor can be demonstrated in preimmunized syngeneic hosts, whereas hepatomas induced by another type of carcinogen lack this property (Baldwin, 1973). In this context, it should be noted that only limited studies have been reported on naturally occurring (spontaneous) tumors, and in general, these tumors are less frequently immunogenic than those induced deliberately by extrinsic agents.

The second point that should be stressed is that tumor cells may express many different types of neoantigens that elicit cell-mediated and humoral immune responses, but not all these neoantigens are able to function efficiently as rejection antigens. That they are not can be exemplified by considering carcinogen-induced tumors, such as 3-methylcholanthrene (MCA)-induced sarcomas, that exhibit so-called "tumor-specific" antigens, these being distinctive for individual tumors, and cross-reactive antigens that have been identified as reexpressed embryonic antigens. The embryonic antigens, however, do not function very effectively, if at all, as rejection antigens, so that immunization against these tumors produces protection only against challenge with cells of the immunizing tumor. Nevertheless, when immune responses to these tumors, especially in the tumor-bearing host, are evaluated using *in vitro* assays such as the microcytotoxicity test of cell-mediated immunity, it is possible to demonstrate reactions to both sets of tumor-associated antigens. This indicates that the *in vitro* assays of tumor immunity are not in themselves predictive of tumor-rejection responses.

II. INITIATION OF TUMOR-IMMUNE RESPONSES

Some of the possible interactions of a tumor cell, or its products, that have been shown to occur, or could theoretically occur, in the induction of tumor-immune responses are outlined in Fig. 1. As is evident from the diagram, this is a highly complex interacting system, and although different aspects of the response can be discussed in turn for the sake of clarity, this interactive aspect should be recognized.

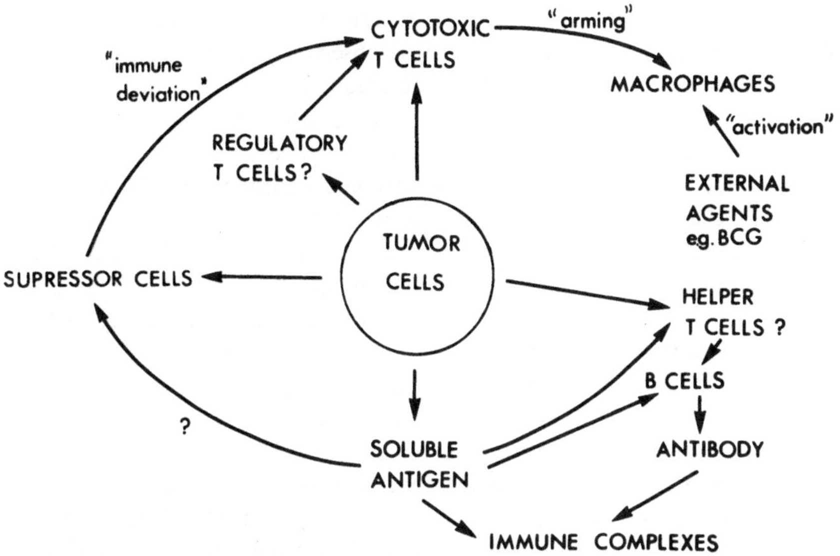

Figure 1. Some possible pathways in the initiation of tumor immune responses.

A. Cell-Mediated Immunity

1. Cytotoxic Lymphocytes

Cell-mediated immunity to tumors in animals has been the subject of many studies, since its importance was shown classically in experiments demonstrating the transfer of tumor immunity to unimmunized recipients by means of lymphoid cells taken from tumor-immune donors (K.E. Hellström and I. Hellström, 1969). For example, immunity to aminoazo dye-induced rat hepatomas can be adoptively transferred using lymph node cells or peritoneal exudate cells from immunized donors, their reactivity being specifically directed toward cells of the immunizing tumor (Baldwin and Barker, 1967; Ishidate, 1967).

In considering the relevance of cell-mediated immunity to tumor cells, it has been emphasized that the host may initiate cell-mediated cytotoxic responses to many different types of neoantigens expressed at the tumor cell surface, but not all these responses necessarily lead to tumor rejection. That they do not may be exemplified by comparing host responses to the individually distinct tumor antigens and cross-reacting embryonic antigens on both carcinogen-induced and naturally occurring rat tumors. Lymph node cells from rats immunized against syngeneic transplants of MCA-induced sarcomas or aminoazo dye-induced hepatomas are cytotoxic *in vitro* for cells of the corresponding tumor (Baldwin and Embleton, 1971; Baldwin *et al.*, 1973c; Zöller *et al.*, 1975). In these examples, the specificity of the *in vitro* lymphocytotoxic responses was comparable to that of the tumor-rejection reaction observed against syngeneically transplanted tumor cells, suggesting, but by no means proving, that the *in vitro* tests were detecting reactions to the tumor-specific rejection antigens. As already noted, these tumors also exhibit cross-reactive antigens at the cell surface that have been identified as reexpressed embryonic components (Baldwin *et al.*, 1974b). In the tumor-bearing host, cell-mediated responses to these tumor-associated embryonic products can also be demonstrated (Zöller *et al.*, 1975). These responses, however, are not specifically directed against cells of the immunizing tumor, since cytotoxic reactions can be demonstrated against even histologically unrelated tumors. In this case, therefore, the *in vitro* cytotoxic reactions with tumor-bearer lymphoid cells are not predictive of the tumor-rejection response. That they are not is consistent with previous studies with naturally occurring rat sarcomas and mammary carcinomas, in which tumor-bearer lymph node cells exhibited tumor-directed cytotoxicity *in vitro*, but these tumors generally lacked tumor-rejection antigens (Baldwin and Embleton, 1974). Again, these responses were identified as being directed toward tumor-associated embryonic antigens, and responses of the tumor-specific type were not detected. In this context, it is pertinent to note that discordant findings have been obtained with other experimental tumor systems when the specificity of the neoantigens involved in tumor-immune rejection responses is compared with those demonstrated by *in vitro* lymphocytotoxicity assays. For example, carcinogen-induced murine bladder carcinomas exhibit individually distinct tumor-rejection antigens, whereas neoantigens detected by *in vitro* lymphocytotoxicity exhibit cross-reactivity (Wahl *et al.*, 1974; Taranger *et al.*, 1972). Similarly, rat colon carcinomas have been shown to express both cross-reacting and organ-specific antigens that have tentatively been identified as embryonic products (Steele *et al.*, 1975), but these antigens function only as weak rejection antigens. Thus, with naturally occurring and chemically induced tumors, cell-mediated immune reactions against embryonic antigens on the tumor cell surface are detectable *in vitro*, although tumor rejection is not normally associated with these reactions.

Many aspects of the initiation of cellular immunity, such as the antigen requirements for stimulation, the cellular response, and the cell–cell interactions involved, are only beginning to be understood. Because of their possible relevance to understanding the genesis and shortcomings of the tumor-immune response, some of these findings will be discussed briefly.

In many tumor systems, the methods available for *in vitro* detection of cell-mediated cytotoxicity, e.g., the microcytotoxicity test, are essentially nonquantitative. In contrast, the ^{51}Cr-release test, when applied to suitable test systems (lymphomas, leukemias, mastocytomas), can yield quantitative comparisons of cytotoxic activity (Cerottini and Brunner, 1971), and this quantitative approach has allowed detailed investigation of the generation of cytotoxic thymus-derived lymphocytes (T cells) in an allogeneic system (Cerottini *et al.*, 1974a,b). Thus, stimulation of spleen cells from normal mice with allogeneic spleen cells under appropriate conditions resulted in production of T cells specifically cytotoxic for target cells bearing the stimulating alloantigen. During prolonged culture, cytotoxic activity decreased, but on restimulation, rapid regeneration of cytotoxic T cells was observed. Separation of cells by velocity sedimentation at 1*g* indicated that cytotoxic cells belonged to a "large" cell population. Interestingly, if a secondary stimulation was performed using cells from primary cultures separated at the time of maximum cytotoxicity, only cultures derived from the "large" (cytotoxic) population gave rise to cytotoxic T cells. These findings indicate that the cytotoxic cell may give rise to memory cells capable of rapid response on restimulation, although another possibility is that the memory cells are derived from a noncytotoxic subpopulation of responsive cells.

An interesting difference between primary and secondary cultures is that intact stimulating cells (irradiated or mitomycin C-treated) are required to initiate a cytotoxic response in previously unsensitized lymphocytes, whereas a secondary response can be provoked with membrane antigen preparations (Cerottini *et al.*, 1974b). These findings may be relevant to the divergent effects produced by immunization of rats with intact tumor cells and membrane antigen preparations (see Section IIB).

Another facet of the cell-mediated response that has not so far been examined in syngeneic tumor systems is that collaboration among subpopulations of T cells has been shown to be necessary for the generation of cytotoxic T cells to allogeneic cells. This necessity was originally indicated by the synergistic effects that could be obtained using mixtures of thymus cells and lymph node cells as responding cells during the generation of cytotoxic cells in mixed lymphocyte culture (Cohen and Howe, 1973; Häyry and Anderson, 1974). By the use of congenic strains differing only at the *Thy-1* locus (the locus that defines an antigen present on T cells, previously known as θ), Cantor and Simpson (1975) were able to show that the cytotoxic cells in the mixed lymphocyte culture were derived from lymph node cells, whereas the regulatory T cells were from thymus cells. Regulatory T cells were also found among a relatively radioresistant and antithymocyte serum-insensitive population of splenic T cells. The concept that distinct sub-populations of specific T cells give rise to cytotoxic cells and regulatory cells has recently been supported by work in mice using the Ly-antigen markers (Kisielow *et al.*, 1975; Cantor and Boyse, 1975).

These findings are mentioned to emphasize that in many tumor systems, our knowledge of the cellular requirements for immune responses is rather unsophisticated, often because of a lack of suitable lymphocyte markers. It is clear, however, that the qualitative and quantitative aspects of presentation of tumor antigen to the immune system will influence the effectiveness of the initiation of cell-mediated cytotoxicity. Thus, the problem is to predict the class of response (cytotoxic T cells, antibody, suppressor cells) that a given form of antigen presentation will provoke, and the effect this response will have on the subsequent reaction presented in other forms.

2. *Suppressor Cells*

The role of suppressor cells in controlling immune responses, and in some types of tolerance, is becoming established (Gershon, 1975; Asherson and Zembala, 1975). It is less clear yet whether suppressor cells are important in tumor immunity, but several recent findings suggest that they might be.

Suppressor cells described so far in tumor systems seem to fall into two main categories:

1. Specific suppressors, which are nonadherent cells, and in some cases have been shown to be T cells.
2. Nonspecific suppressors, which affect a range of responses, even lymphocyte stimulation by mitogens. Non-T cells are usually responsible for suppression of this type.

(a) Specific Suppressor Cells. Suppression of *in vitro* cytotoxic reactions has allowed the detection of suppressor cells in several tumor systems. For example, the cytotoxicity of spleen cells taken from Japanese quails after regression of Rous virus-induced tumors is abolished by admixture with spleen cells from quails bearing progressively growing tumors (Hayami *et al.*, 1972). More recently, it has been reported that lymph node cells from multiparous rats, which recognize embryonic antigens on rat tumor cells, also contain a subpopulation of suppressor cells (Rees *et al.*, 1975a). After fractionation on nylon-fiber columns, nonadherent cells eluted from the column generally lacked cytotoxicity, whereas cells recovered from the column by gentle agitation (retained cells) were cytotoxic. Also, the cytotoxicity of the retained cell population could be suppressed by addition of the eluted cells, and it was suggested that this effect might account for the variable cytotoxic responses when lymph node cell preparations from multiparous rats are tested *in vitro* against target tumor or embryo cells. Whether similar effects occur following sensitization to other types of tumor-associated antigen, especially during the natural development of a tumor, has not yet been resolved. Suppressor cells are produced, however, in rats immunized with isolated tumor antigen preparations, either intact membrane fractions of 3 M KCl–solubilized extracts, from MCA-induced sarcomas (Embleton, 1976a). Immunization with isolated tumor antigen preparations, except under precisely defined conditions, does not induce immunity against a subsequent challenge with tumor, and lymph node cells from immunized donors are frequently not cytotoxic *in vitro* for tumor cells (Baldwin *et al.*,

1973b; Embleton, 1976a). Moreover, addition of lymph node cells from these so-called "deviated" rats to tumor-immune lymph node cells, e.g., from rats rejecting tumor challenge, abolishes the cytoxicity of the latter population, at least when tested *in vitro* on tumor cells.

Specific suppression of tumor immunity by lymphoid cells taken from tumor-bearing hosts has also been reported following *in vivo* studies on immunity to MCA-induced sarcomas (Fujimoto *et al.*, 1976a,b). In this case, suppression was detected by the capacity of tumor-bearer lymphoid cells injected intravenously to abrogate the capacity of tumor-immune mice to reject a challenge with viable tumor cells. When thymus, lymph node, spleen, or bone marrow cells from tumor-bearing mice were injected into the immune recipients, the tumor challenge temporarily grew faster than controls treated with cells from normal donors, and the tumor-specificity of the phenomenon was controlled in tests using lymphoid cells from mice bearing unrelated tumors. The facilitation of tumor growth was not observed if tumor-bearer spleen cells were treated with anti-Thy-1 antiserum and complement, a finding that suggested the involvement of T cells. Suppressive activity was detected as soon as 24 hr after tumor implantation, so this phenomenon represents a very early event in the initiation of the host response to a developing tumor.

Similar effects have also been observed in studies showing that the active immunotherapy of syngeneic transplants of an MCA-induced rat sarcoma can be abrogated by the injection of tumor-bearer lymph node cells (Pimm *et al.*, unpublished observations). In this system, tumors developing from a subcutaneous challenge are completely rejected when the recipients receive a simultaneous contralateral injection of viable tumor cells admixed with Bacille Calmette-Guerin (BCG), provided this mixed inoculum does not grow (Baldwin and Pimm, 1973). This tumor rejection is mediated by a specific response to the individually distinct neoantigens associated with this tumor, since no suppression of tumor growth was obtained when the immunizing tumor inoculum admixed with BCG was not the same as the challenge tumor. Furthermore, the involvement of a lymphocyte-mediated immune response was indicated by the finding that the immunotherapeutic effect was abolished when recipient rats were pretreated with whole-body irradiation (450 rads). The finding that the cell-mediated tumor-rejection response initiated by the contralateral injection of tumor cells admixed with BCG could be abrogated by intravenous injection of tumor bearer lymphoid cells therefore suggests a possible suppressive role for lymphoid cell-associated factors in the tumor-bearing host. Whether the effect of tumor-bearer lymphoid cells is mediated by a suppressor cell or by circulating tumor antigen-containing factors associated with lymphoid cells has not been established.

A similar position has been reached in studies demonstrating suppressor cells in the spleens of rats rendered tolerant to Gross virus (Myburgh and Mitchison, 1976). In this case, spleen suppressor cells were identified by their capacity to prevent spontaneous regression of a highly immunogenic Gross virus-induced lymphoma (C58NT)D. The tumor growth-promoting effect of tolerant spleen cells was sensitive to irradiation, and activity was also abolished by trypsinization of spleen cells.

(b) Nonspecific Suppressor Cells. Spleen cells from mice bearing Moloney sarcoma virus (MSV)-induced tumors do not respond as well as normal spleen cells to DNA synthesis when stimulated with phytohemagglutinin (PHA), but the normal response can be restored by depletion of adherent and phagocytic cells. Furthermore, the PHA response of normal spleen cells was depressed by the addition of tumor-bearer spleen cells, even if this addition was delayed for 16 hr after initiation of cultures, and these studies were interpreted to indicate that subpopulations of these spleen cells function as nonspecific suppressor cells (Kirchner *et al.*, 1974a,b; 1975). The identity of the cell populations involved is still not clearly defined, however, since cells inactivated by antiimmunoglobulin antiserum and complement may also be involved (Gorczynski, 1974b). It is evident, however, that tumor-bearer spleen cells do contain a subpopulation modifying lymphocyte stimulation to tumor-associated antigens and alloantigens, as well as mitogens. For example, spleen cells from rats bearing the (C58NT)D Gross virus-induced lymphoma depressed the proliferative response of spleen cells from tumor-immune rats to stimulation with tumor cells (Glaser *et al.*, 1975). Also, spleen cells from mice bearing transplants of an MCA-induced sarcoma generate less cytotoxicity than normal spleen cells when stimulated with allogeneic cells, but this responsiveness could be restored by removal of adherent cells (Eggers and Wunderlich, 1975).

3. Macrophages

Even though adherent cells (possibly macrophages) can have a negative influence on immune reactions [see Section IIA2(b)], macrophages can also make a positive contribution to tumor immunity. This contribution can occur both in the induction of immune reactions and through the action of macrophages as effector cells after activation by lymphocyte products or exogenous agents such as BCG. Macrophages are important at several stages during the initiation of immune responses (Table I), including antigen-handling, and during lymphocyte collaboration (reviewed by Unanue and Calderon, 1975), although some of these functions may be performed by other adherent cells (Möller *et al.*, 1976). The role of macrophages in antigen-handling is illustrated by studies in which it was shown that cytotoxic lymphocytes could be produced by stimulation with soluble tumor antigen, provided the antigen was added to macrophage monolayers before culture with lymphocytes (Treves *et al.*, 1976).

In addition to the importance of macrophages in the initiation of lymphocyte-mediated responses, they can also become cytotoxic to tumor cells

Table I. Macrophage Activities in Tumor Immunity

Induction	
	Antigen-handling
	T–B collaboration
	Production of lymphocyte-activating factor (LAF)
Cytotoxicity	
	Immune macrophage cytotoxicity
	With immune lymphocytes
	With immune lymphocyte factors (SMAF, MIF)
	With cytophilic antibody
	Activation by exogenous agents (BCG, endotoxin)
	Cytotoxin production

(Table I). Thus, macrophages from tumor-immunized animals can specifically damage cells of the immunizing tumor (Bennett *et al.*, 1964; Granger and Weiser, 1966; Evans and Alexander, 1970). Furthermore, tumor-immune lymphocytes, or supernatants from immune lymphocytes stimulated with antigen, render macrophages from normal animals cytotoxic for the appropriate tumor cell (Evans and Alexander, 1972a). The production of this cytoxicity is envisaged as a two-step process: (1) binding of a lymphocyte product, specific macrophage-arming factor (SMAF), to the macrophage, to give the "armed" stage; (2) "activation" by renewed contact with specific antigen. Activated macrophages are non-specifically cytotoxic. Macrophages may also be rendered cytotoxic by means of cytophilic antibody, and this pathway is distinct from the SMAF arming process (Evans and Alexander, 1972b).

Macrophages may also be initiated to cytotoxicity against tumor cells by a range of stimulants, including BCG, endotoxin, double-stranded RNA, and *Corynebacterium parvum* (reviewed by Levy and Wheelock, 1974), and this cytotoxicity may be the basis of tumor suppression by adjuvant contact, although macrophages activated by, for example, BCG are not universally tumor-suppressive (Nathan and Terry, 1975). The field of macrophage activation and cytotoxicity is a large and controversial one. It remains to be demonstrated whether the different mechanisms of activation outlined above have a common final cytotoxic pathway, or whether different subpopulations of macrophages are involved (Levy and Wheelock, 1974).

B. Humoral Antibody

Host recognition of tumor-associated antigens leading to the induction of humoral antibody responses has been well documented with a wide range of experimental tumors, including those induced by oncogenic viruses (reviewed by

Lamon, 1974) and chemical carcinogens, as well as naturally occurring tumors (Baldwin, 1976; Baldwin and Price, 1975). For example, antibody responses to both the individually specific antigens and the cross-reactive embryonic antigens can be detected in hosts immunized against syngeneic MCA-induced sarcomas and aminoazo dye-induced hepatomas by serum membrane immunofluorescence reactions or complement-dependent cytotoxicity for tumor or embryo cells (Baldwin, 1973; Baldwin *et al.*, 1974b). Similarly, complement-dependent cytotoxicity was demonstrated in the serum of mice after regression of MSV-induced tumors (Tamerius and Hellström, 1974).

It should be noted, however, that antibody reactive with tumor-associated antigens (either specific or cross-reacting) is not generally detected in the tumor-bearing host. That it is not was demonstrated in an early study by Harder and McKhann (1968) with MCA-induced murine sarcomas in which circulating antibody could not be identified in tumor-bearers, but following surgical removal of the tumor, antibody rapidly became detectable. This type of response, involving the appearance of circulating antibody after drastic reduction of tumor load, has been observed in a number of studies (Baldwin *et al.*, 1973c; Thomson *et al.*, 1973; Smith and Leonard, 1974; Prather and Lausch, 1976). One explanation of these findings is that free antibody is neutralized by the tumor or antigen released into the circulation. Thus, when the release of soluble tumor antigen is terminated by tumor removal, the balance between antibody and antigen is disturbed, and antibody becomes detectable. This concept is supported by the demonstration of antibody in the form of immune complexes in the serum of tumor-bearing rats (Baldwin *et al.*, 1973c; Thomson *et al.*, 1973).

Whether free antibody is detected in the circulation will also depend on the degree of stimulation of the antibody response. For example, an ascitic variant of an aminoazo dye-induced hepatoma was shown to stimulate a tumor-specific antibody response very effectively (Robins, 1975). Moreover, free serum antibody was also detected after injection of ascitic hepatoma in rats bearing a subcutaneous tumor derived from the same hepatoma. These studies indicate that antigen and antibody found in the serum will fluctuate interdependently. This is a complicated situation, however, since in some systems, released (soluble) tumor antigen has been shown to be more efficient in eliciting antibody responses than in stimulating cell-mediated immunity. Thus, the balance between cell-mediated and humoral immunity to tumor-associated antigens can be significantly altered when the tumor products are presented in different forms. This point is discussed later in relation to the immune responses elicited by tumor antigen in acellular form compared with those to intact tumor cells. There is as yet, however, little understanding of the fundamental cellular interactions between different subpopulations of lymphocytes and tumor antigen in different forms.

C. Immune Deviation*

As already commented on, the type of immune response to tumor-associated antigen depends on the physical form in which the antigen is presented to the host. Intact tumor cells are usually most effective for inducing tumor-rejection immunity, so that many investigators have used radiation-attenuated tumor cells for this purposes (Sjögren, 1965). In contrast, tumor antigen presented as either isolated membrane fractions or solubilized extracts is not generally so effective (Baldwin *et al.*, 1973b; Pellis and Kahan, 1975), although immunity to tumors in guinea pigs can be elicited by immunization with soluble tumor fractions (Oettgen *et al.*, 1968; Meltzer *et al.*, 1972). With rat sarcomas, for example, tumor-rejection immunity can be induced only when tumor antigen preparations are administered over a restricted dose range, and this response is not so effective as that elicited by irradiated tumor cells. This lesser effectiveness has been shown to be due to an inappropriate type of response to the tumor antigen fractions, which favors the production of tumor-specific antibody rather than cytotoxic lymphoid cells. Furthermore, as already indicated, immunization with tumor antigen in an acellular form leads to the development of a suppressorlike lymphoid cell population that abrogates the cytotoxicity *in vitro* of tumor-immune lymph node cells. This suppressor mechanism also appears to be operative *in vivo*, since rats immunized with membrane fractions or solubilized antigen under conditions that do not provoke any discernible rejection response are no longer responsive to immunization with irradiated tumor cells, which in normal animals confers protection to a subsequent tumor challenge (Baldwin *et al.*, 1973b; Embleton, 1976a). This "immune deviation" is specific, so that rats treated with soluble antigen from one tumor are still able to respond normally to immunization with irradiated cells from a different tumor.

A model system in which both cell-mediated and humoral immunity can be elicited under appropriate conditions has been described by Mackaness and Lagrange (1974). Low doses of SRBC (10^5 cells i.v.) induced cell-mediated immunity detectable as a delayed hypersensitivity reaction to antigen challenge in the footpad, whereas higher doses of antigen (10^8 SRBC i.v.) gave rise to a serum antibody response, but no DH reaction. When animals previously immunized with the high dose of antigen were immunized with the low dose, they also did not develop a DH reaction. These findings appear to parallel those in the tumor model quite closely. A further development in the SRBC system, which

*Abbreviations in this section: (B^{γ}) precursor IgG-producing B cell; (B^{μ}) precursor IgM-producing B cell; (DH) delayed hypersensitivity; (P^{IgG}) IgG-producing plasma cell; (P^{IgM}) IgM-producing plasma cell; (SRBC) sheep red blood cells; (t^c) immature cooperating T cell; (T^c) cooperating T cell; (t^I) immature inhibitory T cell; (T^I) inhibitory T cell; (t^k) immature cytotoxic T cell; (T^k) cytotoxic T cell.

has not so far been attempted in the tumor system, is the "rescue" of antibody-producing mice so that they can mount a DH response. This rescue was achieved by a combination of cyclophosphamide and BCG; after this treatment, the previously unresponsive mice could mount a DH response when immunized with the low dose of SRBC.

The determination of the class of an immune response following antigen stimulation is obviously a very important area for future research. A hypothesis as to how such a determination might be achieved has been put forward by Cohn (1976), who suggested that the class of response is determined by the level of T cooperating activation ($t^c - T^c$). Thus, at low levels of T^c, the maturation of T^k would be stimulated ($t^k - T^k$); at intermediate levels of T^c, the maturation of P^{IgM} would be facilitated ($B^{\mu} - P^{IgM}$), but these higher levels of T^c would suppress the formation of T^k. At the high levels of T^c, P^{IgG} would be formed ($B^{\gamma} - P^{IgG}$), and under these conditions of high T^c, P^{IgM} maturation, as well as the formation of T^k, would be suppressed. It is also suggested that the T^k cell (or T^I), also formed under conditions of low T^c ($t^I - T^I$), would inhibit the maturation $t^c - T^c$, thus allowing a stabilized T^k response within limited conditions of antigen stimulation.

These notions are quite hypothetical at this stage, but they may nonetheless provide a useful conceptual framework for investigating this complicated but very important area.

III. EFFECTOR PHASE OF TUMOR-IMMUNE RESPONSES

It is clear from the data discussed so far that neoantigens expressed on tumor cell surface membranes provoke diverse types of cellular and humoral immune responses (see Fig. 1), which under appropriate conditions can lead to tumor cell stasis or death (Fig. 2). The means by which various arms of the immune response can play a role in tumor rejection will be discussed, but in view of the failure of immune responses to control the growth of immunogenic tumors under many circumstances, attention will also be paid to mechanisms by which the immune responses may be rendered ineffective.

A. Cytotoxic Lymphocytes

Cytotoxic lymphocytes have long been viewed as the main effectors of tumor rejection, since, as already described, tumor immunity can be adoptively transferred with lymphoid cells taken from tumor-immune donors, and in many cases, successful transfer of immunity has been shown to depend on T cells. For example, Gorczynski (1974a) showed that inhibition of the development of

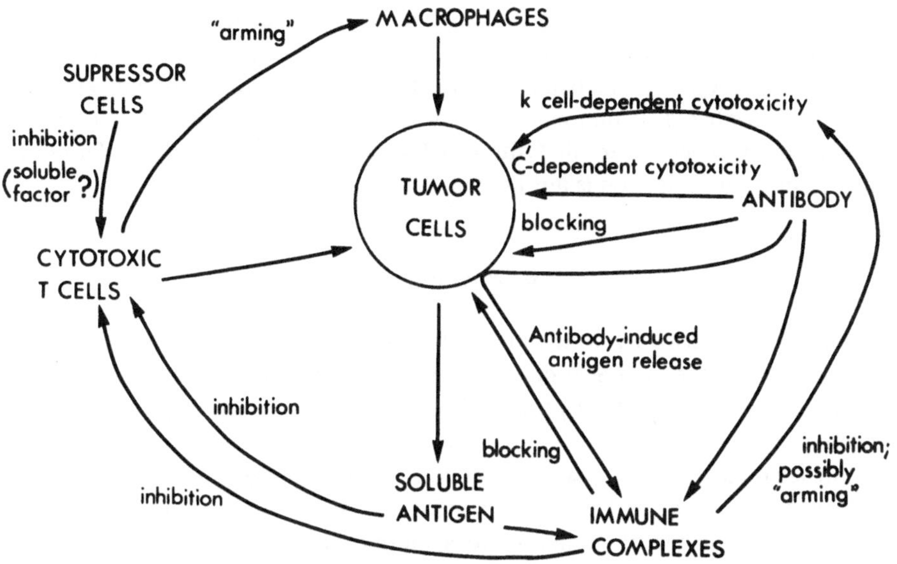

Figure 2. Effector phase of tumor immunity. Shown are some possible antitumor effector mechanisms, and interactions resulting in their neutralization.

MSV-induced tumors by spleen cells from tumor-immune mice is abolished by treatment of the spleen cells with anti-Thy-1 antiserum and complement, but not antiimmunoglobulin antiserum and complement. Similarly, immunity to Simian virus 40 (SV40)-induced tumors (Tevethia *et al.*, 1974; Howell *et al.*, 1974), plasma cell tumors (Rouse *et al.*, 1972), and MCA-induced sarcomas (Kearney *et al.*, 1975) in mice has been shown to depend on T cells. Although characterization of cytotoxic lymphocytes in species other than the mouse is limited by the lack of adequately defined T-cell markers, it has been reported that cell-mediated immunity to MSV-induced sarcomas in rats is mediated predominantly by T cells (Veit and Feldman, 1975). This conclusion is based on the finding that lymphocytes from tumor-bearing rats that are cytotoxic *in vitro* for Moloney sarcoma cells are destroyed by incubation with "T cell-specific" rabbit anti-rat thymocyte serum and complement. Similarly, lysis of the Gross virus-induced rat lymphoma (C58NT)D by lymphoid cells from tumor-immune rats has been shown to depend on T cells (Shellam, 1974). This approach has also been used to characterize lymphocytes cytotoxic for an MCA-induced guinea pig sarcoma, these cells being identified as T cells in view of their susceptibility to complement-dependent lysis by rabbit anti-guinea pig thymocyte serum (Berczi and Sehon, 1975).

All these experimental findings show that the tumor-immune rejection response is T cell-dependent, but they provide only indirect evidence that tumor rejection is mediated by cytotoxic T cells. Thus, the passively immunized recipient in cell-transfer studies could in many cases provide an accessory response to act with the transferred T cells. For example, macrophages could be armed by specific lymphocyte products and activated by contact with tumor antigen. The role of macrophages in tumor rejection will be discussed in more detail, but it should not be overlooked that the exact mechanism by which transferred T cells effect tumor rejection is not known.

B. Macrophages

Some mechanisms by which macrophage cytotoxicity for tumor cells can be initiated were outlined in Section IIA3; several lines of evidence indicate that the cytotoxic macrophages thus generated may play an important part in tumor-rejection responses.

An example of the accessory function of macrophages in tumor rejection may be the requirement for normal peritoneal cells in addition to immune lymphocytes for transfer of immunity to a murine MCA-induced sarcoma (Simes *et al.*, 1975). An important role for macrophages in the tumor–host relationship is also suggested by the demonstration that many animal tumors contain a proportion of cells of host origin, and many of these host cells have the properties of macrophages (Milgrom *et al.*, 1968; Evans, 1972; Wood and Gillespie, 1975). Furthermore, the macrophage content of animal tumors has been shown to relate to immunogenicity, with weakly immunogenic tumors containing a low proportion of macrophages (Eccles and Alexander, 1974). Suppression of the tumor growth on contact with immunological adjuvants such as BCG also depends on macrophages in the tumor (Baldwin, 1976; Baldwin *et al.*, 1976). The host cells present within the tumor have in some cases been shown to be cytotoxic or cytostatic for tumor cells. These antitumor effects are in some cases nonspecific (Evans, 1973; Haskill *et al.*, 1975a), but may also be specific (van Loveren and den Otter, 1974). Cytotoxic cells thought not to be macrophages (and not T cells) have also been demonstrated (Haskill *et al.*, 1975b). These findings indicate that host cells, probably macrophages, that have infiltrated the tumor mass are capable of exerting significant antitumor effects, at least *in vitro*. A role for these effects *in vivo* is suggested by the finding of Wood and Gillespie (1975) that depletion of macrophages from tumor cell suspensions derived from transplanted MCA-induced sarcomas resulted in development of widespread metastases from the injected tumor cells. Control animals injected with tumor cells not depleted of macrophages showed only local tumor growth, with no metastases. These findings are a little surprising, in view of the earlier demonstration that tumors derived from sarcoma cells depleted of macrophages *in vitro* quickly regain their normal proportion of macrophages (Evans, 1972), and might suggest that the macrophages transferred in the control tumor inoculum play a crucial role in the early induction of tumor-immune responses. An experimental approach complementary to that of Wood and Gillespie has been reported by Isa and Sanders (1975). In this approach, the growth of an immunogenic teratoma was enhanced by treatment of tumor recipients with specific antimacrophage serum.

C. Humoral Antibody

Antibody specific for tumor cell surface antigens could exert antitumor effects by at least two mechanisms: in combination with noncommitted Fc receptor-bearing cells in the antibody-dependent cellular cytotoxicitiy reaction, or by fixation of complement. In addition, it should be mentioned that antibody production may change the balance of circulating immune complexes, and this could be very important in relation to the blocking of cell-mediated immune reactions (see Section IVB).

1. Antibody-Dependent Cellular Cytotoxicity

The original demonstration by Möller (1965) that target cells coated with antibody could by lysed by nonimmune lymphoid cells has been followed by numerous studies of antibody-dependent cellular cytotoxicity (ADCC) and related phenomena (reviewed by Perlmann and Holm, 1969; Cerottini and Brunner, 1971). The quantity of antibody required to sensitize target cells is very low, especially in heterologous test systems. For example, lysis of Chang liver cells by blood mononuclear cells from normal individuals could be accomplished with a $1:10^7$ dilution of rabbit antiserum to Chang cells (MacLennan, 1972). IgG antibody, and not IgM, is effective in this system. Effector cells bearing Fc receptors, including lymphocytes, monocytes, and granulocytes, are active in ADCC reactions. Each type of effector cell, however, may cause optimum lysis of different types of target cells. For example, lysis of Chang cells is due to a nonadherent lymphocyte that lacks surface immunoglobulin and is not a T cell (Perlmann *et al.*, 1973), whereas antibody-coated chick erythrocytes are sensitive to lysis by an adherent cell, possibly of the monocyte series (Greenberg *et al.*, 1973). A further point that follows is that the proportion of Fc receptor cells in a population will not necessarily reflect ADCC effector cell activity. Thus, Ortiz de Landazuri *et al.* (1974) showed that antibody-coated Gross virus-induced lymphoma cells can be lysed by blood lymphocytes, but not bone marrow cells, although these two types of cells contain approximately the same proportion of Fc receptor–bearing cells.

Cell-dependent antibody killing has been invoked to account for antitumor effects of antibody in a syngeneic lymphoma system in rats (Hersey, 1973). Animals inoculated with lymphoma cells and injected with allogeneic or xenogeneic antilymphoma antisera showed prolonged survival compared with untreated controls; improved survival correlated well with cell-dependent antibody titers in the sera of treated rats. However, a role for the ADCC mechanism as part of the host rejection response to a wide range of tumors, especially sarcomas and carcinomas, remains to be demonstrated. Antibody capable of inducing ADCC *in vitro* has been demonstrated in the serum of rats bearing an MCA-induced sarcoma (Basham and Currie, 1974). As has already been indicated, however, rats immunized with acellular tumor antigen preparations from MCA-induced sarcomas are unable to resist viable tumor cell challenge, although an antibody response is elicited (Baldwin *et al.*, 1973b). Moreover, syngeneic antibody to these tumors is capable of mediating an ADCC reaction *in vitro* (Baldwin and Fisher, unpublished results). Similarly, passive transfer of serum from tumor-immune rats fails to protect against tumor challenge (Baldwin and Barker, 1967). These findings indicate that the ADCC mechanism may not be effective *in vivo*. There are several possible reasons for this failure, the most likely perhaps being the high sensitivity of the ADCC effect to inhibition by immune complexes, or even high concentrations of immunoglobulin.

2. *Complement-Dependent Cytotoxicity*

Some types of tumors, particularly leukemias and lymphomas, are particularly sensitive *in vitro* to cytotoxic antibody and complement. Thus, the cytotoxic reaction may be complete after as little as 60 min; in contrast, cells from solid tumors such as hepatomas and sarcomas are relatively insensitive, and cytotoxicity is revealed only in assays with long incubation times (Cleveland *et al.*, 1974). This difference may account for the ineffectiveness of antibody in tumor rejection with this type of tumor that was noted above. Another aspect of this problem may be the complement system of the tumor host. For example, significant reduction in tumor could be achieved in AKR mice bearing spontaneous leukemia by infusion of normal mouse serum (Kassel *et al.*, 1973). This effect was ascribed to complement because it was sensitive to heat inactivation and cobra venom factor; also, serum from complement-deficient mice did not give tumor reduction.

Thus, with both complement-dependent and cell-dependent antibody cytotoxicity, the *in vivo* contribution of these cytotoxic mechanisms to the host resistance against antigenic tumor cells may in general not be very great, although under appropriate carefully controlled conditions, they may be beneficial.

IV. FAILURE OF HOST-MEDIATED REJECTION OF TUMORS

Even though the host is able to mobilize various immune responses directed toward the control or destruction of tumor cells, the normal course of events in many cases is for the tumor to grow progressively in the face of this combined tumor-rejection response. Several hypotheses have been proposed to account for the failure of tumor rejection, including:

1. Inadequacy of tumor-specific immunization.
2. Abrogation of tumor immunity by host factors.

A. Inadequacy of Tumor-Specific Immunization

This hypothesis has been described as "sneaking through," and it implies that a nascent tumor may not initially provide a sufficient stimulus to induce an effective immune response, and when host defenses are eventually mobilized, the tumor may already have progressed to a size that is beyond immunological control. Perhaps because of its simplicity, this hypothesis has not received sufficient attention. It should be noted, however, that there are a number of tumors, e.g., the Gross virus–induced lymphoma (C58NT)D, that normally regress when transplanted into syngeneic hosts, and this regression is abrogated by immunosuppressive treatment such as whole-body irradiation or administration of antilymphocyte serum. On the other hand, other types of tumors, such as chemically induced sarcomas, that are often viewed as being "highly immunogenic" grow progressively when transplanted into immunologically competent hosts, and hosts preimmunized to these tumors, e.g., by implantation of radiation-attenuated tumor cells, may reject only modest amounts of tumor, often of the order of 10^6-10^7 cells.

Relevant to the argument that failure of host control of immunogenic tumors may be due in part to a dynamically deficient host response to tumor associated antigens are findings showing that immunostimulation at the time of tumor challenge may result in suppression of tumor growth (Baldwin *et al.*, 1974a). In most instances, however, mere additional stimulation with tumor antigen, e.g., using irradiated tumor cells, is not sufficient, and it is necessary to include an adjuvant. Again, while adjuvant alone may be effective, a more marked response is often achieved when tumor cells and adjuvant are administered together. This more marked response is exemplified by studies with a transplanted MCA-induced rat sarcoma in which a subcutaneous tumor cell challenge is completely rejected when a simultaneous contralateral inoculum of tumor cells admixed with BCG is given (Baldwin and Pimm, 1973). In this model system, however, immune stimulation with BCG alone, as well as specific immunization with irradiated tumor cells, are ineffective. This finding suggests that the immunotherapeutic effect is not due simply to an increase in the rate of host responses to tumor-associated antigens or to a heightening of the responses, but that more qualitative changes may have been induced, perhaps in the lymphoid cell populations recognizing and reacting to produce killer cells. In this context, it is clear that the incorporation of adjuvants into the immunizing inoculum may produce profound changes, especially in the interaction between host lymphocytes and macrophages.

B. Abrogation of Tumor Immunity by Host Factors

The hypothesis that immune responses fail to adequately control tumor growth in the tumor-bearing host through the interaction of factors that diminish the effectiveness of cell-mediated immunity (see Fig. 2) was originally formulated in terms of specific humoral "blocking substances" (I. Hellström and K.E. Hellström, 1969). This hypothesis has been broadened, however, to include a role for both specific and nonspecific humoral factors, and, in addition, suppressor cells (lymphocytes and macrophages) have been implicated.

Specific interference with cell-mediated immunity by serum factors found in the tumor-bearing host has been detected by *in vitro* cytotoxicity tests in several ways. Thus, serum factor may be added to target cells, then removed after incubation, and the susceptibility of the treated target cells to immune lymphoid cell cytotoxicity determined. Abrogation of lymphoid cell cytotoxicity in this type of test has been defined as a *blocking* reaction. Conversely, serum factor may be incubated with normal and immune lymphoid cells, which are subsequently tested after removal of serum for cytotoxicity against previously untreated target cells. Abrogation of immune lymph node cell cytotoxicity under these circumstances is termed *inhibition*. It must be emphasized that these definitions of blocking and inhibition are operational terms that are not meant to imply the mechanism involved in abrogation of cytotoxicity. It is worthwhile to make these distinctions, however, since they give useful information about the factors concerned. For example, hepatoma-bearer serum and hepatoma-immune serum both abrogate immune lymph node cell cytotoxicity when added to the target cell (i.e., blocking); however, immune serum does not affect cytotoxicity when added to the effector cells, but tumor-bearer serum strongly inhibits cytotoxicity (Baldwin and Robins, 1975).

While there are two types of responses that can be envisaged and studied *in vitro*, it is likely that both effects will be operative in the tumor-bearing host. For example, binding of tumor-specific antibody to tumor cell surface antigens may result in marked changes in tumor antigen distribution at the cell surface (e.g., patching, capping) and lead to release of these cell-surface components both in free form and as immune complexes, so that specific inhibition of effector cells can also occur. For example, Hayami *et al.* (1974) showed that incubation of nonblocking serum from Japanese quails after regression of Rous sarcoma virus–induced tumors with Rous sarcoma target cells resulted in the appearance of blocking activity in the culture supernatant. Normal quail serum did not cause the appearance of blocking activity, indicating that antibody-induced shedding of blocking factor had occurred. Because of this interactive aspect, many investigators have not attempted to distinguish between factors that interact with target cells and those that interact with effector cells.

1. Blocking

While the original proposal was that blocking effects were mediated by antibody (I. Hellström and K.E. Hellström, 1969), this interpretation has subsequently been found to be inadequate, and it is thought more likely that immune complexes are involved. For example, serum blocking activity is rapidly lost in animals in which tumors regress spontaneously (I. Hellström and K.E. Hellström, 1969; K.E. Hellström and I. Hellström, 1970) or from which a developing tumor is surgically removed (Baldwin *et al.*, 1973c), and this finding is difficult to interpret in terms of free antibody as the active blocking factor. One of the first indications that blocking factor in tumor-bearer serum may be tumor-specific immune complexes was the finding that the factor in serum of mice bearing MSV-induced sarcomas could be absorbed onto intact tumor cells and then eluted with low-pH buffer. These eluates exhibited blocking when added to cultured Moloney sarcoma cells, preventing cytotoxic responses to sensitized lymph node cells, but when separated at low pH by membrane ultrafiltration into high-molecular-weight (>100,000-dalton) and low-molecular-weight (10,000–100,000-dalton) fractions, individual components lost cytotoxicity, although it was restored on their recombination (Sjögren *et al.*, 1971). More direct evidence that tumor-specific immune complexes protect tumor cells from cytotoxic attack by sensitized lymphoid cells is provided by studies showing that addition of solubilized tumor antigen prepared from a transplanted rat hepatoma to tumor-specific antibody resulted in the development of blocking activity (Baldwin *et al.*, 1972). This activity depended on the presence of appropriate amounts of tumor antigen, however, since no blocking action was observed in antibody or antigen excess. In the latter case, immune complexes will not be able to bind to tumor cells, since antibody reactive to tumor antigen will be fully masked. Interpretation of inadequate blocking by immune complexes in antibody excess is more complicated, and is discussed later.

It should be emphasized that both these approaches indicate that tumor-specific immune complexes are more effective than free tumor-specific antibody in blocking lymphocyte-mediated attack against target tumor cells, but they do not establish conclusively that the same factors are responsible for the effects mediated by tumor-bearer serum.

In studying serum blocking factor from mice bearing MCA-induced sarcomas, however, it was established that the factor(s) could be absorbed onto immunoabsorbent containing Sepharose 4B–linked tumor-specific antibody (Tamerius *et al.*, 1976). The blocking factor was then eluted with 3 M NaSCN and shown by gel-filtration chromatography to separate in the region marked by IgG. From these data, it was concluded that the tumor-bearer serum blocking factor contained immune complexes. Comparably, sequential studies on the appearance of serum blocking factor during growth of a transplanted rat hepatoma (Bowen *et al.*, 1975) showed that the appearance of this activity coincided with the appearance of tumor-specific immune complexes in the serum. In these studies, specific immune complexes were identified by acid dissociation of putative complexes and gel-filtration fractionation under acid conditions to yield components shown to contain tumor-specific antigen and antibody (Baldwin *et al.*, 1973a; Bowen and Baldwin, 1976). It is also relevant to note that the blocking activity of hepatoma-bearing rat serum could be abolished (unblocked) by the addition of tumor-specific antibody, the implication being that antibody neutralization of the antigen moiety of the blocking factor was produced (Robins and Baldwin, 1974).

2. *Inhibition of Lymphoid Cell Reactivity*

Another pathway by which tumor-related factors in the tumor-bearing host may interfere with immunological rejection of tumors is through their effect on cell-mediated immunity. This effect may be produced by specific inhibition of the reactivity of cytotoxic lymphoid cells through interaction with tumor antigen–containing moieties, or tumor-related factors may produce nonspecific depression of cellular immune reactivity.

Considering first the specific effects, circulating tumor antigen–containing moieties may interfere systemically with the tumor-immune response, but it is likely that the factors released in the microenvironment of the tumor will have a more pronounced effect. This effect has been likened to an immunological "camouflage" protecting or inhibiting tumor cells from sensitized lymphoid cells. This camouflage may be particularly relevant in the case of small, progressively growing tumors, with which antigen in the locality of the tumor, but not in the circulation, may induce a localized inhibition of cell-mediated immunity.

Support for the concept that tumor antigen released from a developing tumor may interfere with cell-mediated immunity has been provided by studies showing that the *in vitro* cytotoxicity of sensitized lymphoid cells can be abrogated by brief exposure to tumor antigen. That it can be was initially established in tests with a transplanted rat hepatoma in which particularly well-purified tumor antigen isolated by papain digestion of tumor plasma membrane fractions inhibited the cytotoxicity of lymph node cells from tumor-immune donors for cells of the specific hepatoma (Baldwin *et al.*, 1973d). In these studies, as well as in subsequent tests using tumor antigen preparations isolated by either papain or 3M KCl extraction, it was shown that tumor antigen inhibition was both tumor-specific and dose-dependent (Zöller *et al.*, 1976). For example, appropriate concentrations of extracts prepared from hepatoma D23 inhibited reactivity of hepatoma D23-immune lymph node cells, but not lymph node cells from rats immunized to the immunologically distinct hepatoma D30.

Other studies have supported the view that antigens isolated from tumor may modify the cytotoxicity of sensitized lymphoid cells for tumor cells. With murine sarcoma virus-induced tumors, specific inhibition of cytotoxicity was obtained using 3 M KCl extracts of tumors and either immune spleen cells or purified populations of splenic T cells (Plata and Levy, 1974). It has also been shown that tumor antigen preparations from Gross virus-induced rat lymphomas inhibited the cytotoxicity of sensitized spleen cells. These preparations included crude papain extracts of tumor cell and whole virus, as well as the major virus group specific antigen (P30) (Shellam and Knight, 1974; Shellam *et al.*, 1976). Inhibition of T-lymphocyte cytotoxicity by tumor-associated antigens has also been demonstrated with murine mammary tumor virus-induced tumors, homologous virus completely abrogating the cytotoxicity of sensitized spleen cells (Blair *et al.*, 1975). As already discussed, experimental animal tumors such as carcinogen-induced sarcomas and hepatomas exhibit both individually distinct tumor-specific and cross-reactive embryonic antigens, and cell-mediated immune reactivity to each type of antigen can be inhibited by exposure to the appropriate tissue extract. For example, lymph node cells from rats bearing transplants of MCA-induced sarcomas or aminoazo dye-induced hepatomas contain a population of lymphoid cells sensitized to the tumor-associated embryonic antigens, and the cytotoxicity of these cells can be inhibited by exposure to soluble extracts of embryo tissues (Baldwin *et al.*, 1974b; Zöller *et al.*, 1976).

Comparably, with human tumors, particularly colon carcinomas and melanoma, specific inhibition of peripheral blood effector cell cytotoxicity has been observed after exposure of the lymphoid cells to papain-solubilized tumor membrane fractions (Embleton, 1973; Embleton and Price, 1975) and other crude tumor antigen preparations, including 3 M KCl extracts (Nind *et al.*, 1975).

A possible role for this type of inhibitory response in the tumor-bearing host is suggested, since several studies have also shown that tumor-bearer serum, like the soluble tumor antigen preparations, is able to inhibit the cytotoxicity of lymphoid cells from tumor-immune donors for tumor cells *in vitro* (Baldwin *et al.*, 1973c; Zöller *et al.*, 1975). Similar effects of tumor-bearer serum on lymphoid cell cytotoxicity have been observed with murine tumors induced by the murine sarcoma virus (Plata and Levy, 1974) and the mammary tumor virus (Blair and Lane, 1974). There are also reports that the cytotoxicity of colon carcinoma patients' blood leukocytes for colon carcinoma cells is inhibited by serum from patients with colon carcinoma (I. Hellström *et al.*, 1971; Nind *et al.*, 1975), but interpretation of the human studies is complicated by recent difficulties experienced in interpreting microcytotoxicity tests in human populations (Baldwin and Embleton, 1976).

Circulating tumor antigen and/or immune complexes have been implicated in the inhibitory type of effects observed with tumor-bearer serum, and this hypothesis is supported by the finding that serum activity is rapidly decreased in animals rendered tumor-free, e.g., following surgical resection of tumor grafts, and was not detected in tumor-immune serum (Robins and Baldwin, 1974).

Considering the relevance of these serum-borne factors to the tumor-host relationship, it should be noted that studies with a number of tumors have shown that lymphoid cells taken from tumor-bearers are not reactive, but this activity can be recovered in a number of ways. For example, spleen cells taken from hamsters carrying PARA-7-induced tumors are not cytotoxic *in vitro* for the appropriate target tumor, but they became specifically reactive after *in vitro* incubation overnight at 37°C (Laux and Lausch, 1974). This finding may be interpreted as reflecting removal of inhibitory factors (tumor antigen-containing moieties) following incubation in a fashion comparable to that reported by Currie and Basham (1972), who showed that peripheral blood lymphoid cells from patients with widely disseminated malignant melanoma exhibited cytotoxic reactivity only following extensive washing. However, the prolonged *in vitro* incubation of lymphoid cells in the presence of antigen-containing factors allows for other activation mechanisms. That it does is illustrated by experiments on the *in vitro* stimulation of lymphocytes primed *in vivo* with Gross virus-induced lymphoma cells (Bruce *et al.*, 1976). In these tests, cultures of sensitized lymphocytes (responder cells) with mitomycin C-treated lymphoma cells (stimulator cells) generated effector cells showing a high degree of cytotoxicity to the appropriate target cell. The effector cells emerged from the cultures in a "partially blocked" condition, however, and cytotoxicity was increased by incubation (37°C for 3 hr) followed by washing, this being designed to allow tumor antigen to elute from the effector cells (Bruce *et al.*, 1976).

As already commented on, however, incubation of sensitized lymphoid cell populations in the presence of the appropriate antigen may result in complex changes. That it may is further emphasized by studies on the reactivation of lymphoid cells taken from mice at the advanced stage of tumor growth, i.e., during the so-called "eclipse" phase (Youn *et al.*, 1975). This phase has been defined by Barski and his associates in at least three different mouse tumor systems as the period when lymphoid cells from donors with large tumors became unreactive when tested *in vitro* on the appropriate target tumor cell (Barski and Youn, 1969; Le François *et al.*, 1971; Belehradek *et al.*, 1972). This defect was specific for the tumor, since it was not observed in mice carrying a tumor unrelated to that of the target cells, and the effects have been ascribed partially to mediation by serum factors interacting with the effector cell. It was possible to restore activity to peritoneal exudate cells taken from "eclipsed" donors by transfer to sublethally irradiated (450 rads) syngeneic mice, but for this recovery, it was also necessary to transfer tumor antigen (Youn *et al.*, 1975).

Recovery of cell-mediated cytotoxicity to SV40-induced tumors has also been achieved by treatment of "eclipsed" tumor-bearer lymphocytes with proteolytic enzymes (Blasecki and Tevethia, 1975).

3. *Nonspecific Effects*

Apart from the specific inhibition of lymphoid cell reactivity by tumor antigen-containing factors, other studies have indicated that nonspecific humoral factors may be involved in the tumor-host relationship. For example, serum factors inhibiting stimulation of lymphocytes have been identified in serum from tumor-bearing hosts (Sample *et al.*, 1971; Whitney and Levy, 1975). Also, serum α-globulin fractions with immunosuppressive properties have been implicated in processes of impairment of lymphocyte function (Glasgow *et al.*, 1974; Glaser and Herberman, 1974). These factors have to be considered in accounting for changes in tumor immunity during progressive tumor growth. It is a matter of speculation, however, as to whether they do influence events in the early stages of tumor development, this being the critical period if immunological control is to have relevance. For example, several studies have established that there is no marked immunosuppression during the early period of growth of experimental animal tumors, and it has been clearly shown that tumor-specific cell-mediated immunity can be detected within 2 or 3 days or tumor implantation (Zöller *et al.*, 1975). It has already been emphasized, however, that escape of tumors from host control may reflect relatively minor imbalance, and this escape could easily be achieved through the intervention of some nonspecific factor.

4. *Suppressor Cells*

As already indicated (see Section IIA2), suppressor cell activity may be generated in response to tumor antigens. Evidence is now accumulating suggesting that suppressor cells, especially suppressor T cells, may have an important influence on the host immune response to tumor. In some cases, host T cell deficiency results in retarded tumor growth (Gillette and Fox, 1975; Rotter and Trainin, 1975). The complementary finding of increased tumor growth and metastasis after transfer of T lymphocytes has also been reported (Umiel and Trainin, 1974). Splenectomy may also reduce tumor growth, and this effect has also been attributed to depletion of suppressor T cells (Fujimoto *et al.*, 1976a). The effect of splenectomy may be complex, however, since it has been reported that splenectomized mice may show increased resistance to a large tumor inoculum, but reduced resistance to a small one (Nordlund and Gershon, 1975). Paradoxical effects have also been observed with syngeneic lymphocytes sensitized to tumor cells *in vitro* (Small and Trainin, 1975). Thus, sensitized lymphocytes were cytotoxic *in vitro*, but when injected in admixture with tumor cells, caused enhanced tumor growth; however, when the sensitized lymphocytes were injected systemically, tumor growth was inhibited. Presumably, a suppressor effect not demonstrable under the conditions of the *in vitro* cytotoxicity assay was produced by the *in vitro* sensitization procedure. This may be related to specific stimulatory effects on tumor growth *in vitro* that have been observed after *in vitro* sensitization of normal lymphocytes to tumor antigens (Kall and Hellström, 1975).

A further interesting aspect of the *in vivo* and *in vitro* suppressor effects is the possibility that they may be due to the synthesis of blocking factors (K.E. Hellström and I. Hellström, 1976). Thus, supernatants from cultures of spleen cells from tumor-bearing mice specifically blocked cell-mediated cytotoxicity to the appropriate tumor (Nelson *et al.*, 1975a). Further studies of the production of this blocking factor indicated that protein synthesis was necessary for release of blocking factor into the supernatant (Nelson *et al.*, 1975c). Investigation of the cellular requirements for production of blocking factor revealed that T cells were obligatory, whereas removal of plasma cells did little to affect production (Nelson *et al.*, 1975b). The view that the synthesis of blocking factor is a T-dependent B-cell activity is supported to some extent by the partial restoration of synthesis of blocking factor in T-depleted populations by addition of T cells from normal mice (Nelson *et al.*, 1975b). These findings form an interesting link between studies of suppressor T cells and humoral blocking factors, and it is tempting to speculate that these two areas of study are merely different aspects of the same basic phenomenon.

The experiments discussed in this section emphasize the complexity of interactions between various aspects of the immune response and the control of the growth of tumor. This complexity suggests that in order for *in vitro* sensitization to tumor antigens, or indeed any procedure designed to increase tumor immunity, to be of benefit, a full understanding of the requirements for stimulation of each aspect of the response must be attained.

V. IMMUNOBIOLOGICAL EFFECTS OF CIRCULATING TUMOR ANTIGEN IN THE TUMOR-BEARING HOST

The studies on the influence of tumor-bearer serum on the *in vitro* cytotoxicity of sensitized lymphoid cells reviewed herein establish several pathways whereby serum-borne factors may modify cell-mediated immunity to tumors. The establishment of these pathways does not, however, establish any *in vivo* relevance, and this lack has led to a number of studies designed to correlate the appearance of serum blocking/inhibitory factors with the stage of tumor growth, the implication being that early events are likely to have most relevance. Since these effects are viewed as being mediated by tumor antigen–containing moieties, several investigations have also been carried out to determine serum levels of tumor antigen and immune complexes.

As preface to comment on these studies, it should be recognized that serum levels of tumor-associated factors will reflect a number of phenomena, including the rate of tumor antigen release and also the rate of its elimination from the circulation (Price and Baldwin, 1976). Each of these processes will also be affected by complex changes associated with the type of tumor, the nature of the tumor-associated antigen, and the stage of the disease. Release of tumor-associated antigen in soluble form into the extracellular environment may occur, for example, as a consequence of tumor cell death due to inadequate nutrient supply or induced by cytotoxic factors, followed by fragmentation and autolysis of cell constituents. Metabolic turnover of tumor cell surface membranes may be more important, however, and this "shedding" will represent several processes, including release of plasma membrane by a process of "pinching-off" of microvilli and synthesis and release of cell-surface products. These processes may be enhanced (or inhibited) by cellular and humoral reactions with the cell surface–expressed tumor antigens (Nicolson, 1976; Price and Baldwin, 1976); for example, interaction with antibody leads to surface antigen redistribution, "patching," and "capping" effects. The rate of elimination of circulating tumor antigen and/or specific immune complexes will also be influenced by a number of factors, one of the most important probably being the effectiveness of the host immune response. This response, again, will involve several components, including antibody and the reticuloendothelial system.

From these considerations, it is not surprising that the pattern of release of tumor antigen and immune complexes varies with different tumor systems, and also with the type of neoantigen analyzed. This variation is exemplified by comparative studies on the release into serum of tumor-specific and tumor-associated embryonic antigens during subcutaneous growth of a transplanted rat hepatoma (Bowen *et al.*, 1975; Rees *et al.*, 1975b). Tumor-specific antigen was detected in serum within 7–10 days after tumor implantation, but with further progressive growth, the antigen became undetectable (Fig. 3). At this stage, however, tumor-specific immune complexes were identified, suggesting that the decrease in free antigen levels reflected the development of a tumor-specific immune response. Then, in the terminal phase of tumor growth, it was possible to detect circulating tumor-specific antibody, but again in the presence of specific immune complexes. The pattern of release into serum of the embryonic antigen associated with this tumor differed in that circulating antigen together with immune complexes were detected at all stages of tumor growth, apart from the initial period when the tumor was becoming established. Several factors may be considered in accounting for these differences, but one important point is thought to be the relative instability of the embryonic component within the tumor cell surface membrane. This is indicated, for example, by the ease with which embryonic

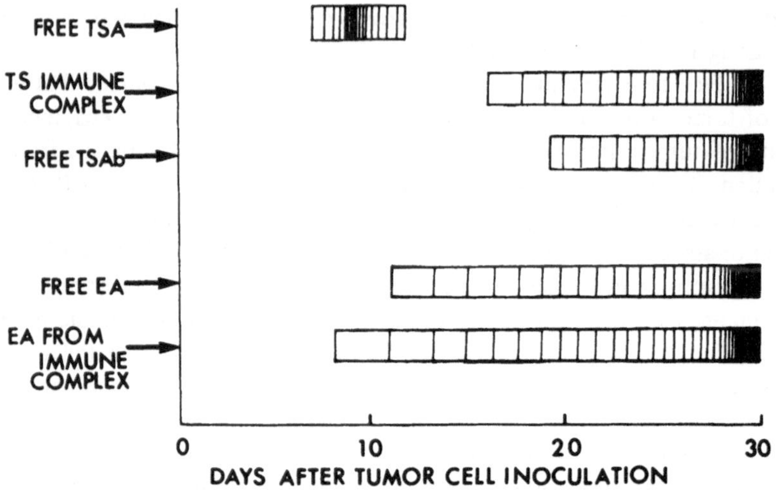

Figure 3. Diagrammatic representation of the serum factors detected during the subcutaneous growth of aminoazo dye–induced rat hepatoma D23. Free circulating tumor-specific antigen (TSA) was demonstrable during the early phase of growth of hepatoma D23 (between days 7 and 11), while at later stages (from about day 16), free antibody (TSAb) was detectable. Tumor-specific (TS) immune complexes were detected before free antibody activity was evident, although both factors then persisted in the serum throughout tumor development. Immune complexes containing hepatoma-associated embryonic antigen (EA) were identified after about 1 week following tumor cell inoculation, this being accompanied by the appearance of free circulating embryonic antigen activity shortly afterward, which remained in excess during tumor growth. Data compiled from Bowen *et al.* (1975) and Rees *et al.* (1975b).

antigens can be released from ruptured tumor cells, and these antigens have been shown to be rapidly released *in vitro* from tumor cells following binding to specific antisera (Price and Baldwin, 1976). In comparison, the tumor-specific product is firmly incorporated into the cell surface membrane so that its release requires degradative treatment, e.g., papain digestion or 3 M KCl extraction, and this component shows greater stability at the cell surface even following cell-antibody binding.

Although there are quite marked variations in the pattern of release into serum of tumor-associated products during growth of different experimental tumors, a common finding is that tumor antigen appears during the early phase of tumor growth. As already described, this appearance occurs with rat hepatomas implanted subcutaneously, and similar effects are obtained with this tumor developing either intraperitoneally or in pulmonary tissue following intravenous challenge (Bowen and Baldwin, 1976). Similarly, tumor-specific antigen is detected during the early phase of growth of a transplanted rat sarcoma, and progressive growth is accompanied by a continuous increase in serum antigen levels (Thomson *et al.*, 1973; Thomson, 1975). These and other studies in which serum factors have been identified by their influence *in vitro* in cell-mediated immune reactions (Poupon *et al.*, 1974; Robins and Baldwin, 1974; Bray *et al.*, 1975) suggest that tumor antigen released during the early phase of tumor growth may be of paramount importance in abrogating cell-mediated rejection of tumor. As already emphasized, however, this effect may operate primarily in the local environment of the tumor, in which case the serum factors may be taken to indicate only local effects.

Few attempts have been made as yet to verify the validity of the concepts developed from studies on the abrogation of *in vitro* lymphocyte cytotoxicity for tumor cells, and the evidence, as presented, is open to several alternative explanations. For example, studies monitoring serum blocking activity have frequently shown a correlation between their decrease and the success of immunotherapy (Bansal and Sjögren, 1972; Embleton, 1976b). This finding could be simply interpreted, however, as a measure of circulating tumor antigen-containing moieties that should decrease following tumor destruction, and it can in fact be demonstrated by immunochemical evaluation (Thomson, 1975; Bowen and Baldwin, 1976).

There are similar difficulties in interpreting studies designed to influence tumor growth either positively or negatively by alteration of the spectrum of serum factors. For example, administration of tumor immune serum under conditions in which the blocking activity of tumor-bearer serum was neutralized has been shown to result in an inhibition of tumor growth (Bansal and Sjögren, 1972). Interpretation of these results in terms of "unblocking" is not entirely satisfactory, however, since transferred immune serum may act more directly on the tumor through complement- or cell-dependent antibody-mediated cytotoxic effects. Similar problems are also evident in interpreting studies on rat sarcomas in which the active development of a tumor immune cell-mediated response that causes rejection of tumor, e.g., by contralateral immune stimulation with tumor cells admixed with BCG, can be abrogated by simultaneous intraperitoneal administration of solubilized tumor antigen (Baldwin, 1976). This abrogation can be interpreted according to the hypothesis derived from *in vitro* studies as being mediated by the enhanced production of circulating tumor antigen thus interfering with cell-mediated immunity. As already discussed, however, stimulation with soluble tumor antigen may produce a number of effects, including the formation of suppressor cells.

Acknowledgment

This work was supported by a block grant from the Cancer Research Campaign to Professor R.W. Baldwin.

VI. REFERENCES

Asherson, G.L., and Zembala, M., 1975, *Curr. Top. Microbiol. Immunol.* **72**:55.
Baldwin, R.W., 1973, *Adv. Cancer Res.* **18**:1.
Baldwin, R.W., 1976, *Transplant. Rev.* **28**:62.
Baldwin, R.W., and Barker, C.R., 1967, *Int. J. Cancer* **2**:355.
Baldwin, R.W., and Embleton, M.J., 1971, *Int. J. Cancer* **7**:17.
Baldwin, R.W., and Embleton, M.J., 1974, *Int. J. Cancer* **13**:433.
Baldwin, R.W., and Embleton, M.J., 1976, *Int. Rev. Exp. Pathol.*, in press.
Baldwin, R.W., and Pimm, M.V., 1973, *Br. J. Cancer* **28**:281.
Baldwin, R.W., and Price, M.R., 1975, *Cancer: A Comprehensive Treatise* (F.F. Becker, ed.), Vol. 1, Plenum Press, New York, p. 353.
Baldwin, R.W., and Robins, R.A., 1975, *Curr. Top. Microbiol. Immunol.* **72**:21.
Baldwin, R.W., Price, M.R., and Robins, R.A., 1972, *Nature (London) New Biol.* **238**:185.
Baldwin, R.W., Bowen, J.G., and Price, M.R., 1973a, *Br. J. Cancer* **28**:16.
Baldwin, R.W., Embleton, M.J., and Moore, M., 1973b, *Br. J. Cancer* **28**:389.
Baldwin, R.W., Embleton, M.J., and Robins, R.A., 1973c, *Int. J. Cancer* **11**:1.
Baldwin, R.W., Price, M.R., and Robins, R.A., 1973d, *Int. J. Cancer* **11**:527.
Baldwin, R.W., Cook, A.J., Hopper, D.G., and Pimm, M.V., 1974a, *Int. J. Cancer* **13**:743.
Baldwin, R.W., Embleton, M.J., Price, M.R., and Vose, B.M., 1974b, *Transplant. Rev.* **20**:77.
Baldwin, R.W., Hopper, D.G., and Pimm, M.V., 1976, *Ann. N. Y. Acad. Sci.*, in press.
Bansal, S.C., and Sjögren, H.O., 1972, *Int. J. Cancer* **9**:490.
Barski, G., and Youn, J.K., 1969, *J. Nat. Cancer Inst.* **43**:111.
Basham, C., and Currie, G.A., 1974, *Br. J. Cancer* **29**:189.
Belehradek, J., Barski, G., and Thonier, M., 1972, *Int. J. Cancer* **9**:461.
Bennett, B., Old, L.J., and Boyse, E.A., 1964, *Transplantation* **2**:183.
Berczi, I., and Sehon, A.H., 1975, *Int. J. Cancer* **16**:665.
Blair, P.B., and Lane, M.A., 1974, *J. Immunol.* **112**:439.
Blair, P.B., Lane, M.A., and Yagi, M.J., 1975, *J. Immunol.* **115**:190.
Blasecki, J.W., and Tevethia, S.S., 1975, *Int. J. Cancer* **16**:275.
Bowen, J.G., and Baldwin, R.W., 1976, *Int. J. Cancer* **17**:254.
Bowen, J.G., Robins, R.A., and Baldwin, R.W., 1975, *Int. J. Cancer* **15**:640.
Bray, A.E., Holt, P.G., Roberts, L.M., and Keast, D., 1975, *Int. J. Cancer* **16**:607.
Bruce, J., Mitchison, N.A., and Shellam, G.R., 1976, *Int. J. Cancer* **17**:342.
Cantor, H., and Boyse, E.A., 1975, *J. Exp. Med.* **141**:1376.
Cantor, H., and Simpson, E., 1975, *Eur. J. Immunol.* **5**:330.
Cerottini, J.-C., and Brunner, K.T., 1971, *In Vitro Methods in Cell-Mediated Immunity* (B.R. Bloom and P. Glade, eds.), Academic Press, New York, p. 369.
Cerottini, J.-C., Engers, H.D., MacDonald, M.R., and Brunner, K.T., 1974a, *J. Exp. Med.* **140**:703.
Cerottini, J.-C., MacDonald, H.R., Engers, H.D., and Brunner, K.T., 1974b, *Progress in Immunology II* (L. Brent and J. Holborow, eds.), Vol. 3, North-Holland Publishing Company, Amsterdam, p. 153.
Cleveland, P.H., McKhann, C.F., Johnson, K., and Nelson, S., 1974, *Int. J. Cancer* **14**:417.
Cohen, L., and Howe, M.L., 1973, *Proc. Nat. Acad. Sci. U.S.A.* **70**:2707.
Cohn, M., 1976, *Molecular Approaches to Immunology, Miami Winter Symposium* (E.E. Smith and D.W. Ribbons, eds.), Vol. 9.
Currie, G.A., and Basham, C., 1972, *Br. J. Cancer* **26**:427.
Eccles, S.A., and Alexander, P., 1974, *Nature (London)* **250**:667.
Eggers, A.E., and Wunderlich, J.R., 1975, *J. Immunol.* **114**:1554.

Embleton, M.J., 1973, *Br. J. Cancer* **28**, *Suppl. I*, 142.
Embleton, M.J., 1976a, *Int. J. Cancer* (abstract), in press.
Embleton, M.J., 1976b, *Br. J. Cancer*, **33**:584.
Embleton, M.J., and Price, M.R., 1975, *Behring Inst. Mitt.* **56**:157.
Evans, R., 1972, *Transplantation* **14**:468.
Evans, R., 1973, *Br. J. Cancer* **28**, *Suppl. I*, 19.
Evans, R., and Alexander, P., 1970, *Nature (London)* **228**:620.
Evans, R., and Alexander, P., 1972a, *Nature (London)* **236**:168.
Evans, R., and Alexander, P., 1972b, *Immunology* **23**:627.
Fujimoto, S., Greene, M.I., and Sehon, A.H., 1976a, *J. Immunol.* **116**:791.
Fujimoto, S., Greene, M.I., and Sehon, A.H., 1976b, *J. Immunol.* **116**:800.
Gershon, R.K., 1975, *Transplant. Rev.* **26**:170.
Gershon, R.K., Carter, R.L., and Kondo, K., 1967, *Nature (London)* **213**:674.
Gillette, R.W., and Fox, A., 1975, *Cell. Immunol.* **19**:328.
Glaser, M., and Herberman, R.B., 1974, *J. Nat. Cancer Inst.* **53**:1767.
Glaser, M., Kirchner, H., and Herberman, R.B., 1975, *Int. J. Cancer* **16**:384.
Glasgow, A.H., Nimberg, R.B., Menzoian, J.O., Saproschetz, I., Cooperband, S.R., Schmid, K., and Mannick, J.A., 1974, *N. Engl. J. Med.* **291**:1263.
Gorczynski, R.M., 1974a, *J. Immunol.* **112**:533.
Gorczynski, R.M., 1974b, *J. Immunol.* **112**:1826.
Granger, G.A., and Weiser, R.S., 1966, *Science* **151**:97.
Greenberg, A.H., Shen, L., and Roitt, I.M., 1973, *Clin. Exp. Immunol.* **15**:251.
Harder, F.H., and McKhann, C.F., 1968, *J. Nat. Cancer Inst.* **40**:231.
Haskill, J.S., Proctor, J.W., and Yamamura, Y., 1975a, *J. Nat. Cancer Inst.* **54**:387.
Haskill, J.S., Yamamura, Y., and Radov, L., 1975b, *Int. J. Cancer* **16**:798.
Hayami, M., Hellström, I., Hellström, K.E., and Yamanouchi, K., 1972, *Int. J. Cancer* **10**:507.
Hayami, M., Hellström, I., Hellström, K.E., and Lannin, D.R., 1974, *Int. J. Cancer* **13**:43.
Häyry, P., and Anderson, L.C., 1974, *Eur. J. Immunol.* **4**:145.
Hellström, I., and Hellström, K.E., 1969, *Int. J. Cancer* **4**:587.
Hellström, I., Sjögren, H.O., Warner, G.A., and Hellström, K.E., 1971, *Int. J. Cancer* **7**:226.
Hellström, K.E., and Hellström, I., 1969, *Adv. Cancer Res.* **12**:167.
Hellström, K.E., and Hellström, I., 1970, *Annu. Rev. Microbiol.* **24**:373.
Hellström, K.E., and Hellström, I., 1974, *Adv. Immunol.* **18**:209.
Hellström, K.E., and Hellström, I., 1976, *Ann. N. Y. Acad. Sci.* **276**:176.
Hersey, P., 1973, *Nature (London) New Biol.* **244**:22.
Howell, S.B., Dean, J.D., Esber, E.C., and Law, L.W., 1974, *Int. J. Cancer* **14**:662.
Isa, A.M., and Sanders, B.R., 1975, *Transplantation* **20**:296.
Ishidate, M., 1967, *Nature (London)* **215**:184.
Kall, M.A., and Hellström, I., 1975, *J. Immunol.* **114**:1083.
Kassel, R.L., Old, L.J., Carswell, E.A., Fiore, N.C., and Hardy, W.D., 1973, *J. Exp. Med.* **138**:925.
Kearney, R., Basten, A., and Nelson, D.S., 1975, *Int. J. Cancer* **15**:438.
Kirchner, H., Chused, T.M., Herberman, R.B., Holden, H.T., and Lavrin, D.H., 1974a, *J. Exp. Med.* **139**:1473.
Kirchner, H., Herberman, R.B., Glaser, M., and Lavrin, D.H., 1974b, *Cell. Immunol.* **13**:32.
Kirchner, H., Muchmore, A.V., Chused, T.M., Holden, H.T., and Herberman, R.B., 1975, *J. Immunol.* **114**:206.
Kisielow, P., Hirst, J.A., Shiku, H., Beverley, P.C.L., Hoffman, M.K., Boyse, E.A., and Oettgen, H.F., 1975, *Nature (London)* **253**:219.
Lamon, E.W., 1974, *Biochim. Biophys. Acta* **355**:149.

Laux, D., and Lausch, R.N., 1974, *J. Immunol.* **112**:1900.

Le François, D., Youn, J.K., Belehradek, J., and Barski, G., 1971, *J. Nat. Cancer Inst.* **46**:981.

Levy, M.H., and Wheelock, E.F., 1974, *Adv. Cancer Res.* **20**:131.

Mackaness, G.B., and Lagrange, P.H., 1974, *J. Exp. Med.* **140**:865.

MacLennan, I.C.M., 1972, *Transplant. Rev.* **13**:67.

Meltzer, M.S., Oppenheim, J.J., Littman, B.H., Leonard, E.J., and Rapp, H.J., 1972, *J. Nat. Cancer Inst.* **49**:727.

Milgrom, F., Humphrey, L.J., Tønder, O., Yasuda, J., and Witebakey, E., 1968, *Int. Arch. Allergy* **33**:478.

Möller, E., 1965, *Science* **147**:873.

Möller, G., Lemke, H., and Opitz, H.-G., 1976, *Scand. J. Immunol.* **5**:269.

Myburgh, J.A., and Mitchison, N.A., 1976, *Transplantation* **22**:236.

Nathan, C.F., and Terry, W.D., 1975, *J. Exp. Med.* **142**:887.

Nelson, K., Pollack, S.B., and Hellström, K.E., 1975a, *Int. J. Cancer* **15**:806.

Nelson, K., Pollack, S.B., and Hellström, K.E., 1975b, *Int. J. Cancer* **16**:539.

Nelson, K., Pollack, S.B., and Hellström, K.E., 1975c, *Int. J. Cancer* **16**:932.

Nicolson, G.L., 1976, *Biochim. Biophys. Acta* **458**:1.

Nind, A.P.P., Matthews, N., Pihl, E.A.V., Rolland, J.M., and Nairn, R.C., 1975, *Br. J. Cancer* **31**:620.

Nordlund, J.J., and Gershon, R.K., 1975, *J. Immunol.* **114**:1486.

Oettgen, H.F., Old, L.J., McLean, E.P., and Carswell, E.A., 1968, *Nature (London)* **220**:295.

Ortiz de Landazuri, M., Kedar, E., and Fahey, J.L., 1974, *J. Nat. Cancer Inst.* **52**:147.

Pellis, N.R., and Kahan, B.D., 1975, *J. Immunol.* **115**:1717.

Perlmann, P., and Holm, G., 1969, *Adv. Immunol.* **11**:117.

Perlmann, P., Wigzell, H., Goldstein, P., Lamon, E.W., Larsson, A., O'Toole, C., Perlmann, H., and Svedmyr, E.A.J., 1973, *Adv. Biosci.* **12**:71.

Plata, F., and Levy, J.P., 1974, *Nature (London)* **249**:271.

Poupon, M.-F., Lespinats, G., and Kolb, J.-P., 1974, *J. Nat. Cancer Inst.* **52**:1127.

Prather, S.O., and Lausch, R.N., 1976, *Int. J. Cancer* **17**:380.

Price, M.R., and Baldwin, R.W., 1976, *Cell Surface Reviews* (G. Poste and G.L. Nicolson, eds.), Vol. III, North-Holland Publishing Co., Amsterdam, in press.

Rees, R.C., Bray, J., Robins, R.A., and Baldwin, R.W., 1975a, *Int. J. Cancer* **15**:762.

Rees, R.C., Price, M.R., Shah, L.P., and Baldwin, R.W., 1975b, *Transplantation* **19**:424.

Robins, R.A., 1975, *Br. J. Cancer* **32**:21.

Robins, R.A., and Baldwin, R.W., 1974, *Int. J. Cancer* **14**:589.

Rotter, V., and Trainin, N., 1975, *Transplantation* **20**:68.

Rouse, B.T., Rollinghoff, M., and Warner, N.L., 1972, *Nature (London) New Biol.* **238**:116.

Sample, W.F., Gertner, H.R., and Chretien, P.B., 1971, *J. Nat. Cancer Inst.* **46**:1291.

Shellam, G.R., 1974, *Int. J. Cancer* **14**:65.

Shellam, G.R., and Knight, R.A., 1974, *Nature (London)* **252**:330.

Shellam, G.R., Knight, R.A., Mitchison, N.A., Gorczynski, R.M., and Maoz, A., 1976, *Transplant. Rev.* **29**:249.

Simes, R.J., Kearney, R., and Nelson, D.S., 1975, *Immunology* **29**:343.

Sjögren, H.O., 1965, *Prog. Exp. Tumor Res.* **6**:289.

Sjögren, H.O., Hellström, I., Bansal, S.C., and Hellström, K.E., 1971, *Proc. Nat. Acad. Sci. U.S.A.* **68**:1372.

Small, M., and Trainin, N., 1975, *Int. J. Cancer* **15**:962.

Smith, H.G., and Leonard, E.J., 1974, *J. Nat. Cancer Inst.* **53**:187.

Steele, G., Sjögren, H.O., and Price, M.R., 1975, *Int. J. Cancer* **16**:33.

Tamerius, J.D., and Hellström, I., 1974, *J. Immunol.* **112**:1987.
Tamerius, J., Nepom, J., Hellström, I., and Hellström, K.E., 1976, *J. Immunol.* **116**:724.
Taranger, L.A., Chapman, W.H., Hellström, I., and Hellström, K.E., 1972, *Science* **176**:1337.
Tevethia, S.S., Blasecki, J.W., Waneck, G., and Goldstein, A., 1974, *J. Immunol.* **113**:1417.
Thomson, D.M.P., 1975, *Int. J. Cancer* **15**:1016.
Thomson, D.M.P., Eccles, S., and Alexander, P., 1973, *Br. J. Cancer* **28**:6.
Treves, A.J., Schechter, B., Cohen, I.R., and Feldman, M., 1976, *J. Immunol.* **116**:1059.
Umiel, T., and Trainin, N., 1974, *Transplantation* **18**:244.
Unanue, E.R., and Calderon, J., 1975, *Fed. Proc. Fed. Amer. Soc. Exp. Biol.* **34**:1737.
Vaage, J., 1971, *Cancer Res.* **31**:1655.
van Loveren, N., and den Otter, W., 1974, *J. Nat. Cancer Inst.* **53**:1057.
Veit, B.C., and Feldman, J.D., 1975, *Int. J. Cancer* **15**:367.
Wahl, D.V., Chapman, W.H., Hellström, I., and Hellström, K.E., 1974, *Int. J. Cancer* **14**:114.
Whitney, R.B., and Levy, J.G., 1975, *J. Nat. Cancer Inst.* **54**:733.
Wood, G.W., and Gillespie, G.Y., 1975, *Int. J. Cancer* **16**:1022.
Youn, J.K., Le François, D., Hue, G., Santillana, M., and Barski, G., 1975, *Int. J. Cancer* **16**:629.
Zöller, M., Price, M.R., and Baldwin, R.W., 1975, *Int. J. Cancer* **16**:593.
Zöller, M., Price, M.R., and Baldwin, R.W., 1976, *Int. J. Cancer* **17**:129.

Cytotoxic T Lymphocyte Membrane Components: An Analysis of Structures Related to Function

Arthur K. Kimura and Hans Wigzell

Department of Immunology
University of Uppsala Biomedical Center
Box 582, S-751 23 Uppsala, Sweden

I. INTRODUCTION

Linus Pauling once stated that "life is the harmony between molecules and not the property of any one." As immunologists concerned with the "disharmony between molecules," we seek to unravel and understand the complexities of cellular recognition of disturbing structures, cellular activation, and finally the relief of the disharmony by the various effector mechanisms of the immune system.

In transplantation systems, several types of lymphoid cells have been shown to possess tissue-destructive activities against histoincompatible grafts. Among these types of cells are the cytotoxic thymus-dependent "T" lymphocyte, the antibody-dependent "K" cell, and the "armed" macrophage. Each of these effector cell systems appear to represent the direct cytotoxic action of immune lymphoid cells without the participation of complement factors. One of the most widely studied lymphoid cells in this respect has been the thymus-dependent T lymphocyte. The physiological importance of T lymphocytes in allograft rejection and cytolytic activity against some virus-modified syngeneic cells has received considerable acclaim. T cells appear to function autonomously at all stages of immune reactivity against allogeneic cells, and in the absence of antibody, only T lymphocytes have been shown to be capable of specific killing. This cellular compartment of the immune system represents a fascinating biological model for examining the phenomena of specific antigen-recognition, differentiation, and the striking capacity of these cells to destroy the histoincompatible cells to which they were initially activated.

The realization that lymphoid cells can perform tissue-destructive activities against incompatible cells without secretion of detectable amounts of toxins, and yet accomplish this destruction in an immunologically specific manner, has led us to examine T cell membrane components that could be expected to possess important components relating to these activities.

Since the molecular characteristics that define a cytotoxic T lymphocyte (CTL) and the mechanisms through which killing is exerted remain obscure, we have focused our efforts on the analysis of those cell-surface membrane components that play a relevant role in the ability of CTLs to exert their cytolytic activity. One of the most appealing systems for the analysis of membrane structures related to cytolytic function would be one correlating the appearance of new membrane structures found only on fully differentiated CTLs with the ability to express immunologically specific cytolytic function. Our system of analyzing the functional relevance of various membrane components has employed a large battery of antisera against components of cytotoxic T lymphocyte membranes and the subsequent effect of such antisera to interfere with specific cell-mediated cytolysis in the absence of complement. We have analyzed the distribution of various antigenic and functional membrane components on selected subpopulations of purified CTLs to distinguish active compartments of T cell reactivity at the effector stage, trying to understand the types of interactions CTLs can have with target cells. Finally, we have undertaken biochemical analysis of unique membrane components found on populations of cytotoxic T lymphocytes, and have tried to correlate their presence with the ability of CTLs to exert cytolytic function.

The principal aim of this review is to summarize the approaches we have taken to analyze the relevance of various CTL membrane components as necessary for killing to be exerted. We do not intend to cover the extensive literature that forms the basis of our present understanding of CTLs, and have made every attempt to save the reader time by avoiding undue speculation.

II. FRACTIONATION AND SENSITIZATION PROCEDURES USED IN OBTAINING "HIGHLY PURIFIED" POPULATIONS OF CTLs

Since much of the interpretation and evaluation of the work to be discussed in this article is based on the purity of the various cell populations we have examined, a discussion of our fractionation procedures and criteria for "highly purified CTLs" is warranted. We have employed a variety of experimental fractionation procedures as well as *in vitro* and *in vivo* proliferative pressures to achieve highly purified populations of cytotoxic T lymphocytes. Much of the experimental detail on cell fractionation has been recently reviewed (Wigzell and Häyry, 1974), but will be dealt with briefly in the following sections.

A. Specific Selection of Responding T Cells by Affinity Fractionation

Highly purified populations of "T" lymphocytes can be easily obtained from peripheral lymphoid tissue by filtration of the cells through glass-bead or degalan-bead columns first coated with mouse immunoglobulin (Ig), followed by a heterologous (rabbit) anti-mouse Ig serum (Wigzell *et al.*, 1972). Such an affinity column removes cells with surface immunoglobulin due to their interaction with free antigen-binding "arms" of the rabbit anti-mouse Ig sera; retains cells bearing Fc receptors which combine with the immune complexes formed on the beads; and to a large extent removes adherent cells, presumably via the electrostatic features of the glass or plastic surfaces. Thus, we can easily achieve starting populations of "T" cells of purity in excess of 98%, as judged by their susceptibility to anti-Thy 1 + complement cytotoxicity or immunofluorescent staining. "T" cells prepared in this manner have been routinely used as the starting (responding) cell population in all these studies.

B. *In Vitro* and *in Vivo* Conditions for the Generation of Specifically Cytotoxic T Lymphocytes

The positive selection of a "clone" of antigen-reactive T lymphocytes reactive to a given set of alloantigens can easily be accomplished *in vitro* or *in vivo* by sensitization across a suitable histocompatibility barrier. Using populations of "T" cells prepared by fractionation on Ig-anti-Ig columns, we have routinely used the two methods described below for the generation of CTLs.

1. Mixed Leukocyte Culture (MLC) Sensitization

Spleens from donor mice to be used as the responding cell population were carefully teased apart on a stainless steel wire mesh to produce a single cell suspension. The cells were washed twice in phosphate-buffered saline (PBS) + 5% fetal calf serum (FCS), and the final cell pellet was resuspended in 0.84% NH_4Cl to lyse the red cells (Boyle, 1968), and washed an additional time in PBS + FCS. "T" cells were then obtained by filtration of the cell suspension through an Ig-anti-Ig column and washed twice in PBS + FCS. The cells were then adjusted to a concentration of 2×10^6/ml in modified Eagle's-Hanks' amino acid-supplemented medium (Peck and Bach, 1973) containing 10^{-5} M 2-mercaptoethanol, 20 mM *N*-2-hydroxyethyl-piperazine-*N'*-2-ethanesulfonic acid (Hepes), antibiotics, and 5% FCS. After receiving 2000 R X-irradiation, stimulating cells were washed twice and resuspended to the same concentration in the tissue culture medium described above + FCS. The cells were mixed at a ratio of 1:1 and cultured in upright Falcon flasks (No. 3013) for a period of 5-6 days at 37°C in an atmosphere of 5% CO_2 in air.

2. *Sensitization in Lethally Irradiated Allogeneic Hosts*

Populations of Ig-anti-Ig-purified "T" lymphocytes were prepared as described above and used as the source of responding cells. Allogeneic hosts irradiated with 800 R were injected intravenously with $2.5\text{-}3.0 \times 10^7$ allogeneic T cells and maintained an antibiotic supplemented drinking water (polymyxin B sulfate, 125 mg/liter) for the 5-6 day period of sensitization. At the end of this period, the spleens were harvested under aseptic conditions, red cells were lysed with NH_4Cl, and the cells were washed twice in PBS.

C. Unit-Gravity Velocity Sedimentation of the Cytotoxic T Lymphocytes

During the course of sensitization and depending on the culture or *in vivo* conditions, there are at least two selective pressures operating that favor the proliferation and maturation of a given antigen-reactive population of T lymphocytes: (1) positive selection for the rapidly proliferating antigen-specific T lymphocyte precursors; (2) the gradual *in vitro* dying off of the unstimulated small lymphocytes with reactivities against other antigenic specificities. At the peak of the primary cytotoxic response, the activated "T" blasts display restricted specificity toward the sensitizing set of allo-antigens, and this restriction is expressed and improved on repeated restimulation of the memory T cells (L.C. Andersson and Häyry, 1974; Cerottini *et al.*, 1974). These rapidly dividing lymphocytes induced by antigenic stimulation display phenotypic characteristics of "blast" cells (L.C. Andersson, 1973), in sharp contrast to the surviving nonreactive small T lymphocytes of unrelated antigenic specificities. One can take advantage of the blast characteristics of the antigen-activated clone of T cells for a final purification of the cytotoxic T lymphocyte population. This has been done by velocity sedimentation at 1g in a linear 15-30% serum gradient (Miller and Phillips, 1969; L.C. Andersson and Häyry, 1975; Wagner and Röllinghoff, 1976). By employing these fractionation and selective pressures, we obtain populations of CTLs that are highly efficient in cell-mediated cytotoxicity and possess the restricted memory for that given set of alloantigens. Some of the surface characteristics of CTLs prepared by these procedures are summarized in Table I.

Table I. Characteristics of "Highly Purified" Populations of CTL Blasts

	Sensitized:	
Surface markers	*In vitro*	*In vivo*
Thy-1.2	98%	98%
Ig	<0.01%	< 0.5%
H-2 donor genotype	>97%	>95%
Phagocytic[a]	1%	1–2%

[a]Phagocytic cells were determined by ingestion of sensitized (7 S antibody) coated erythrocytes or Zymosan particles (Huber and Wigzell, 1975). The frequency of such cells can be greatly reduced (100-fold) by a combination of carbonyl iron + magnetism treatment and adherence at 37°C to plastic or glass surfaces.

III. CHARACTERISTICS OF T CELL-MEDIATED CYTOLYSIS

A. Requirements for Initiation and Propagation of the Lytic Cycle

Attempts to inhibit the activity of specifically cytotoxic T lymphocytes by various reagents draw from and expand on our present understanding of the steps and mechanisms involved in the lytic cycle. Although we are far from an understanding of the molecular components that effect target cell destruction by CTLs, certain features and requirements of the interaction have been studied in detail (for reviews, see Berke and Amos, 1973; Henney, 1973; Golstein and Smith, 1976a).

The first event initiating the lytic cycle of CTLs is a Mg^{2+}-dependent binding of killer and target cell (Stulting and Berke, 1973; Golstein and Smith, 1976b). This binding is relatively temperature-dependent, proceeding optimally at 37°C, and is dependent on an intact microtubule system (Henney and Bubbers, 1973). After appropriate binding of the CTL to the target cell, and under optimal conditions of pH, temperature, and presence of Ca^{2+}, the target cell is "programmed to die" in an irreversible manner. This step has been referred to as the "lethal hit." Very little is known regarding the molecular events that occur during the induction of the lethal hit. After specific binding of the CTL, the induction of the lethal hit is very rapid, and the further presence of the aggressive T lymphocyte appears to be unnecessary. Thus, the CTL can be removed by alloantisera and complement or dissociated from the target cell with EDTA and further reassociation prevented by the addition of highly viscous media (Martz and Benacerraf, 1973), yet these early events are sufficient to cause ^{51}Cr release from the target cell. Current estimates of the time necessary to elicit this message are less than a minute (MacDonald, 1975), and completion of the lytic cycle resulting in the destruction of the target cell within 10 min (Berke and Amos, 1973; MacDonald, 1975). The effector T cell is not consumed in this reaction (Berke *et al.*, 1972; Cerottini and Brunner, 1974; Martz, 1976) and goes on killing many cells, propagating the lytic cycle.

B. Where Are the Potential Sites of Inhibition by Antibody?

The two steps in the lytic cycle that offer potential as sites for antibody-induced inhibition of cytotoxicity would thus appear to be those related to specific recognition-binding function and those involved in the delivery of the lethal hit. The membrane components on CTLs participating in these functions will be collectively referred to as "killing-relevant" structures. That the two functions can be dissociated on the basis of divalent cation requirements may suggest that they represent the activities of independent membrane moieties; however, a certain interrelationship is suggested. A successful "ligand-type" binding appears to be a necessary prerequisite in the delivery of a lethal hit. Evidence supporting this interrelationship comes from a number of studies in which highly efficient CTLs can be brought into cell–cell contact with irrelevant target cells by centrifugation, yet there is no delivery of a lethal hit. Once a binding is promoted either by specific antigen receptors or artificially with certain lectins (PHA), a lethal hit will be delivered to the target cell (Forman and Möller, 1973). The possible interrelationship between surface structures that achieve specific binding and those responsible for the lethal hit is fascinating, but awaits more investigation.

C. The Assay System

Under our conditions of assaying cytolysis, we have taken great care to maintain optimal conditions of pH, temperature, and serum concentration (Berke and Amos, 1973) for maximum efficiency and linearity of the response. The assays were performed in V-bottom Cooke microtiter plates (220M-25AR) as a modification of the microsystem previously used (Kimura and Clark, 1974). Such a system offers a number of advantages for the processing of hundreds of triplicate samples and economy in the number of cells needed. The plates can be directly centrifuged, which enables controlled initiation and termination of the assay. Assays were routinely performed at doubling dilutions of CTLs at effector–target cell ratios between 12:1 and 0.75:1 ($1.2 \times 10^5:10^4$ to $7.5 \times 10^3:10^4$). Control values for each ratio were determined using normal spleen or thymocyte preparations at identical concentrations.

1. Conditions of Antiserum Treatment of CTLs

(a) Pretreatment. Test antisera at various dilutions were preincubated with serial dilutions of CTLs directly in the microtiter wells for 1 or 2 hr at 4°, 20°, or 37°C. After the incubation period, the plates were centrifuged, the supernatants were removed, and each well was washed an additional two times in PBS + 2% FCS. The cell pellets were finally resuspended with the suspension of ^{51}Cr-labeled target cells in a volume of 100 μl and taken through the cytotoxicity assay. Rapid initiation of the cytotoxic response for all groups was achieved by centrifugation of the plates at 300*g* for 4 min. As a control for the efficiency of washing, the entire supernatant from the second wash could not be shown to bind to target cells in a sensitive radioimmunoassay using ^{125}I-labeled protein A (Dorval *et al.*, 1974), or to confer any protection to target cells in the presence of untreated CTLs. Viability tests after antisera pretreatment were always performed and compared with normal serum as well as FCS values. This procedure also served as a convenient check to ensure that any measurable inhibition of cytolytic function was not due to a nonspecific agglutination of effector cells, preventing them from interacting in a free manner with target cells.

(b) Continued Presence of Antisera. For assays in which test sera were present during the assay, 50 μl of target cells were added directly to the CTL–serum pretreatment mixture and taken through the cytotoxicity assay. Under such procedures of continued presence of antisera, we can maximize the chances of antibody interaction with potentially relevant structures. The use of low numbers of effector cells and short-term assays also serves to detect weak activities in various sera.

At given times (usually 1.5–3 hr), the assays were terminated by the addition of 100 μl ice-cold PBS to each of the wells with a Hamilton repeating syringe. The plates were spun at 600*g* in an X-3 Wifug (Winkle-Centrifug, Stockholm) for 6 min at 4°C. Aliquots (0.1 ml) of the supernatant were collected and counted in a gamma scintillation spectrometer, and the percentage of ^{51}Cr released was calculated as before (Kimura, 1974). Using highly purified CTLs in this assay system, we can detect significant differences in the amount of cytolysis if CTLs are temporarily paralyzed by an antiserum treatment creating a lag time of 15 min, or if as little as 20% of the population are completely inhibited by antiserum treatment.

IV. ANALYSIS OF DEFINED SURFACE STRUCTURES AS POSSIBLE PARTICIPATING COMPONENTS IN THE EXPRESSION OF T CELL-MEDIATED CYTOLYSIS

Of the approaches used to assess or ascribe a functional role to a specific membrane component, the interference with function by specific antisera is the most appealing. Several consequences have been reported to occur as a result of antibody binding to cell-surface components: (1) antibody-induced redistribution of cell-membrane proteins into "patches" or "caps," followed by their endocytotic removal from the cell surface (Taylor *et al.*, 1971); (2) antibody-induced shedding of cell-surface components (Unanue and Karnovsky, 1973); and (3) time-dependent covering or masking of cell-surface determinants. The consequences of each of these three types of antibody binding would result in the loss of function attributable to these structures until cellular mechanisms can regenerate and restore the cell-surface integrity.

We have employed a large number of antisera with specificities against most of the defined structures reported to be present on the membranes of cytotoxic T lymphocytes. The various antisera were tested for inhibitory activity in pretreatment assays under both capping and noncapping conditions. Experiments were also performed in which antisera were present during the entire assay (with and without pretreatment) and at a wide range of effector-target cell ratios, using relatively short-term assays of 1.5-3 hr to permit the detection of even a weak effect of a given antiserum.

In the previous section, the characteristics of cell-mediated cytolysis were discussed along with the conditions and factors that affect the interaction of CTL and target cell. It should be realized, however, that once optimal environmental conditions for cytolysis are established, it is extremely difficult to interfere with this function with a variety of antisera against cell-surface components of the CTL. This difficulty is readily seen in a summary chart of our efforts to block the activity of such aggressor cells in the absence of complement (Table II). The positive control of antiserum + complement treatment demonstrates the presence of the various determinants on CTLs and in sufficient quantity to achieve antibody + complement lysis. The extent of inhibition of cytotoxicity by CTLs was directly proportional to the concentration of the sera, and thus to the percentage of CTLs lysed. The serologically defined antigens of the *H-2D* and *K* region, *Thy-1*, and the Ly antigens are indeed useful surface markers for some studies, but do not appear to have any active involvement in the effector mechanisms of CTLs.

The K_a antigen described by Sullivan *et al.* (1973) was an interesting prospect for a structure possibly related in some way to cytolytic function. This antiserum was produced by immunization of rats with mouse immune peritoneal exudate lymphocytes obtained shortly after the rejection of an intraperitoneal tumor allograft. After extensive adsorptions, this antiserum could be shown by serological methods to contain reactivity against a component found on the CTL membrane. Adsorption protocols indicated that this determinant must be distinct from the antigens of the Ly series, *Thy-1*, and *H-2*. However, all of our attempts to achieve an inhibition with such serum were negative, which is consistent with the findings of Sullivan (personal communication).

Table II. Cell-Surface Antigens on Cytotoxic T Lymphocytes

Antigen	Reagents tested for blocking activity	Conditions: Pretreat-ment	Conditions: Incubated with	Effect on subsequent cytolytic T-cell activity: (–) Complement	Effect on subsequent cytolytic T-cell activity: (+) Complement[a]
H-2K, D	Hyperimmune Alloantisera[b]	+	+	None	Abolished
Thy-1 (θ)	Anti-Thy-1.2 Rabbit anti-BAT[c]	+	+	None	Abolished
β_2-Micro-globulin	Rabbit Anti-β_2-microglobulin[d]	+		None	ND[e]
Ly-2.2 -3.2	Anti-Ly sera[f]	+	+	None	Abolished
K_a	Rat anti-K_a sera[g]	+	+	None	Abolished
Fc re-ceptors	Aggregated IgG[h] Ag–Ab complexes[i]	+	+	None	ND[e]
Ig	Polyvalent rabbit Anti-mouse Ig	+	+	None	None

[a] Fresh rabbit and guinea pig sera were adsorbed with mouse tumor cells according to the method of Boyse *et al.* (1970), and served as the complement source for these studies.
[b] Hyperimmune alloantisera against the H-2 genotype of the effector T cell were produced by repeated immunization of mice syngeneic to the target cell with lymphoid cells of the effector T cell genotype. Sera were titered for activity and adsorbed against the target cells before use.
[c] Rabbit anti-brain associated theta was produced by footpad injection of CBA brain in Freund's complete adjuvant, boosted intravenously with CBA thymocytes 7 days later, and bled 5 days following the last injection. The serum was extensively adsorbed with AKR bone marrow cells and characterized as reactive with T lymphocytes.
[d] Rabbit anti-β_2-microglobulin was kindly provided by Dr. P.A. Peterson.
[e] Not done.
[f] Anti-Ly 2.2 and 3.2 were not available for these studies, but are included as the consistent finding of several investigators (Sullivan, 1973; Shiku *et al.*, 1975; Cantor and Boyse, 1975).
[g] Kindly provided by Dr. K.A. Sullivan. Antisera were produced by intraperitoneal immunization of Lewis rats with mouse immune peritoneal exudate lymphocytes following tumor allograft rejection. For details on adsorption protocols and serological characteristics, see Sullivan *et al.* (1973).
[h] DEAE-purified, heat-aggregated human and mouse IgG were tested.
[i] Ovalbumin-antiovalbumin soluble immune complexes were formed in antibody excess.

The physical association of β_2-microglobulin with the serologically defined products of the *D* and *K* regions of the *H-2* complex (Rask *et al.*, 1974), as well as other closely linked gene products such as the allogeneic effect factor (Armerding *et al.*, 1975) and the thymus leukemia antigen (Östberg *et al.*, 1975), made β_2-microglobulin an interesting target to examine in our assays. The presence of β_2-microglobulin on CTLs was established, and the serum was standardized in radioimmunoassay (Welsh *et al.*, 1975). Again, the inability of rabbit anti-β_2-microglobulin to interfere with CTLs gave us no positive information as to relevant surface components needed to exert cytolysis.

A polyvalent rabbit anti-mouse Ig serum with activity against the various heavy-chain classes as well as anti-light-chain activity had no effect on the ability of CTLs to function with or without the presence of complement. These results are consistent with a number of our other observations and those of others that conventional Ig is not an inherent membrane component of T lymphocytes.

Possible criticisms regarding the strength of alloantisera as a reason for the failure to detect inhibitory activities are largely overshadowed by our studies using very powerful heterologous antisera. Using either a rabbit anti-brain associated theta or hyperimmune rabbit antithymocyte serum, we can demonstrate strong reactivity against CTLs in radioimmunoassays or antibody + complement cytotoxicity, and yet there is no measurable effect on the ability of CTLs to exert their function.

Despite the series of unsuccessful attempts to block CTL activity with defined antisera, these studies bring out at least one point worth considering: CTLs can perform without measurable handicap even when a considerable amount of antibody is bound to their cell surfaces. Depending on the weight one is willing to devote to negative effects, these results would emphasize that positive blocking antisera (see Section VI) very likely react with killer-relevant structures, and do not exert their activity merely by irrelevant steric hindrance.

V. DISTINGUISHING CELL-SURFACE CHARACTERISTICS OF CELLS WITHIN PURIFIED POPULATIONS OF CTLs–ARE THESE CHARACTERISTICS IMMUNOLOGICALLY ADVANTAGEOUS?

Within highly purified preparations of CTLs, a further division of these cells can be made by distinguishing cell-surface characteristics. The existence of subpopulations of cells carrying surface markers not present on all the cells at once raises the question whether a functional advantage (or disadvantage) is conferred to the cells bearing these structures. We have examined the functional properties of two such subpopulations of cells by direct isolation or deletion with antisera + complement.

A. Fc Receptor–Bearing CTLs

A variety of cells of the immune system possess membrane components that bind homologous and heterologous IgG (Basten *et al.*, 1972; Paraskevas *et al.*, 1972; Dickler and Kunkle, 1972). The binding of IgG to these structures is specific for the Fc fragment, and the structures have therefore been termed *Fc receptors* (FcRs). Within recent years, a great deal of effort has been spent on understanding the biological role, if any, of these structures. One of the most interesting systems relating this structure to a biological function seems to be found among a small population of lymphoid cells called *K cells*, which are functionally defined by their ability to become cytotoxic to IgG antibody-coated target cells (Perlmann and Holm, 1969). K-cell activity in human systems has been shown to be a property of several cell types, including monocytes (Greenberg *et al.*, 1973), granulocytes (Shin *et al.*, 1974), and small lymphocytes that do not appear to carry surface markers characteristic of typical T or B lymphocytes (Perlmann *et al.*, 1975).

The earliest report on the presence of FcR on antigen-activated T lymphocytes (Yoshida and Andersson, 1972) drew attention to the increasing list of lymphoid cells bearing these receptors. Using populations of T lymphocytes (thymocytes) as responding cells in irradiated allogeneic recipients, these workers were able to demonstrate the presence of large amounts of FcR-positive cells within the killer cell population found in the spleen 5 days later. By analysis of overlapping percentages of FcR-positive cells, it was concluded that activated T cells do indeed bear FcR. These types of studies have been repeatedly confirmed in a variety of systems and in other species (Van Boxel and Rosenstreich, 1974; Andersson and Grey, 1974; Fridman and Golstein, 1974; Rubin and Hertel-Wulff, 1975). The biological significance of these FcRs, however, remains elusive (Rubin and Hertel-Wulff, 1975).

As seen in Table II, the addition of aggregated IgG or soluble antigen-antibody complexes to block the FcR on CTLs does not interfere with the cell's ability to function in "classical" T-cell-mediated cytotoxicity. The results of these types of experiments, however, do not rule out the possibility that FcRs may be important under a different set of conditions.

Concentrating on a functional role of the FcR on cytotoxic T lymphocytes, we have sought analogy to the observations found in the K-cell cytotoxic systems (Kimura *et al.*, 1976a,b). A number of experimental results suggested that the presence of FcR may provide a mechanism for specifically activated T killer cells to interact with target cells having IgG antibody coating their surfaces. It has been shown that for *in vitro* assays of cell-mediated killing, alloantibody coating of target cells protects them from subsequent cell-mediated cytotoxicity, presumably due to masking of serologically defined target-cell antigens (Möller, 1965; Brunner *et al.*, 1968). Other studies (Forman and Möller, 1973) have indicated that specifically antigen-activated T killer cells can kill nonspecifically, provided contact with an unrelated target cell is somehow accomplished, in their case through the use of PHA. In a recent report (Berke and Fishelson, 1975), the formation of effector T-cell–target-cell specific conjugates could be detected under conditions in which pretreatment of target cells with hyperimmune alloantisera could be expected to at least partially mask the target-cell antigens. Such populations of effector T lymphocytes derived from the peritoneal cavity after tumor allograft rejection have been shown to contain extremely high percentages of FcR-positive cells (Kimura and Andersson, unpublished results). We therefore felt that the FcR may provide the necessary means of interaction with the target cell under conditions in which classic T-cell-mediated killing was prevented by the coating of the target cell antigens with alloantibody. Once the binding of the CTL to the target cell has occurred, the induction of the lethal hit may proceed as in classical T-cell–mediated killing.

One of our earliest observations was that under our conditions for the generation of CTLs *in vitro*, the percentage of FcR-positive cells never exceeded a few percent of the total purified blast population, nor were they present in the small-lymphocyte fraction. Since most of the reports demonstrating the existence of FcR-positive killer T cells involved sensitization *in vivo*, we then compared the *in vitro* and *in vivo* sensitized populations of killer T cells for the presence of FcRs. In Fig. 1, the dichotomy in the percentage of FcR-positive killer T cells obtained by these two types of sensitization procedures can be seen. Since our selection process of responding cells is the same for these two types of sensitization, namely, Ig–anti-Ig-purified spleen cells devoid of Ig and Fc receptor-bearing cells (see Section IIA), we feel that the initial selection process against all FcR-bearing cells (including the FcR-positive T cells) in the responding cell population will not permit the generation of FcR-positive cells under our culture conditions. It appears, however, that *in vivo* a different set of

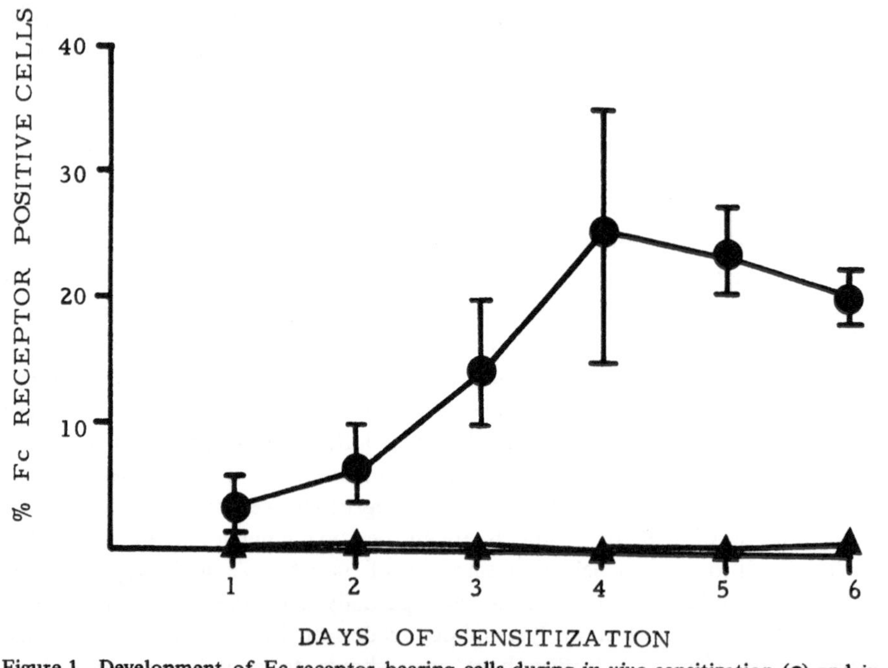

Figure 1. Development of Fc receptor–bearing cells during *in vivo* sensitization (●) and *in vitro* MLC sensitization (▲). FcR-positive cells were quantitated by rosette formation with IgG-coated SRBCs. Vertical bars represent the ranges observed in 5 individual animals or *in vitro* cultures.

environmental factors are operating to yield a population of killer T cells with membrane receptors for the Fc portion of IgG. Whether these environmental factors relate to passively adsorbed serum components or represent actively synthesized membrane structures induced by the *in vivo* state are currently being studied.

Quantitative studies were then performed, focusing on this *in vivo* population of FcR-positive CTLs to compare their efficiency to the FcR-negative killer cell population in two types of cell-mediated cytotoxic systems: (1) classical T-cell-mediated killing, as discussed in Section III, and (2) antibody-dependent cellular cytotoxicity ("K"-cell cytotoxicity).

The FcR-positive T killer blasts were detected first by batch rosette formation with IgG antibody-coated SRBCs, and then isolated from the non-rosette forming T blasts by 1*g* velocity sedimentation as depicted in Fig. 2. With such a procedure, it is possible to obtain a highly enriched population of FcR-positive T killer blasts with little or no overlap from the non-rosette forming T killer blasts, due to the different sedimentation rates of the rosetted vs. the nonrosetted T killer blasts. Analysis of the "T" natures of the rosetted cells was determined by immunofluorescence using a directly fluoresceinated anti-Thy-1.2 antiserum and a fluoresceinated rabbit anti-mouse Ig serum (Table III).

The FcR-positive and FcR-negative blasts were then tested for their ability to perform as cytotoxic effector cells against the relevant ^{51}Cr-labeled target cells and against IgG antibody-coated target cells. As can be seen in Fig. 3, the FcR-positive and FcR-negative killer blasts functioned to approximately the

Table III. Immunofluorescence Staining of EA Rosette- and Non-Rosette-Forming CTL Blasts

	Percentage positively stained cells with[a]:	
	Anti-Thy-1.2[b]	Rabbit anti-mouse Ig
FcR-positive blasts[c]	98	0
FcR-negative blasts	97.5	<0.5
Normal CBA spleen cells	44.3	50.2

[a] Values are the average percentages from two independent experiments.
[b] Directly fluorescein-labeled anti-Thy-1.2 and Fl.-Rab.anti-mouse Ig were generously provided by Dr. C. Janeway.
[c] EA_{7S}-rosetted blasts were isolated by 1*g* velocity sedimentation, and SRBCs were lysed with 0.84% NH_4Cl. The cells were washed twice in cold PBS and prepared for fluorescent staining. Fluorescence was read with a Leitz Microscope (Leitz SM-Lux microscope with a ploem fluorescence-illuminator).

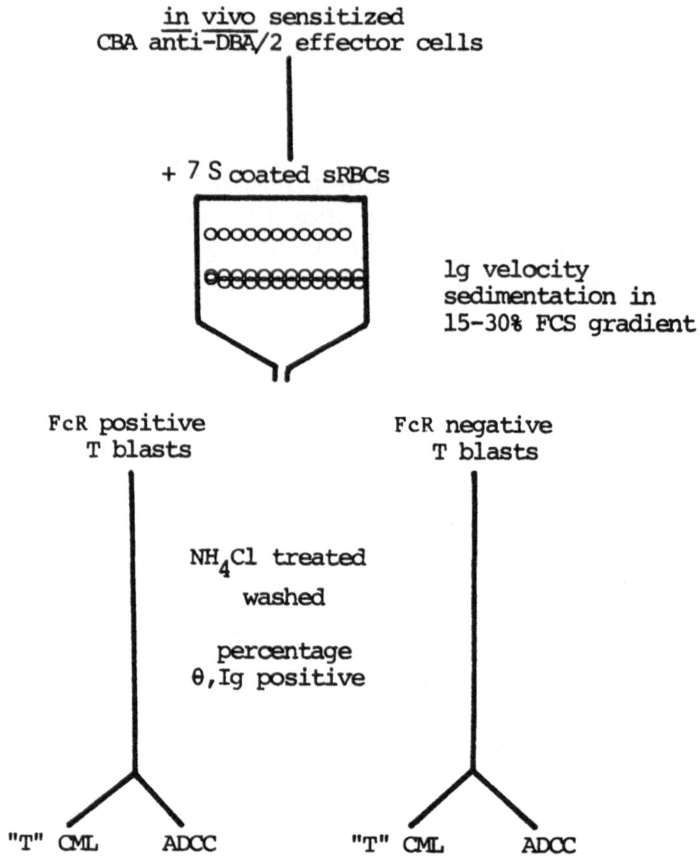

Figure 2. Protocol for the isolation and testing of FcR-positive and FcR-negative T blasts obtained from *in vivo* sensitization.

same extent against their respective target cell in "classical" T-cell–mediated cytotoxicity, while the capacity to kill antibody-coated target cells was confined to the FcR-positive population of T blasts (Fig. 4).

Other studies were performed using the DEAE-purified IgG fraction of alloantisera against the target cell to see whether the FcR-negative blasts were more readily inhibited than the FcR-positive ones by such a treatment. As can be seen in Fig. 3 and Table IV, they were so inhibited. However, the inhibition of the FcR-negative T cells by IgG antibodies against the target cells was only partial, and may suggest incomplete saturation of the target-cell antigens. These results would suggest that IgG alloantibody against the target cell can be either protective to the target cell by covering serologically defined target cell antigens or deleterious by the induction of "K"-cell cytotoxicity in the FcR-positive T blasts.

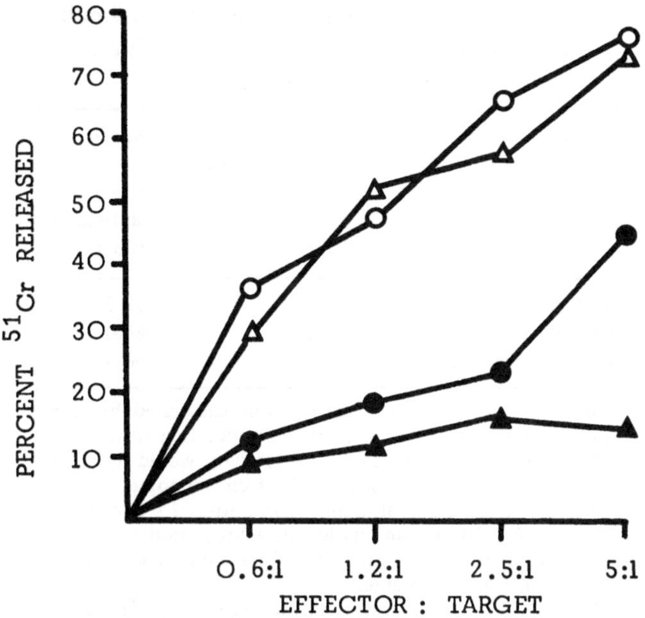

Figure 3. Comparison of the efficiency of FcR-positive and FcR-negative T blasts in cell-mediated cytolysis. The influence of IgG anti-target cell antibodies was also examined. (○) FcR^+ T blast killing of P815; (△) FcR^- T blast killing of P815; (●) FcR^+ T blast killing of P815 + IgG anti-target cell antibodies; (▲) FcR^- T blast killing of P815 + IgG anti-target cell antibodies. The IgG antibodies of *CBA* anti-*DBA/2* hyperimmune alloantisera were purified by gel-filtration and DEAE chromatography.

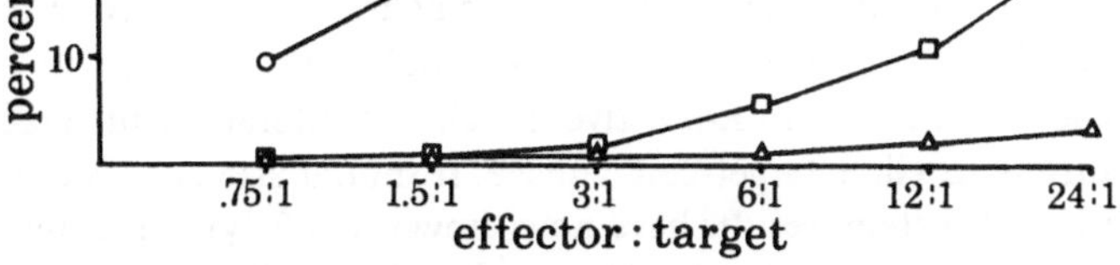

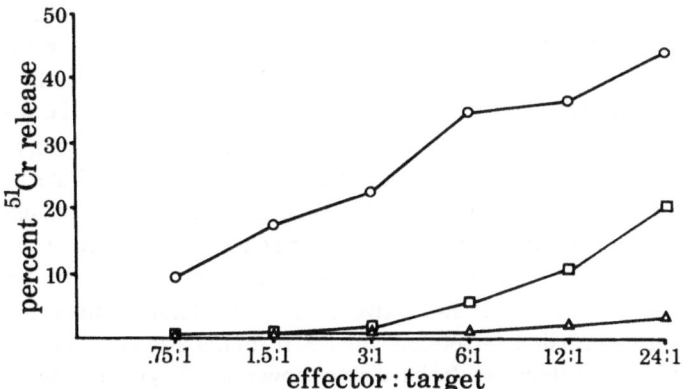

Figure 4. K-cell cytolytic activities of FcR^+, FcR^-, and normal CBA spleen cells against antibody-coated chicken RBCs. (○) FcR^+ T blasts; (△) FcR^- T blasts, (□) normal spleen cells.

Table IV. Effect of Anti-Target Cell IgG Antibodies on the Ability of FcR⁺ or FcR⁻ T Killer Blasts To Express Cytotoxicity

	Percentage ^{51}Cr released from[a]:	
Effector cell	*P815*	*P815* + anti-target IgG antibodies[b]
FcR^+ blasts[c]	90.4	89.5
FcR^- blasts[c]	86.5	66.0
Normal spleen cells	1.1	-0.5

[a] The percentage of ^{51}Cr released was calculated by using FcR^- thymocytes as a control cell population so that possible background effects of K-cell activity would not cover an observed effect in even normal spleen cell populations.

[b] The IgG from hyperimmune *CBA* anti-*P815* alloantisera was purified by a combination of gel-filtration and DEAE chromatography, and used at a final dilution of 1:20 of the original serum volume.

[c] *CBA* anti-*DBA/2* effector T cells were sensitized *in vivo* and fractionated into FcR-positive and FcR-negative T blasts by EA_{7S} rosette formation, followed by 1*g* velocity sedimentation.

These observations are consistent with the hypothesis that FcR-positive CTLs can, under appropriate conditions, react with and kill antibody-coated target cells. The implications of such an alternate mechanism for the interaction of specifically cytotoxic T lymphocytes with target cells is especially exciting with regard to the *in vivo* mechanisms governing enhancement and rejection of grafts. We are certainly aware, however, that our procedures for the selection of FcR-positive T blasts may also favor contaminating "K" cells and macrophages, although the possible degree of contamination is low (see Table III). We are now focusing on assays at the single-cell level in hopes of further clarifying this point. Using a recently developed plaque assay for K-cell cytotoxicity (Biberfield *et al.*, 1975), techniques for the formation of specific conjugates with mixed populations of target cells, and microcinematography to follow the lytic behavior of FcR-positive blasts with mixed target-cell populations, we hope to answer the question whether a single FcR-positive T cell can interact with target cells via two mechanisms to elicit target-cell damage. It should also be mentioned that in the human K-cell system, results have now shown that T lymphocytes as defined by SRBC or lectin markers may express K-cell function (Permann, personal communication).

B. The Ia-Bearing Subpopulation Within CTL Preparations

The rapidly accumulating data on genetically controlled immune responsiveness mapping within the *IA*, *B*, and *C* regions of the *H-2* complex prompted us, first, to look for the presence of these antigens on purified populations of CTLs and, second, to assess the relevance of these structures as necessary in either recognition or subsequent steps in the lytic cycle of specifically activated T effector cells.

Using either various genetic crosses or *I* region recombinant mice, it is possible to make antisera against part or all the serologically defined products of the *I* region. Using an *A.TL* anti-*A.TH* serum (s*kkk*kd anti-sssssd), we have performed radioimmunoassays with ^{125}I-protein A to examine the binding of such anti-Ia^s sera to thymocytes, spleen cells, and purified populations of CTLs from both *A.SW* (ssssss) and *CBA* (k*kkk*kk). The results are shown in Table V. The specificity of the antiserum for spleen cells of the *H-2^s* genotype and negative binding to *H-2^k*, as well as the negative binding to thymocytes, are in accord with previous reports on the genetic and lymphoid distribution of cells bearing

Table V. Radioimmunoassay of Anti-Ia^s Binding to Normal and Cytotoxic T Lymphocytes

Target cell type	[^{125}I] pA bound (cpm) after treatment with[a]: *A.TL* anti-*A.TH*[b]	Normal *A.TL*[b] serum	[^{125}I]pA alone
H-2^s (ssssss)			
A.SW spleen cells	3229 ± 262	300 ± 49	240
A.SW thymocytes	220 ± 23	169 ± 10	265
A.SW anti-*DBA/2* CTL blasts[c]	3018 ± 45	1032 ± 159	530
H-2^k (k*kkk*kk)			
CBA spleen cells	294 ± 14	374 ± 24	339
CBA thymocytes	203 ± 23	219 ± 17	229
CBA anti-*DBA/2* CTL blasts[c]	1414 ± 54	1568 ± 32	944

[a] For each test, 7.5 × 10^5 cells from the indicated cell preparations were reacted with an equal volume of anti-Ia^s or preimmune *A.TL* serum (diluted 1 : 1 with PBS) and incubated for 45 min at 4°C. The cells were washed 3 times with PBS + 10 mM NaN_3 and incubated for 45 min with ^{125}I-protein A. The cells were again washed 3 times in PBS + NaN_3, and counted in a gamma scintillation counter.

[b] Sera were centrifuged at 150,000*g* for 1 hr in an MSE 65 ultracentrifuge to remove large aggregates. Then, 4/5 of the supernatant was carefully removed and immediately used in these studies.

[c] MLC-generated CTLs were isolated by 1*g* velocity sedimentation in a 15–30% FCS gradient and washed 3 times in PBS.

Table VI. Autoradiographic Distribution of Ia-Bearing Cells of Normal and Immune Cell Preparations[a]

	Percentage positively stained cells with:		
	A.TL anti-*A.TH*	Normal *A.TL* sera	Anti-*Thy-1.2*
A.SW spleen	19	1	37.2
A.SW thymus	0	0.2	96
A.SW anti-*DBA/2* MLC blasts	8	0	97
CBA spleen	3	1	35.0
CBA thymus	1	0	98
CBA anti-*DBA/2* MLC blasts	1	1	96

[a]The cells used for radioimmunoassay in Table V were resuspended in a 20% BSA-PBS solution and cytocentrifuged onto precleaned microscope slides. The slides were prepared for autoradiography using AR 10 fine-grain stripping film and exposed for various time periods.

these antigens (Hämmerling *et al.*, 1974, 1975; Shreffler and David, 1975). The 3-fold preferential binding of the anti-Ia^s sera to *A.SW* CTLs was of considerable interest, in view of proposed theories regarding T-cell receptors as gene products of the *I* region. Whether this substantial binding represented a low expression of Ia specificities on all the activated T blasts or a small population was then determined by autoradiography. These results are shown in Table VI. In normal *A.SW* spleen preparations, the positively stained Ia-bearing cells were relatively homogeneous in their grain distribution, and represented 19% of the total cell population. A background level of 3% was noted in the *CBA* spleen cell preparation, although this preparation was less intense in grain count. The strong binding of the anti-Ia^s sera to the CTLs of the *A.SW* genotype seen in radioimmunoassay was confined to only 8% of the blast cells. These results posed the question whether this 8% represented a unique or highly reactive subset of CTLs. Two approaches were used for the functional analysis of these Ia-bearing cells. An intact functional role of *Ia* structures within the T-cell membrane could be assessed by pretreating our effector T cells with the sera and leaving it in during the cytotoxic assay to maximize the chances of antibody interaction with possibly relevant structures. The results of this experiment are presented in Table VII.

The lack of any effect in the system described above would disfavor the possibility of *Ia* structures detected by this sera as being active components of the CTL effector mechanism. However, the possibility that such a cell population bearing *Ia* antigens may represent an unusually highly reactive killer cell population was investigated in the following type of experiment: Purified popu-

Table VII. Effect of Anti-Ia Sera on the Expression of T Cell-Mediated Cytotoxicity

			Percentage ^{51}Cr released in the presence of[b]:		
Effector T cell[a]	CTL: target ratio	Final reciprocal serum dilution	Normal *A.TL* serum[c]	*A.TL* anti-*A.TH*[c]	FCS[c]
A.SW anti-*DBA/2* (sssssss)	10:1	4	38.9	41.2	45.6
		8	41.6	43.7	46.2
		16	42.0	39.9	44.6
		32	40.8	41.8	43.8
CBA anti-*DBA/2* (k*k*kkkk)	10:1	4	52.1	54.3	56.7
		8	53.0	58.7	56.2
		16	51.6	57.5	58.5
		32	54.7	58.1	57.1

[a] CTLs were sensitized *in vitro*, and the T blasts were isolated by 1*g* velocity sedimentation in a 15–30% FCS gradient.
[b] Percentage ^{51}Cr released in 2 hr.
[c] Doubling dilutions (25 μl) of normal *A.TL* preimmune sera, *A.TL* anti-*A.TH*, or FCS were mixed with 25 μl effector T lymphocytes (10^5 cells) and incubated for 1 hr at 4°C. At the end of the incubation period, 25 μl (10^4 cells) ^{51}Cr-labeled target cells were added and taken through the assay.

lations of *A.SW* anti-*DBA/2* and *CBA* anti-*DBA/2* CTLs were pretreated with either *A.TL* anti-*A.TH* serum or the preimmune *A.TL* serum and lysed by the addition of adsorbed rabbit complement. The remaining cells were then tested against ^{51}Cr-labeled target cells. The results of this experiment can be seen in Fig. 5. No evidence was found that would suggest that Ia-positive CTLs are more efficient than average. Whether they are in fact CTLs at all cannot be answered because of their low percentage of the total population.

The possible expression of *Ia* structures as a surface characteristic of CTL memory cells was also investigated. The CTL blast population remaining after treatment of the cells with anti-Ia^s or normal serum + complement was allowed to revert in culture to small lymphocytes. After 3 days, the blasts had reverted to morphologically small lymphocytes, and were then restimulated with irradiated *DBA/2* cells and tested for cytotoxicity against ^{51}Cr-labeled target cells 32 hr later. Again, no difference could be detected as a consequence of treatment with anti-Ia^s + complement (Table VIII).

Taken together, these data would thus favor the idea that the Ia-positive cells within preparations of CTL T blasts represent a group of cells that have either a normal or no active part in T-cell-mediated cytotoxicity, and that Ia

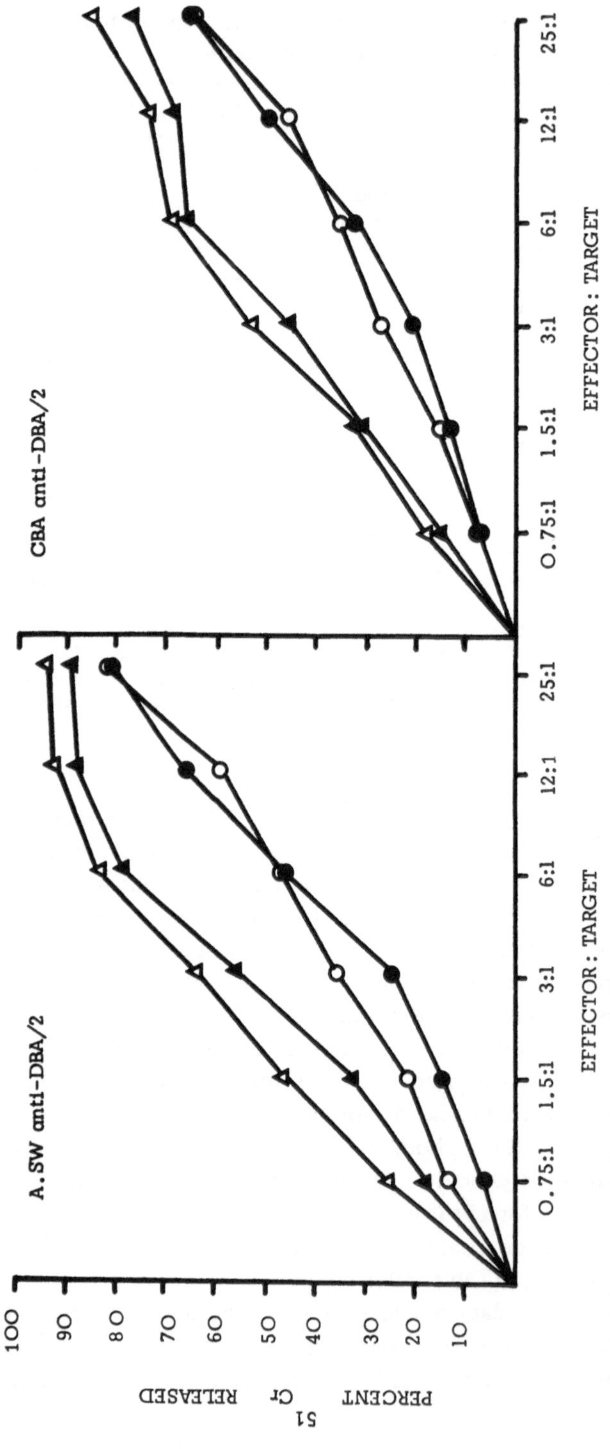

Figure 5. Effect of anti-Ia^{s} (*A.TL* anti-*A.TH*) sera + complement on the ability of CTLs to effect T cell-mediated cytotoxicity. Open symbols: anti-Ia^{s} + complement; closed symbols: preimmune *A.TL* normal serum + complement. Circles: ^{51}Cr released after 1.5 hr; triangles: release after 3 hr.

Table VIII. Effect of Anti-Ia Serum + Complement (C) on the Development of CTLs upon Restimulation in MLC

	Treatment			Percentage ^{51}Cr released at effector: target cell ratios of[a]:			
	A.TL anti-*A.TH* + C	Normal *A.TL* serum + C	C alone	10:1	5:1	2.5:1	1.2:1
A.SW anti-*DBA/2*[b]	+			40.3	22.7	14.8	8.2
		+		41.5	21.1	11.4	7.7
			+	42.6	20.9	12.6	9.3
CBA anti-*DBA/2*	+			33.1	18.6	8.1	3.0
		+		32.4	20.2	11.4	5.3
			+	34.5	19.7	9.8	4.4

[a]Percentage ^{51}Cr released in 2 hr from 10^4 target cells. Values are the averages of duplicate samples.
[b]CTLs from MLC were purified by 1*g* velocity sedimentation and treated with anti-Ia^s + C, normal *A.TL* serum + C, or C alone. The remaining blasts were allowed to revert to small lymphocytes in culture (3 days), and were restimulated with irradiated *DBA/2* spleen cells. The cytolytic activity of these cells was determined against ^{51}Cr-labeled target cells (P815) 32 hr later.

determinants detected by this serum are not actively involved in the effector mechanism of the CTL.

VI. APPLICATION OF ANTI-CTL SERA IN THE STUDY OF "KILLER-RELEVANT" MEMBRANE COMPONENTS

The approach taken thus far has carried the benefit of using both allo- and heteroantisera with rather well-defined specificities and of sufficiently high titer to sequentially assess the relevance of certain membrane structures in the crucial interaction of killer and target cell. These antigenic and functional markers (see Table II), however, are not restricted in their distribution to the activated CTLs that carry the differentiated function we measure. Yet such an approach was important if any of these membrane-associated determinants participated in the buildup of a cytolytic, functional complex. All our attempts with defined antisera and complexed immunoglobulin have failed to have any impact on the ability of CTLs to exert killing. This finding stressed the importance of the alternate approach—the use of CTLs as immunogens across a species barrier in hopes of characterizing antigenic determinants thus far undefined and perhaps more directly related to the cytolytic function of these cells.

A number of experimental observations exist that support the contention that activated T lymphocytes possess qualitatively unique membrane determinants. These observations have come from studies of lymphocyte stimulation against mitogen-induced autologous blasts (Bluming *et al.*, 1975), through serological approaches using heteroantisera against cytotoxic T lymphocytes (Sullivan *et al.*, 1973; Kimura, 1974; Kimura *et al.*, 1975), and by direct biochemical analysis of membrane glyco-proteins (Gahmberg *et al.*, 1976). Thus, by using purified populations of CTLs presumably bearing the membrane structures of interest as immunogens, one would be more hopeful of obtaining sera capable of interacting and interfering with the relevant structures necessary to exert target-cell lysis.

In the original investigations and in the present experiments as well, rabbits were immunized against mouse "killer" T lymphocytes obtained by sensitization across an *H-2* barrier (Kimura, 1974). Such antisera could be shown to exert two functions: (1) a strong general anti-killer cell activity affecting mouse killer cells of a wide range of specificities, and (2) a weaker anti-killer cell activity of "anti-idiotypic" nature, selectively affecting killer cells of a given antigenic specificity. Our rabbit anti-mouse CTL sera were highly successful in blocking mouse killer-cell function in pretreatment, washout assay not involving complement, whereas conventional antithymocyte sera fail to do so (see Section IV). This finding suggested the usefulness of the former reagents in the analysis of "killer-relevant" structures on the activated, immune mouse T cells.

A. T Cell Membrane Components Associated with Recognition of Antigen

The rationale employed in the search for antibodies in the rabbit antisera against recognition units on effector lymphocytes is schematically depicted in Fig. 6. Using essentially a clone of reactive CTLs with restricted specificity as immunogens, one would hope to raise antisera with components of reactivity against either the specific combining region responsible for antigen-specific interaction with the relevant target cell or against determinants of more "constant-type" structures in such receptors. Removal of the great majority of antibodies against "constant-type" surface antigenic determinants could then be accomplished by adsorption of the antisera against syngeneic effector cells directed against another antigenic specificity. It has been our experience that the remaining activity against the relevant CTL has been low, but frequently functions specifically to block cell-mediated cytolysis in the absence of complement. Results of an experiment demonstrating both the general and antigen-specific inhibitory activities of this type of sera are shown in Table IX. Evidence that killer T lymphocytes do indeed express idiotypic receptors has also been ob-

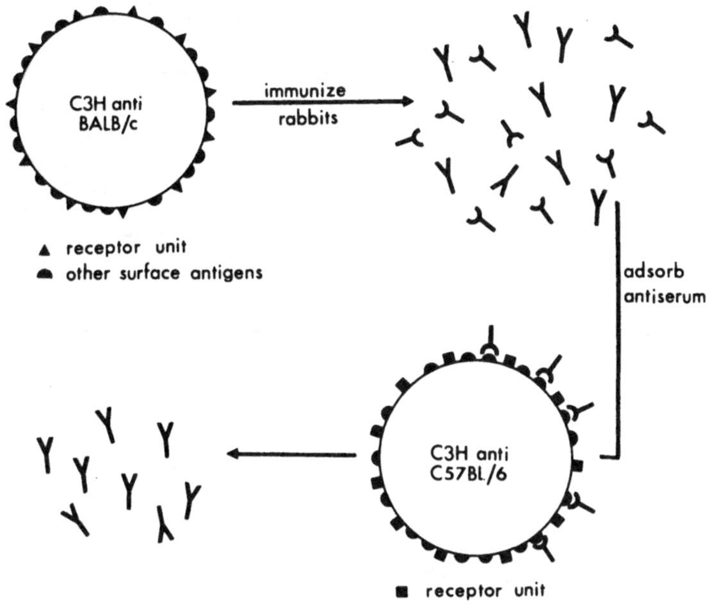

Figure 6. Schematic representation of immunization and adsorption protocols for the detection of anti-recognition structure antibodies.

tained using antiidiotypic antibodies raised within the species (Binz and Wigzell, 1975).

Using heteroantisera adsorbed in such a manner, we have attempted quantitative radioimmunoassays of IgG binding to the relevant CTL to further examine this restriction in specificity. Using a *functionally* specific antiserum (with regard to blocking of cytotoxic T cells), we have tested its direct binding capacity to several syngeneic and unrelated mouse CTL preparations. Such binding assays have failed to demonstrate the restriction seen in functional assays (Fig. 7). These results, which were at first surprising to us, suggested the presence of substantial amounts of other antibodies remaining after adsorption but apparently insufficient in themselves for a functional blockade of the unrelated killer T cells. Such diverging results when using different assays are troublesome, but we now know that they are frequently encountered when trying to obtain functionally reactive (blocking) antisera raised across a species barrier.

However, this troublesome "background" against killer cells that remains after adsorption is even more prominent in unadsorbed sera. This finding raised the question whether the general "anti-killer cell" activity represented other equally important components of these sera. The reactivity against killer T cells in the unadsorbed sera may thus carry components of reactivity against CTL-specific determinants and "killing-relevant" structures.

Table IX. General and Antigen-Specific Inhibitory Activities of a Rabbit Anti-CTL Serum

CTL[a]	Antiserum preadsorbed against[b]:	Effector to target ratio	Percentage ^{51}Cr released against relevant target cells after pretreatment of the CTLs with[c]: *EL-4*[d] NRS	*EL-4*[d] AS[e]	*P815*[d] NRS	*P815*[d] AS
CBA anti-*BALB/c*	–	25:1			40.2	2.6
		12:1			26.3	1.8
		6:1			15.3	0.1
CBA anti-*C57BL/6*	–	25:1	38.4	3.1		
		12:1	22.1	2.2		
		6:1	13.8	1.8		
CBA anti-*BALB/c*	*CBA* anti-*C57BL/6*	25:1			40.2	8.4
		12:1			26.3	5.5
		6:1			15.3	3.1
CBA anti-*C56BL/6*	*CBA* anti-*C57BL/6*	25:1	38.4	32.7		
		12:1	22.1	19.8		
		6:1	13.8	9.5		

[a] CTLs used in this experiments were sensitized *in vivo*.
[b] Sera were twice adsorbed on ice at a vol/vol ratio of 2:1 (serum:packed cells). CTLs used for adsorption were also generated *in vivo*.
[c] CTLs (25 μl; 2.5×10^5–6.0×10^4 cells) were preincubated with 25 μl of either normal rabbit serum (NRS) or rabbit anti-CTL serum (AS) diluted 1:5. After 1.5 hr at room temperature, the cells were washed twice with PBS + 5% FCS, and the final cell pellet was resuspended in 100 μl (10^4 cells) of ^{51}Cr-labeled target cells. Values represent the percentage of ^{51}Cr released from triplicate samples in a 3-hr assay.
[d] *EL-4* is the syngeneic leukosis of *C57BL/6* (*H-2*^{b}) and *P815* is the *DBA/2* mastocytoma (*H-2*^{d}) which represent the specific targets for *CBA* anti-*C57BL/6* and *CBA* anti-*BALB/c* effector cells, respectively.
[e] Rabbit anti-CTL serum was produced by 7 iv injections of *in vivo* sensitized CBA anti-BALB/c CTLs.

B. General Anti-Killer T Cell Activity—A Marker for CTLs?

Using several unadsorbed antisera from the various bleedings, we then came to realize that hyperimmune heteroantisera obtained from rabbits after many immunizations with mouse CTLs frequently carried a strong reactivity against CTLs in general, but very low activity against other types of nonimmune T cells from normal mice.

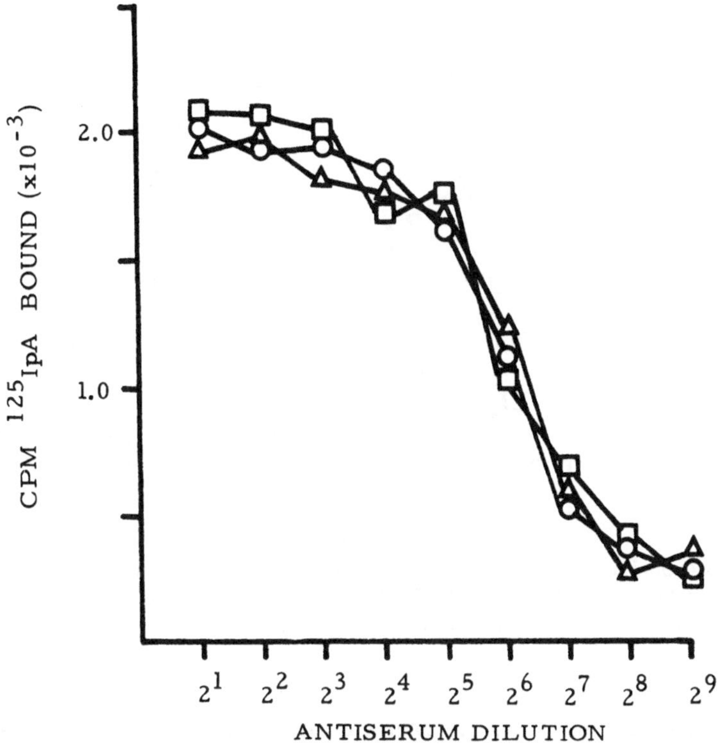

Figure 7. IgG-binding profiles of a functionally specific rabbit anti-(*CBA* anti-*BALB/c*) antiserum. The antiserum was twice adsorbed against *CBA* anti-*C57BL/6* CTLs (as in Table IX) and tested for IgG binding to various CTL preparations using ^{125}I-labeled protein A. Values are the mean counts per minute of triplicate samples of ^{125}I-protein A-binding to 10^6 *CBA* anti-BALB/c CTLs (□), *CBA* anti-*C57BL/6* CTLs (○), and *A.CA* anti-*C57BL/6* CTLS (△).

Using an unadsorbed rabbit antiserum made against *CBA* anti-*C57BL/6* CTLs, we first examined its quantitative binding characteristics to three preparations of *CBA* "T" cells. Lymphoid cell suspensions were prepared from normal *CBA* thymus, *CBA* spleen, and *CBA* anti-*C57BL/6* effector T cells obtained by alloimmunization of purified "T" cells into lethally irradiated *C57BL/6* recipients. "T"-cell preparations were then obtained by passage of these three cell preparations through Ig-anti-Ig columns (see Section IIA), and monitored for "T"-cell purity by their sensitivity to anti-Thy-1.2 + complement, which was greater than 95% for each preparation. For the binding assay, 25 μl (2×10^6 cells) of each of the three preparations of T cells described above was mixed with 25-μl serial dilutions of the rabbit antiserum and incubated for 1 hr at 4°C, washed, and reacted with ^{125}I-labeled protein A (Dorval *et al.*, 1974) to measure the amount of surface bound IgG. The results of such an experiment are shown

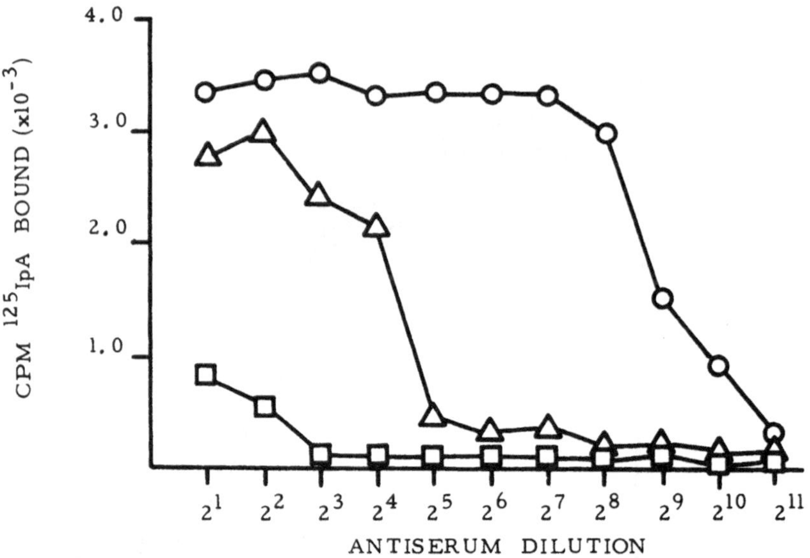

Figure 8. IgG-binding profiles of an unadsorbed rabbit anti-CTL serum to normal and immune T cells. (○) *CBA* anti-*C57BL/6* CTLS; (△) purified T cells from normal spleen; (□) *CBA* thymocytes. All preparations were purified in Ig–anti-Ig columns.

in Fig. 8. The differential binding characteristics of this antiserum to the various T-cell preparations displayed a preference for the antigen-activated CTLs, with moderate binding to purified spleen T cells, and only slight binding to thymocytes. That this difference in IgG binding is not simply due to blast characteristics of the effector cells is known from the binding patterns seen when either alloantisera or anti-Thy-1.2 are reacted with various T-cell preparations as done above.

The strong inhibitory activity of this serum in functional assays of cell-mediated cytotoxicity and the strong and "restricted" binding to CTLs suggested a possible interrelationship of "structures related to function" that might allow further characterization of killing-relevant structures found on these cells.

C. Gel-Precipitation of a Killer "T" Relevant Membrane Component

In an attempt to isolate membrane structures distinguishing CTLs from normal T cells, we began reacting various rabbit anti-effector T cell sera with NP-40 detergent–solubilized membrane preparations from normal and immune T lymphocytes in hopes of selectively precipitating structures found only on the activated T lymphocytes.

On standardizing the conditions for direct membrane precipitations in gels

(Kimura *et al.*, 1975), we found that many of the later bleedings from rabbits repeatedly immunized with effector T lymphocytes displayed sharp precipitin lines that were visible without staining. These precipitation reactions were specific for CTL-membrane preparations regardless whether they were sensitized *in vivo* or *in vitro*. As can be seen in Fig. 9, this reaction is one of identity, and is apparently unrelated to the genotype of the effector T lymphocyte. Our attempts to obtain precipitin reactions against PHA or LPS mitogen-stimulated lymphoblasts have thus far been unsuccessful.

With such a membrane component in the precipitin line—a component that, it was hoped, was killer T cell-specific—antiserum against the mouse component of the line was produced by back-immunization of the precipitin line into normal rabbits. With antiserum against this membrane component, one could then begin to assess its relevance in T cell-mediated killing, and also confirm its presence on the cell membrane. Membrane precipitates were extensively washed against several changes of 0.5 M NaCl, pooled, cut out, emulsified in Freund's complete adjuvant, and injected intramuscularly into normal rabbits. The rabbits

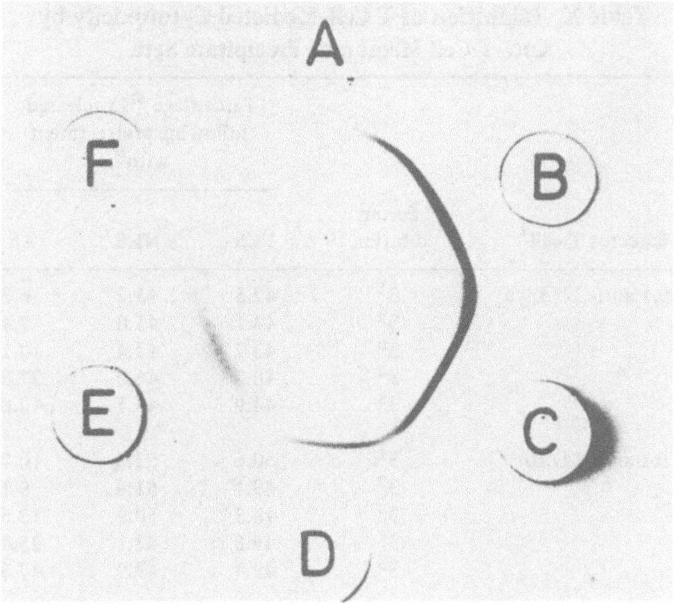

Figure 9. Direct precipitation reactions of a rabbit anti-(*CBA* anti-*C57BL/6* CTL) antiserum with NP-40 detergent-solubilized membrane preparations from normal and immune T cells. Center well: unadsorbed rabbit anti-(*CBA* anti-*C57BL/6*) serum; outer wells: (A) normal *CBA* spleen T cells; (B) *CBA* anti-*C57BL/6* CTLs; (C) *CBA* anti-*DBA/2* CTLs; (D) *A.CA* anti-*C57BL/6* CTLs; (E) *C57BL/6* anti-*DBA/2* CTLs; (F) normal (*CBA* × *C57BL/6*)F_1 T cells.

were boosted twice, once subcutaneously and intramuscularly in incomplete Freund's adjuvant, and finally intravenously in PBS. Sera were collected 7 days following the last immunization, heat-inactivated at 56°C for 30 min, sterile-filtered, and kept at -20°C.

Anti-membrane precipitate sera made in this manner have been used in the unadsorbed state to test for their functional capacity to interact with CTLs in a short-term assay of cell-mediated cytotoxicity. To eliminate the possibility of antibody interaction with the target cells, effector T cells were pretreated with various dilutions of antiserum, washed, and taken through the cytotoxicity assay immediately after the addition of the ^{51}Cr-labeled target cells. Under these pretreatment and washout assays, we were able to measure quite significant blocking activity of the aggressor T lymphocytes. The results of these experiments (Table X) show significant inhibitory capacities at serum pretreatment dilutions out to 1:81. The final supernatant of the washed effector cells could not be shown to contain any detectable anti-target cell antibodies, as measured

Table X. Inhibition of T Cell–Mediated Cytotoxicity by Anti-T Cell Membrane Precipitate Sera

		Percentage ^{51}Cr released following pretreatment with[b]:		
Effector T cell[a]	Serum dilution	FCS	NRS	AS
CBA anti-*C57BL/6*	3^1	42.5	45.2	6.2
	3^2	44.1	41.0	7.4
	3^3	43.7	43.4	10.1
	3^4	40.2	46.2	27.8
	3^5	44.9	43.1	40.8
CBA anti-*BALB/c*	3^1	50.6	52.3	10.7
	3^2	49.1	51.8	9.1
	3^3	48.3	50.9	13.6
	3^4	48.8	48.1	25.4
	3^5	49.4	49.9	47.3
A.CA anti-*BALB/c*	3^1	38.1	40.2	15.2
	3^2	36.0	34.6	16.9
	3^3	39.3	38.3	21.0
	3^4	37.4	38.9	32.4
	3^5	36.8	36.4	25.8

[a] Effector T cells were sensitized *in vivo* and further purified by passage through Ig–anti-Ig columns.
[b] Values are the means of triplicate samples.

in a highly sensitive radioimmunoassay, or to confer any protection to target cells when reacted with untreated effector T cells. Thus, antisera obtained against killer T cell membrane precipitates interact with the outer membrane of mouse killer T cells, since pretreatment of the cells in the absence of complement, followed by washing, was sufficient to inhibit the cytolytic activity of these lymphocytes against their corresponding target cells. As a result, the killer T cells could be shown to remain viable, not agglutinated, but inhibited with regard to cytolytic function.

The fate of these structures defined by the antisera, whether internalized, shed, or simply blocked at the surface of the cell, is unknown. Prolonged killer assays (7-9 hr) do show the revival of killer-cell activity to normal (and once at slightly accentuated) rates, indicating that the inhibition obtained with antiserum pretreatment is reversible with time.

That our rabbit antisera could distinguish antigenic determinants of CTLs by a simple, insensitive gel-precipitation in agarose led us to examine other, more sensitive biochemical methods for a further test of their restricted representation on CTLs.

VII. BIOCHEMICAL ANALYSIS OF CYTOTOXIC T LYMPHOCYTE MEMBRANE COMPONENTS

A. Enzyme-Catalyzed Radiolabeling of Cell-Surface Glycoproteins for the Detection of "Unique" Membrane Determinants

We have employed the galactose oxidase-tritiated sodium borohydride technique of Gahmberg *et al.* (1976) for the selective radiolabeling of cell-surface glycoproteins of various mouse lymphocyte preparations. Briefly, this labeling procedure involves the enzyme-catalyzed oxidation of exposed terminal galactosyl and *N*-acetyl galactosaminyl residues to the corresponding C6 aldehyde by galactose oxidase, which is then reduced with tritiated sodium borohydride. In these studies, sialic acids were removed by mild treatment of the cells with neuraminidase (*Vibrio cholerae*, 25 U/ml per 10^7 cells) to achieve a greater efficiency of labeling, as suggested by Gahmberg *et al.* (1976). Under these conditions of neuraminidase treatment, there was no diminution whatsoever in the viability or functional capacity of effector T cells.

The labeled cells were then solubilized for 20 min on ice with a 0.5% solution of NP-40 in PBS containing protease inhibitors [1 mM phenylmethylsulfonylfluoride (PMSF), soybean trypsin inhibitor, and a 1% saturated solution of ϵ-amino caproic acid]. The membrane-rich fractions were obtained by centrifugation at 12,000g for 30 min, and immediately either used for indirect precipitations or processed for molecular-weight determinations in polyacrylamide slab gels.

We have made two types of comparisons for the evaluation of unique membrane glycoproteins on CTLs. If cell-surface glycoproteins arise as a consequence of the antigen-driven maturation of cytotoxic T lymphocyte precursors, they should (1) be a feature of CTLs and absent on nonimmune T lymphocytes and thymocytes and (2) not be a property of any highly metabolic, rapidly dividing T cell blast lacking cytotoxic capacity.

Ig–anti-Ig-purified *CBA* thymocytes, *CBA* spleen cells, and MLC-induced *CBA* anti-*BALB/c* CTLs were prepared, labeled with NaB^3H_4, and solubilized with NP-40 as described above. The membrane-rich fractions containing approximately 76–80% of the incorporated label and radiolabeled marker proteins were run in linear 5–15% polyacrylamide–sodium dodecyl sulfate (SDS) gels in a discontinuous buffer system according to the method of Laemmli (1970). The gels were fixed overnight in an acetic acid–isopropanol–water mixture (1.2 : 3.1 : 8), and processed for fluorographic autoradiography using the highly sensitive method of Bonner and Laskey (1974), which incorporates the fluor 2,5-diphenyloxazole (PPO) into the gel. The slab gels were dried by heating and vacuum suction, overlayered with RP X-Omat X-ray film, wrapped in aluminum foil, and exposed at −70°C for a period of 2–10 days. Figure 10 shows the com-

Figure 10. NaB^3H_4-labeling patterns of the cell-surface glycoproteins from normal and immune T cells. NP-40-solubilized, NaB^3H_4-labeled membrane preparations were run in a 5–15% acrylamide–SDS slab gel and processed for fluorographic autoradiography. (A) *CBA* thymocytes; (B) *CBA* splenic T cells; (C) *CBA* anti-*DBA/2* T killer blasts.

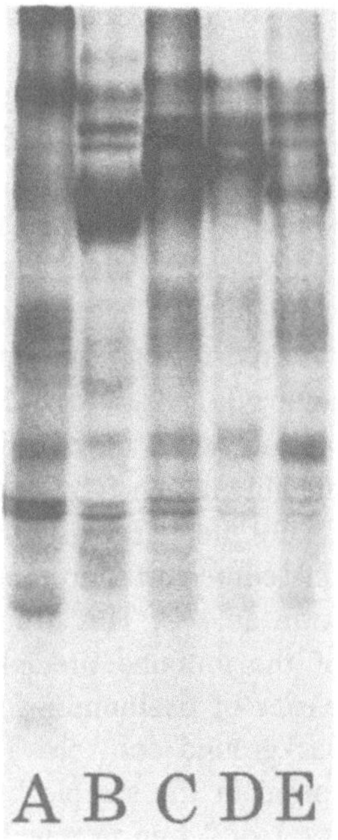

Figure 11. NaB^3H_4-labeling patterns of the cell-surface glycoproteins from T and B cell blasts. Blast cells were isolated by 1*g* velocity sedimentation, labeled with NaB^3H_4, solubilized with NP-40, and run in 5–15% acrylamide–SDS gels and processed for fluorographic autoradiography. (A) *CBA/J* LPS blasts; (B) *AKR* thymoma; (C) secondarily restimulated *CBA* "T" killer blasts; (D) MLC-induced *CBA* anti-*DBA/2* T killer blasts; (E) CBA ConA blasts.

parison in the labeling patterns of these cell preparations. Qualitatively, it is clear that CTL blasts express similarities as well as differences in glycoprotein labeling pattern when compared with normal resting T lymphocytes or thymocytes. The crucial comparison, however, is how well these differences hold up when compared with other rapidly proliferating T and B cell blasts. Four preparations of lymphoblasts were prepared to examine the labeling pattern of glycoproteins among T and B cell blasts. Each preparation of cells was first purified by 1*g* velocity sedimentation into a blast-cell fraction of greater than 98% viability, labeled with NaB^3H_4, and solubilized with NP-40. As can be seen in Fig. 11, the patterns of the three T blast preparations are roughly similar, but distinctly different from the B cell blast. In addition to the distinct glycoprotein bands of the ConA blasts (E) and syngeneic thymoma (B), the MLC-induced killer T cells (C,D) again could be distinguished by the diffuse band of cell-surface glycoprotein(s), which is heavily labeled and covers the molecular-weight range of approximately 150,000–160,000. This glycoprotein band is a consistent feature of CTLs obtained by either MLC or *in vivo* sensitization (D), and is present with similar intensity on secondarily restimulated CTLs (C). This finding is in direct confirmation of the results reported by Gahmberg *et al.* (1976), and probably corresponds to their molecule of 165,000 daltons.

B. Indirect Precipitations with Anti-CTL Sera

Cellular immunologists have long awaited specific membrane markers that would make identification of CTLs possible. These high-molecular-weight glycoproteins offer promise as such specific markers. It was of considerable interest for us to examine the molecular-weight characteristics of the T cell membrane component(s) precipitated with the rabbit anti-CTL sera for comparison with these "unique" glycoproteins.

Preparations obtained from secondarily stimulated CTLs, ConA blasts, tumor T cells, and LPS blasts were either labeled with NaB^3H_4 or internally labeled with 50 μCi [^{3}H]leucine and solubilized as described above. The membrane-rich fractions were then reacted with the rabbit anti-CTL serum, and finally precipitated with a swine anti-rabbit Ig. Immune precipitates formed by this coprecipitation were disrupted by sonication (25 KHz) and allowed to re-form at 4°C. This procedure was repeated twice to obtain a thorough washing of the immune precipitates. Material brought down by the nonspecific complexes of ovalbumin–antiovalbumin and remaining after the washings served as background controls. The final immune precipitates were again sonicated, dissolved in the sample buffer containing 1% SDS and 2-mercaptoethanol, boiled for 1 or 2 min in a water bath, and run in parallel gel slots with marker proteins for molecular-weight determinations. Preliminary experiments have shown that the rabbit anti-CTL serum precipitates two distinct bands of radioactivity of apparent molecular weights 155,000 and 145,000 in the surface-labeled (NaB^3H_4) preparation of CTLs, and one of approximately 155,000 in the ConA preparation. Very similar patterns are seen in the internally labeled preparations of CTLs and ConA blasts. It is extremely interesting to note that the two bands of radioactivity precipitated in the CTL preparation are within the diffuse area of "unique" glycoproteins found only on CTLs. We are now further investigating this very interesting family(?) of glycoproteins found in the heavily labeled region of our gels with modified gradient gel systems combined with parameters of fractionation other than molecular weight.

VIII. SUMMARY AND CONCLUDING REMARKS

Specifically cytotoxic T lymphocytes effect target-cell destruction in a manner that leaves no telltale clues as to the molecular mechanisms involved. The direct cytotoxic action of these immune cells is a rapid process that cannot be explained on the basis of release of nonspecific toxic factors. Furthermore, the studies of Golstein and Gomperts (1975) provide evidence disfavoring the concept that CTLs perform target-cell destruction via "classic" secretory-type processes. The use of Ca^{2+} ionophores to drive Ca^{2+} into the cell does not produce increased lytic activity of the cells, which points to the possibility that the critical need for Ca^{2+} in the induction of the lethal hit may be, for the most part, extracellular. Previous studies with internally labeled ([^{3}H]leucine) effector cells and target cells (Kimura and Welsh, unpublished results) could give no positive evidence that effector T cells either (1) deposit an internally labeled product on the target cell or (2) pull off labeled target-cell antigens that might be expected to be found on the surface of the CTL. Thus, it would seem that the important components necessary for the induction of target-cell lysis might be found to be inherent properties and components of the T cell membrane itself.

A. Serological Approaches

Our method for the functional analysis of various membrane components has brought to mind several important considerations regarding the "effector" activity of CTL membrane components. Through the use of antisera against all the structures of the CTL membrane thus far defined (Thy-1, *H-2D* and *K*, Ka, Ly), we must conclude that these antigens are not associated with the killing-relevant structures of cytotoxic T lymphocytes (see Table II). *In vitro* systems allow us to follow the activity of CTLs "loaded" with these antibodies, and yet they function with normal efficiency. Similarly, Ia antigens that have received considerable attention as potential immunoregulatory gene products do not appear to be of any need during the late stages of this T cell immune response, the expression of cell-mediated cytotoxicity. Our results would suggest that the proportion of cells in CTL preparations bearing these antigens (1) have either a normal part or no active part in T cell-mediated cytotoxicity (see Fig. 5), and (2) are not the sole carriers of T cell memory function (see Table VIII). Further, our results suggest that (3) the Ia antigens themselves are not active components in the effector mechanism (see Fig. 5 and Table VII). That only 8% of the purified killer blast population express Ia specificities would question whether these are in fact killer T cells at all.

B. FcR-Bearing CTLs

The presence of FcRs on activated T lymphocytes could easily be the subject of extensive speculation. However, firm results for a single function of such a structure are lacking. Our preliminary experiments show that a killer T cell population endowed with specific cytolytic activity may use these FcRs under certain conditions as an "auxiliary" means of interacting and killing antibody-coated target cells (see Fig. 4). An analysis of the activity of these cells has been performed by direct isolation of the FcR-positive T killer blasts. We have found that within this isolated population (98% Thy-1 positive), the functions of "classical" T-cell-mediated and antibody-dependent cellular cytotoxicity (Fig. 4) are readily measurable. The question whether a "single" killer T cell performs these two functions and whether the means of inducing a lethal hit are the same is unknown.

C. Application of Rabbit Anti-CTL Sera

Results obtained thus far have demonstrated the usefulness of rabbit antisera against CTLs for the study of "killing-relevant" membrane structures. That such antisera can block T-cell-mediated killing in pretreatment, washout assays in the absence of complement makes them unique reagents. In addition to the results reported here obtained in the mouse systems, essentially identical anti-killer T cell activity has been obtained with rats, using anti-sera made in rabbits against rat CTLs (Welsh, personal communication) under the same pretreatment, washout type assays. These sera against CTLs in both the mouse and rat systems have shown that the serological reactivity (radioimmunoassays and antibody + complement cytotoxicity) against CTLs parallels the inhibitory capacity of such sera in functional assays of cell-mediated cytotoxicity (see Table IX). These sera can be shown to recognize components not detectable on normal cells (see Figs. 8 and 9), and, conversely, heteroantisera against normal cells do not contain this type of reactivity against CTLs. Adsorption and adsorption–elution studies of the anti-CTL sera using normal and immune T cells have also demonstrated this restricted specificity (Welsh, personal communication).

Antisera against precipitated T killer membrane structures further demonstrate the existence of membrane components relevant for killing to be effected (see Table X).

D. Biochemical Studies

The selective radiolabeling of surface glycoproteins with the NaB^3H_4 technique of Gahmberg *et al.* (1976) has provided another approach for the study of membrane components. These biochemical approaches will serve as a powerful means of analysis when combined with serological and, most important, functional tests. Our studies consistently show the presence of a high-molecular-weight glycoprotein (or glycoproteins) (145–155,000 daltons) present on purified CTLs, but absent on normal T or B cells, as well as T and B cell blasts obtained by mitogen stimulation. Immune precipitations of labeled CTL membrane components with the functionally inhibitory anti-CTL sera brings down two distinct bands of radioactivity clearly in the region of these "CTL-unique" glycoproteins. Experiments having the potential to firmly establish a structure-function relationship are currently in progress.

ACKNOWLEDGMENTS

Many of the experimental results reported here have stemmed from exciting discussions and very close collaboration with Drs. K.I. Welsh, Leif C. Andersson, and Jan Andersson, and their major contributions are gratefully acknowledged. We thank Dr. K. Sullivan for the generous gift of her anti-K_a sera for comparison in our studies, and Dr. David Sachs for the anti-Ia^s sera.

Arthur K. Kimura's work is supported by a postdoctoral fellowship (1 F22 CA02355-01) from the National Cancer Institute, National Institutes of Health.

Hans Wigzell's work is supported by the Swedish Cancer Society and by the N.I.H. contract NO1-CB-33859.

IX. REFERENCES

Andersson, C.L., and Grey, H.M., 1974, *J. Exp. Med.* **139**:175.
Andersson, L.C., 1973, *Scand. J. Immunol.* **2**:75.
Andersson, L.C., and Häyry, P., 1974, *Scand. J. Immunol.* **2**:107.
Andersson, L.C., and Häyry, P., 1975, *Transplant. Rev.* **25**:121.
Armerding, D., Kubo, R.T., Grey, H.M., and Katz, D.H., 1975, *Proc. Nat. Acad. Sci. U.S.A.* **72**:4577.
Basten, A., Miller, J.F.A.P., Sprent, J., and Pye, J., 1972, *J. Exp. Med.* **135**:610.
Berke, G., and Amos, D.B., 1973, *Transplant. Rev.* **17**:71.
Berke, G., and Fishelson, Z., 1975, *J. Exp. Med.* **142**:1011.
Berke, G., Sullivan, K.A., and Amos, D.B., 1972, *Science* **177**:433.
Biberfield, P., Wåhlin, B., Perlmann, P., and Biberfield, G., 1975, *Scand. J. Immunol.* **4**:859.
Binz, H., and Wigzell, H., 1975, *J. Exp. Med.* **142**:197.
Bluming, A.Z., Lynch, M.J., Kavanah, M., and Khiroya, R., 1975, *J. Immunol.* **114**:717.
Bonner, W., and Laskey, R.A., 1974, *Eur. J. Biochem.* **46**:83.
Boyle, W., 1968, *Transplantation* **6**:761.
Boyse, E.A., Hubbard, L., Stockert, E., and Lamm, M.E., 1970, *Transplantation* **10**:446.
Brunner, K.T., Mauel, J., Cerottini, J.C., and Chapuis, B., 1968, *Immunology* **14**:181.
Cantor, H., and Boyse, E.A., 1975, *J. Exp. Med.* **141**:1376.
Cerottini, J.C., and Brunner, K.T., 1974, *Adv. Immunol.* **18**:67.
Cerottini, J.C., Engers, H.D., MacDonald, H.R., Robson, H., and Brunner, K.T., 1974, *J. Exp. Med.* **140**:703.
Dickler, H.B., and Kunkle, H.G., 1972, *J. Exp. Med.* **136**:191.
Dorval, G., Welsh, K.I., and Wigzell, H., 1974, *Scand. J. Immunol.* **3**:405.
Forman, J., and Möller, G., 1973, *J. Exp. Med.* **138**:672.
Fridman, W.H., and Golstein, P., 1974, *Cell. Immunol.* **11**:442.
Gahmberg, C., Häyry, P., and Andersson, L.C., 1976, *J. Cell Biol.* **68**:642.

Golstein, P., and Gomperts, B.D., 1975, *J. Immunol.* **114**:1264.
Golstein, P., and Smith, E.T., 1976a, *Contemporary Topics in Immunobiology*, Vol. 7, Plenum Press, New York, in press.
Golstein, P., and Smith, E.T., 1976b, *Eur. J. Immunol.* **6**:31.
Greenberg, A.H., Shen, L., and Roitt, I.M., 1973, *Clin. Exp. Immunol.* **15**:251.
Henney, C.S., 1973, *Transplant. Rev.* **17**:37.
Henney, C.S., and Bubbers, J.E., 1973, *J. Immunol.* **110**:63.
Huber, C., and Wigzell, H., 1975, *Eur. J. Immunol.* **5**:432.
Hämmerling, G.J., Deak, B.D., Mauve, G., Hämmerling, U., and McDevitt, H.O., 1974, *Immunogenetics* **1**:68.
Hämmerling, G.J., Mauve, G., Goldberg, E., and McDevitt, H.O., 1975, *Immunogenetics* **1**:428.
Kimura, A.K., 1974, *J. Exp. Med.* **139**:888.
Kimura, A.K., and Clark, W., 1974, *Cell. Immunol.* **12**:127.
Kimura, A.K., Welsh, K.I., and Wigzell, H., 1975, in: (V. Eijsvogel, ed.), *Proceedings of the 10th Leukocyte Culture Conference*, Academic Press, New York.
Kimura, A., Andersson, L.C., and Wigzell, H., 1976a, *Clin. Immunol. Immunopathol.*, in press.
Kimura, A., Andersson, L.C., and Rubin, B., 1976b, submitted for publication.
Laemmli, U.K., 1970, *Nature (London)* **227**:680.
MacDonald, H.R., 1975, *Eur. J. Immunol.* **5**:251.
Martz, E., 1976, *Transplantation* **21**:5.
Martz, E., and Benacerraf, B., 1973, *J. Immunol.* **111**:1538.
Miller, R.G., and Phillips, R.A., 1969, *J. Cell. Physiol.* **73**:191.
Möller, E., 1965, *J. Exp. Med.* **122**:11.
Östberg, L., Rask, L., Wigzell, H., and Peterson, P.A., 1975, *Nature (London)* **253**:735.
Paraskevas, F., Lee, S.T., Orr, K.B., and Israels, L.G., 1972, *J. Immunol.* **108**:1319.
Peck, A.B., and Bach, F.H., 1973, *J. Immunol. Methods* **3**:147.
Perlmann, P., and Holm, G., 1969, *Adv. Immunol.* **11**:117.
Perlmann, P., Perlmann, H., Larsson, A., and Wåhlin, B., 1975, *J. Exp. Med.* **141**:287.
Rask, L., Lindblom, J.B., and Peterson, P.A., 1974, *Nature (London)* **249**:833.
Rubin, B., and Hertel-Wulff, B., 1975, *Scand. J. Immunol.* **4**:451.
Shiku, H., Kisielow, P., Bean, M.A., Takahashi, T., Boyse, E.A., Oettgen, H.F., and Old, L.J., 1975, *J. Exp. Med.* **141**:227.
Shin, H., Hayden, M.L., and Gately, C.L., 1974, *Proc. Nat. Acad. Sci. U.S.A.* **71**:163.
Shreffler, D.C., and David, C.S., 1975, *Adv. Immunol.* **20**:125.
Stulting, R.D., and Berke, G., 1973, *J. Exp. Med.* **137**:932.
Sullivan, K.A., 1973, Ph.D. thesis, Duke University, Durham, North Carolina.
Sullivan, K.A., Berke, G., and Amos, D.B., 1973, *Transplantation* **16**:388.
Taylor, R.B., Duffus, W.P.H., Raff, M.C., and de Petris, S., 1971, *Nature (London) New Biology* **233**:225.
Unanue, E.R., and Karnovsky, M.J., 1973, *Transplant. Rev.* **14**:184.
Van Boxel, J.A., and Rosenstreich, D.L., 1974, *J. Exp. Med.* **139**:1002.
Wagner, H., and Röllinghoff, M., 1976, *Eur. J. Immunol.* **6**:15.
Welsh, K.I., Dorval, G., and Wigzell, H., 1975, *Nature (London)* **254**:67.
Wigzell, H., and Häyry, P., 1974, *Curr. Top. Microbiol. Immunol.* **67**:1.
Wigzell, H., Sundqvist, K.G., and Yoshida, T.O., 1972, *Scand. J. Immunol.* **1**:75.
Yoshida, T.O., and Andersson, B., 1972, *Scand. J. Immunol.* **1**:401.

Index